ADVANCED DESIGN IN NURSING RESEARCH

SECOND EDITION

ADVANCED DESIGN IN NURSING RESEARCH

SECOND EDITION

PAMELA J. BRINK

MARILYNN J. WOOD

SAGE Publications
International Educational and Professional Publisher
Thousand Oaks   London   New Delhi

For information:

SAGE Publications, Inc.
2455 Teller Road
Thousand Oaks, California 91320
E-mail: order@sagepub.com

SAGE Publications Ltd.
6 Bonhill Street
London EC2A 4PU
United Kingdom

SAGE Publications India Pvt. Ltd.
M-32 Market
Greater Kailash I
New Delhi 110 048 India

Printed in the United States of America

Library of Congress Cataloging-in-Publication Data

Main entry under title:

Advanced design in nursing research / edited by Pamela J. Brink,
  Marilynn J. Wood — 2nd ed.
      p. cm.
  Includes bibliographical references and index.
  ISBN 0-8039-5800-5 (cloth: acid-free paper)
    1. Nursing—Research—Methodology. I. Brink, Pamela J.
  II. Wood, Marilynn J.
  RT81.5.A38   1998
  610.73'072—dc21   97-33824

This book is printed on acid-free paper.

          01 02 03 10 9 8 7 6 5 4

Acquiring Editor:	Dan Ruth
Editorial Assistant:	Anna Howland
Production Editor:	Sanford Robinson
Production Assistant:	Karen Wiley
Copy Editor:	Linda Gray
Typesetter/Designer:	Janelle LeMaster
Indexer:	Paul Corrington
Print Buyer:	Anna Chin

Contents

Preface to the First Edition

In our first text, *Basic Steps in Planning Nursing Research: From Question to Proposal,* we organized the entire volume according to three levels of research based on knowledge of the topic. To help the beginner to plan research accurately, these levels of knowledge were presented throughout that text, from "how to ask a researchable question" to "how to write a research proposal." We acknowledge that these three levels of research could be further subdivided into many designs, but we believe the three-level approach is useful for the novice to learn the essential decision-making rules for planning research.

The current work follows that primary theme of three major designs based on knowledge: exploratory-descriptive, survey, and experimental. In this book, however, we subdivide each of these three designs into two further levels and acknowledge that there are undoubtedly other levels as well, but those presented do cover the major designs used in nursing research and contribute an extremely useful way to classify research designs. Beginning with the experimental design, in which the researcher has the most control over the variables and their action, each subsequent design is contrasted with this model, and its strengths and weaknesses are viewed in relation to the classic or "true" experiment. Subsequent designs derive from the experimental design in logical order. Ordinal scales are known to be inexact, and this one is no exception. We do, therefore, provide research approaches from nursing and other disciplines at the end of the text to explain how one uses and/or critiques designs that do not fit the presented model.

This text is offered to the advanced student or the teacher who used *Basic Steps in Planning Nursing Research* in their earlier days and found this schema useful but not sufficiently detailed to use as a graduate text and reference. We hope this text fills that need.

We would like to acknowledge the assistance of Gail Ardery, who critiqued our chapters for content and rhythm. Having used *Basic Steps*, she was thoroughly familiar with the Brink and Wood style of writing, thinking, and teaching nursing research. With her doctorate in linguistics, she was an invaluable asset to us. We would also like to thank the reviewers who critiqued the book, gave us invaluable advice, and encouraged us to go on. Finally, we thank the many students in Iowa and California who asked questions at each step along the way.

Preface to the Second Edition

In the first edition of this text, we followed the basic organizational scheme of our text *Basic Steps in Planning Nursing Research.* We added, at the end, chapters on the historical method and the epidemiological method as well as a chapter on instrumentation. These chapters have not been changed from the original edition. They have, however, been moved. The epidemiology and the instrumentation chapters have been placed in the section on Descriptive Survey Designs, and the historical chapter has been placed in the Exploratory-Descriptive Design section. The chapter on the pilot study, which has been revised, has been placed in the Exploratory-Descriptive section to highlight its function—to pretest instruments or to explore the feasibility of doing a study. It is not a study but the preliminary or exploratory work for a subsequent study. Although the study may be an experimental design, its pilot study does not meet the criteria for an experiment. Also in the second edition, we have added a chapter on theory testing through structural equation modeling using existing data sets, and the section on Experimental Designs now includes a new chapter on within-subject designs and the earlier chapter on evaluation research designs. No serious researcher interested in theory development or theory testing can ignore either of these avenues of data exploration.

Part I

Introduction

1

Introduction

PAMELA J. BRINK
MARILYNN J. WOOD

This text is based on the premise that theory and research are inextricably intertwined. Neither is useful in advancing nursing knowledge without the other. Theory provides explanations for why things happen the way they do. Research provides the means to test theory to determine whether its explanations hold true, and it simultaneously leads to new ideas for theory construction. Accordingly, for research to be of value in the advancement of knowledge, it must be closely and appropriately melded into the process of theory development. The basic principle put forth in this text is that the level of knowledge available on a research topic determines the level of design that can be used to study that topic. This principle cannot be overemphasized. Fawcett and Downs (1986), in *The Relationship of Theory and Research,* exemplify this principle by including in their appendixes research reports representing the three basic levels of knowledge.

The function of this reader is to describe a number of research designs useful in nursing research. Each design is described using a standard format. The classical design is presented, along with its usual variations. One to three examples of the design, as they have appeared in the nursing literature, are provided. Strengths and weaknesses of each design in sampling, methods, reliability, validity, data analysis, and issues related to the use of human subjects are discussed. Finally, each chapter discusses issues that must be dealt with in relation to human subjects, proposal writing, and critiquing.

Two major concepts provide the basic organization of this text. The first is that research designs are based on the level of knowledge (and therefore the level of theory) about the topic being studied. The second is that research designs can be categorized according to the degree of control each offers over the research situation. The designs in this book are ordered from the most highly controlled, or those in which a great amount of knowledge exists on the topic being researched, to the least controlled designs, or those in which little knowledge exists on the topic. *Control* refers to investigator regulation of the research variable(s). In other words, a *controlled* research variable is not allowed to interfere with the action of other variables. The investigator has sufficient knowledge about the actions and interactions of variables that they can be isolated and studied in precise ways, all of which are established by the investigator at the outset of a study. In other words, variables can be controlled during the data collection phase or the data analysis phase, but the decision as to when a variable will be controlled is made in advance of data collection. When a variable is controlled, it does not vary in any way other than the way the investigator has predetermined it to vary. When a variable varies by itself and the investigator only observes the variance and documents it, the situation or the variable is in control of the research situation, not the investigator.

TYPE OF RESEARCH DESIGN AND TERMINOLOGIES

Research studies may be described or classified in a variety of ways. Although all such classifications have their failings, taken together, they provide a handy tool for identifying particular characteristics of each level of research. The following sets of terms, adapted from Nieswiadomy (1987), will be used throughout the text.[1]

Qualitative and Quantitative

The terms *qualitative* and *quantitative* refer both to the *method* of data collection and to the *type* of data collected. The distinguishing feature is whether the data to be collected are already enumerated, whether they can be collected and enumerated, or whether they must remain verbal descriptions. Data that are structured in the form of numbers or that can be immediately transposed into numbers are considered *quantitative.* Data that cannot be structured in the form of numbers are considered *qualitative.* Measurement—whether at the nominal, ordinal, interval, or ratio level—is the hallmark of quantitative designs. Quantitative methods attempt to measure phenomena on a numeric scale of some kind, producing data that reflect at least the *frequency* with which a phenomenon occurs and, at most, an exact measure of the *amount* of the phenomenon occurring under prescribed circumstances. By nature, quantitative methods require substantial knowledge of the phenomena under study, for tools to be available to measure these phenomena. In contrast, qualitative data collection methods are flexible and unstructured, capturing verbatim reports or observable characteristics and yielding data that usually do not take a numerical form. Words, film, postcards, art, and all sensory data are considered qualitative data unless they are transformed into some numeric system. Qualitative data can serve as the bases for insights, grounded theories, categorizations, taxonomies, processes, or outcomes. (For further reading in qualitative nursing research, see Field & Morse, 1985; Leininger, 1985; Morse, 1988; Munhall & Oiler, 1986; Parse, Coyne, & Smith, 1985; Stern, 1980, 1985; Swanson & Chenitz, 1986; Wilson, 1985, 1986.)

The choice between qualitative and quantitative methods is based on the type of research design. Exploratory designs primarily use flexible, open-ended qualitative data collection methods, whereas descriptive designs combine qualitative and quantitative methods. All other designs may incorporate qualitative data collection as an enhancement to the data but not as a primary data collection method. Although the qualitative-quantitative distinction is widely used to classify research, it provides only two vast categories, each containing numerous designs. We find it more useful to place designs on a continuum based on the amount of theory and knowledge each requires. By doing this, it becomes possible to envision a research program or a given topic moving along this continuum as knowledge and theory in that topic area evolve.

The Concept of Time in Relation to the Design

A number of design terms refer to the researcher's temporal perspective looking back in time or looking forward: retrospective, prospective, ex post facto, historical, longitudinal, and cross-sectional. *Retrospective* (or ex post facto) designs measure phenomena that have occurred earlier in time. Designs in which the outcome or dependent variable is known and the independent or causal variable is sought are correlational retrospective designs. All historical studies are also retrospective. *Prospective* designs, on the other hand, measure variables that will be occurring during the study. All experimental studies are prospective because they are based on predictive hypotheses. Time-series designs are also prospective. *Longitudinal* is a term used, particularly by epidemiologists, to describe a prospective design that follows a cohort or group of study participants over time. The term *cross-sectional* describes designs conducted in the present time to examine what currently exists. The fundamental characteristics of cross-sectional designs is that all data are collected at one time period. (See Polit & Hungler, 1987, for a more complete description of these concepts in relation to design.)

In some cases, the use of these terms is redundant. In describing an experimental design, one would not add that it is prospective just as one would not add that a historical design was retrospective or that a correlational design was cross-sectional. These terms are assumed by the nature of the design. In a comparative design, however, it would be important to add the time element so that others would know immediately whether the sample would be compared either on the dependent or on the independent variable.

Location or Setting

Research may also be described according to location or setting, generally differentiating between laboratory and field studies.

Laboratory studies are conducted in controlled settings particularly suited to the experimental design. In addition to the traditional settings used by basic scientists, laboratory sites include clinical research units within hospitals, rooms equipped with two-way mirrors or video equipment for studies of behavior, and facilities equipped with physiological monitoring equipment for studies of human physiological responses. In contrast, most observational nursing research is conducted in the "real" world or the "field." Although it is certainly possible to conduct a descriptive observational study in a laboratory setting, this is a more expensive method of conducting such a study and raises questions about the validity of the findings.

Field studies occur in natural settings, where people are behaving as they usually do. Data are collected in the field primarily by means of observation and questioning. Additional information is obtained through available data, photography, and so on. *Field settings* include not only Pacific islands and African villages but hospital wards, classrooms, nursing homes, and clinics. Nurses do field research when they observe nurse-patient interactions in health care institutions, document student-teacher interactions in classrooms, or describe staffing patterns in hospitals. The type of setting chosen for a study depends on the research design. For example, an exploratory or descriptive study of the type and amount of foods people eat should be observed in a natural setting so that daily food choices, methods of preparation, and social setting for eating are as "usual" as possible. In contrast, a laboratory setting in which all foods are prepared and eaten under highly controlled circumstances would be useful if precise measurement of food intake was sought. Studies of the relationship between nutritional intake and weight reduction lend themselves nicely to highly controlled experiments conducted in clinical laboratory settings. Because field studies have less control, it is important for the researcher to describe the field in detail as part of the setting in which the study occurred.

Applied Versus Basic Research

Another major distinction is made between applied and basic research. *Basic* research is undertaken for the sake of learning something new, of building knowledge, without concern for whether or not the knowledge can be used directly. Its purpose is simply a desire to know, or to study the phenomenon, not to change human circumstances. The knowledge gained may or may not be directly usable and applicable to a present-day problem.

In contrast, the major purpose of *applied* research is to use the knowledge derived from the research in the practice situation. Applied research is undertaken to test whether some specified change can be effected and whether that change will be permanent (Foster, 1969). Searching for the causes of diseases such as cancer or AIDS is basic research. Testing interventions (or treatments) is *applied research*. Most nursing care research is applied. Any clinical experimental or comparative design that tests one nursing intervention technique against another is essentially an applied research study. Its purpose is to change something, to improve the human condition in some way, to improve the delivery of nursing care, or to alter some aspect of the patient environment. Not all experimental designs, however, are applied. Some experiments are conducted to increase knowledge only, to see what will happen in a controlled setting when variables are manipulated. Within a practice discipline such as nursing, however, most research will eventually be applicable to practice, although many different studies involving several levels of research may be required before application is possible.

Deductive Versus Inductive

Some texts use the terms *deductive* and *inductive* to designate whether research contributes to theory testing or theory building. The main thrust of theory testing is deductive. Experimental designs are by their very nature deductive or derived from theory. Their purpose is to test theory. On the basis of data obtained in an experiment, an investigator either accepts or rejects a research hypothesis. Rejection entails "deducing" either that the theory was in error or that the experiment did not directly test the theory. Acceptance entails both deducing that the theory was correct and assuming that the experiment directly tested the theory. Deductive studies are usually empirical, more specific, fact based or "hard" data based, and not abstract.

Inductive studies, by contrast, are more abstract and general in scope, based on "soft" data, less specific, usually using exploratory or descriptive designs and qualitative data collection methods for the purpose of building or creating theory. The process of deriving theory from an in-depth qualitative data collection project has been called "grounded theory" (Glaser & Strauss, 1967; Hutchinson, 1986, Stern, 1980, 1985; Swanson & Chenitz, 1986; Wilson, 1986). These studies develop concepts from the data that are then used to develop theory. Inductive studies using phenomenological inquiry frequently result in a description of an experience. Correlational studies, although usually deductive, can also be inductive when significant relationships between variables lead to insight regarding cause-and-effect linkages. Descriptive designs can be either deductive or inductive.

Process Versus Content

Research endeavors may also be described as either *process* or *content* studies. Studies of grieving, dying, maturing, and crisis, for example, all examine a process, whereas studies of the incidence of disease, measurement of health attitudes, or the opinions of nurses regarding professional practice are content studies. The process-content distinction parallels the distinction between purely descriptive designs and purely exploratory designs. Most exploratory studies focus on process in an attempt to explain the phenomena under study. Descriptive studies, even longitudinal studies, describe phenomena or populations at a particular time period. Although descriptive data can be collected at several points in time, each data collection period constitutes a distinct cross-sectional study, because data are collected at one moment in time. Consequently, descriptive research findings neither describe a process nor explain how or why it works. Process studies frequently attempt to discover the stages people go through in response to a threat or particular stressor. For example, dying can be conceptualized as a process of moving from social life and living to social dying and eventual death. Bereavement has been studied as the process a person goes through in coping with death or other loss (Saunders, 1983). *Culture shock* (Brink & Saunders, 1976) refers to the process of adapting to a move from a familiar to an unfamiliar environment. The discovery of one's sexual identity has been considered a stressor to which the individual must adjust (Kus, 1985). Adjustment, of course, is a process. In process studies, therefore, the process is the content. Process studies examine how people adjust or adapt to change. Content studies in these areas might examine the numbers of persons failing to resolve the crisis encountered through the death of a significant other, comparisons of the adaption of men versus women to a move to an unfamiliar environment, or the numbers of persons in particular occupational groups who identify themselves as homosexual versus heterosexual. These cases simply examine a phenomenon as it exists either in different populations or within one population.

Experimental Versus Nonexperimental

Many texts label research studies as either experimental or nonexperimental. *Experimental* designs involve manipulation of the independent variable, whereas *nonexperimental* designs do not manipulate variables. This classification system is very limited, considering the enormous number of possible nonexperimental designs. In addition, this distinction is derived from, and tends to perpetuate, the belief that only experimental designs are "real" or "scientific" research.

THE DESIGN LABELS USED IN THIS BOOK

The design taxonomy used in this book is based on the principle of control, or the degree to which the investigator is able to prevent any untoward variance among the variables under study. Control itself is based on the current level of knowledge about the topic. The paradigm enumerated previously by Brink and Wood (1978, 1983, 1988, 1994) presents three basic levels of design—experimental, survey, and exploratory-descriptive—each of which contains two sublevels. These are carried forward into this book as follows:

- Level III: Experimental designs
  a. Experimental
  b. Quasi-experimental
- Level II: Survey designs
  a. Comparative
  b. Correlational
- Level I: Exploratory-descriptive designs
  a. Descriptive
  b. Exploratory

Ideally, at successively higher levels of design, the degree of control and the level of knowledge about the variables increases. The level of knowledge about pertinent variables should be the greatest at the level of the experiment and is expected to be most limited at the exploratory level.[2] Accordingly, the choice of an appropriate design is based on the current level of knowledge (or theory) about the research topic. The current level of knowledge and theory about a topic must be thoroughly examined prior to entering into an experimental design. Two methods of examining existing theory on any well-studied topic is either to do a conceptual mapping of the literature to determine what is missing, what is conflicting, and what is causal or to perform meta-analysis of the published literature to determine if there are conclusions that can be drawn and applied or whether further work is needed to explain contradictions or omissions. When a causal relationship between variables can be both predicted and ethically *tested*, experimental or quasi-experimental designs are warranted. If a researcher believes research variables are related and can predict the outcome of their interaction but cannot ethically manipulate the independent variable, a comparative design may be used to test theory and safeguard living subjects at the same time. If the researcher has a basic descriptive knowledge about the individual research variables but does not know whether they are related, the design is best formulated at the correlational level. If, on the other hand, a variable or concept has been discovered through exploration but no information is available about its existence in particular populations, a descriptive design is appropriate. Finally, if very limited or no knowledge about the topic is available, an exploratory design is most appropriate. Control of variables and prediction of their action require extensive knowledge. If the outcome of an experiment cannot be predicted and supported with theory, it is unethical to conduct that experiment on living subjects.[3] Level of design is based, therefore, on knowledge about the operations of the variables in the topic and on the degree of control that can be exercised over these variables in the research process itself.

Theory is built and supported at each level of knowledge so that when we speak of a knowledge base for research, we automatically assume a theory base. Because theory is built on accepted knowledge to explain what is known, theory changes as knowledge changes. And because a careful building of facts is prerequisite to developing and testing theory, all levels of research design are needed to advance theory development in nursing. Moreover, theory building might require moving back and forth across the continuum of research designs, because acquiring knowledge might require returning to explore further topics once thought to be well understood.

Level III. The experimental level of research is designed to test theory in laboratory settings or in controlled clinical trials. The greater the degree of control in the research setting, the greater the confidence that the research findings are accurate.

The *experimental design*, the most highly controlled of all research designs, is amenable to laboratory study, entails manipulation of the independent variable(s), and requires control of all intervening variables. On the basis of theory developed from previous research, each step in the experiment requires a predictive hypothesis regarding the effect of the independent on the dependent variable(s). All assumptions are spelled out and are either verified by previous research or tested by the current research. All logical steps between cause and effect are specified. The key issue for this design is *internal validity*, or the assumption that changes in the dependent variable are actually due to the independent variable. Experimental and control groups are created by random assignment. Ethical concerns for the protection of human and animal subjects are the most restrictive. Experimenters, more than any other kind of researchers, are required to establish that all subjects' rights are protected to the greatest degree possible and that potential harmful effects are counterbalanced by potential benefits. Data collection is quantitative and prospective. Data analysis is designed to discriminate between and among experimental and control groups. Although experimental studies are the most directly applicable to nursing practice because of their controlled samples, they are the least widely generalizable in and of themselves. This is simply due to the controlled narrowness of the study and sample. Experiments are designed to be repeated on many samples with small variations in the independent variable over time. A single experiment on a single small sample adds to the test of a part of the theory but not of the entire theory. Many experiments with different samples may be required to increase generalizability to the point where findings can be widely applied in practice.

The *quasi-experimental design* is distinguished from the true experiment by the lack of random assignment of participants to groups. This lack of control limits confidence in the internal validity of the study. Otherwise, the design is exactly the same as the experimental design. Data are predominantly quantitative, and data analysis distinguishes between and among treatments and among treatment groups. Many field experiments actually use a quasi-experimental design when the assignment of participants to the various experimental and control groups cannot be controlled by the researcher. For example, a researcher may want to use an in-patient hospital population in an experiment, but physicians control who is admitted to the hospital. A nurse, therefore, may not have control over extraneous or intervening variables in the available population, in which case a quasi-experiment in appropriate.

The *within-subject experimental design* has been a neglected area in nursing research, but it deserves some attention. There are times, particularly in clinical studies, when the best control can be achieved only by having participants randomly assigned to order of treatment rather than to groups. A basic assumption in these studies is that the study participants themselves provide the best control group. It is then possible to use very small, unique clinical populations for whom there would otherwise be no adequate control group. In the case of toxic shock, for example, there were only five deaths. The population was small and unique. No adequate control group would be possible.

Another design type is the *evaluative design*. Many clinical and educational programs have attempted to change something in the current system, improve some practice, or enhance a problem-solving mechanism. All these programs need to be evaluated in some consistent fashion. Evaluative research is both descriptive, seeking to describe what has occurred, and experimental, testing the effect of some manipulation or change. Data can be either qualitative or quantitative, and usually, both are included.

Level II. At the survey level of research, prior research findings are available in the literature. These studies yield a statistical analysis of the relationships between and among variables.

The *comparative design* is used when a cause-and-effect relationship can be predicted between variables on the basis of previous research findings. This design subjects a theory to testing without manipulation of the independent variable. Comparative designs usually occur in field studies. The sample is selected on the basis of the presence or absence of the independent variable, thus creating comparative groups at the beginning of the study. There are times, however, when the groups are established during data analysis. Data are predominantly quantitative, and data analysis differentiates between and among groups. This design is used in both basic and applied research, often when the independent variable cannot be manipulated due to ethical constraints. For example, if the researcher wanted to study the cause-and-effect relationship between smoking and lung cancer, it would be unethical to create a research design according to the type of substance smoked (cigarette, cigar, pipe) or length of time the study participant smoked before the onset of lung cancer. In this situation, the researcher would be deliberately creating a malignancy.

The *correlational design* examines the relationship between two or more variables when no previous research findings support a prediction of cause and effect. This design simply allows one to study the relationship of two or more variables based on hunches or logical assumptions. The design is also appropriate when one is searching for possible causative variables or for a particular outcome variable. Although specific variables may be "assumed to be" independent or dependent on the basis of their temporal occurrence, their actual relationship can be determined only through correlational data analysis. Correlational designs are usually field studies rather than laboratory studies, basic rather than applied, cross-sectional rather than longitudinal, and either prospective or retrospective. They are based on quantitative data collection from large samples. Control is increased through reliability and validity testing of data collection instruments, sample selection procedures, and data analysis. The central issue in these studies is to establish generalizability or *external validity*.

Epidemiological designs tend to mix elements of other designs, most frequently using correlational designs but not limited to them. They can vary greatly in control over variables and level of knowledge. Their primary goal is to document health, illness, and disease patterns for the purpose of establishing prevention, intervention, or maintenance programs for health problems.

The *methodological* study is used to develop and test data collection instruments. Although this area has been neglected in nursing research until recently, it is evolving into a specialty area. The methodological study can be part of a research project at any level, because its major purpose is to develop reliable and valid instruments. In instrument development, researchers often make use of all three levels of research, analyzing a concept at the exploratory level, and then developing and testing an instrument to measure this concept through the other levels. In the process, theory may be developed and tested as it relates to the concept. In this book, the major discussion of reliability and validity of measurement will be found in Chapter 10 on methodological research.

Level I. At the exploratory-descriptive level of research, usually little or no theory or prior research has addressed the specific variable under study. Alternatively, prior research on the variable may have been conducted but only in populations other than the one currently under study. The phenomena under study are either unknown or understudied, or because of recent happenings, a reexploration is indicated. By using flexible approaches to discovery, these studies attempt to provide either a total or "in-the-round" description of a variable or an exploration of some process.

The *descriptive design* is used to describe a single variable or population completely, accurately, and thoroughly. Descriptive studies usually involve cross-sectional field research using both qualitative and quantitative data collection techniques. Examples include anthropological ethnographies and population surveys such as the U.S. census. Data analysis includes a mixture of content analysis, taxonomies, and descriptive statistics. External validity is a major issue in descriptive studies of known populations that do not use the total available population. Because many descriptive studies are of unknown or understudied populations, representativeness is always an issue.

The *exploratory design* is the least controlled design. Its central purpose is to develop valid definitions of a concept, describe a process, or yield beginning theories that explain the phenomenon under study. Data are collected in depth and over time to increase the validity of the concept being developed. Consequently, samples are usually quite small (from 1-20). Data are most frequently collected by means of a qualitative field study subjected to inductive analysis. Examples include phenomenological studies examining processes according to the perspective of the individuals undergoing the process and the grounded theory or field study approach, using participant observation with intensive interviewing to observe and analyze a process as it occurs in order to explain why it occurs the way it does.

Historical research is nonexperimental and is based on available written data, artifacts, or oral histories, all of which are usually qualitative data. Historiography can be cross-sectional or longitudinal. Depending on the question asked, the study may be comparative, correlational, descriptive, or purely exploratory. A critical step in historiography is establishing whether the data are primary or secondary, hearsay or eyewitness accounts, and true or falsified documents and whether the data sources are biased or objective observers of the times. The process of data analysis involves a great deal of interpretation on the part of the researcher, and in this way is similar to the exploratory study. The variables under study, however, may be well-known in the present day. The researcher has no control over the way in which the original data were collected but a great deal of control over which data are included in the study and how these are interpreted. Although historical studies are just beginning to appear in the nursing research literature, their legitimacy is indisputable.

The last chapter is devoted to the *pilot study*. Frequently equated with exploration but rarely described in any detail, pilot studies are assumed to be the first step in any research plan and are sometimes published in the literature. The difference between using exploratory designs as beginning stages of a planned program of research and pilot projects is critical.

This book has emerged as a result of our many years of looking for a good resource for graduate courses in advanced design. We hope that others will find this approach useful in helping them make decisions about the design of a research project.

NOTES

1. This classification of nursing research studies has been adapted from Nieswiadomy (1987, pp. 39-54).

2. We expect ethical researchers to have a great deal of knowledge about the effects on human subjects of the manipulation of the independent variable prior to inflicting the independent variable on them. For this reason, we state that knowledge at this level should be the highest, because we are intervening in people's lives. Although there may be an enormous knowledge base in survey designs, these designs are still descriptive, even when using complex statistical techniques.

3. One of the reasons there are such strict guidelines on the protection of human subjects in the United States today is that in the past many experiments were conducted on humans as "fishing expeditions"—to find out what would happen if this or that were manipulated. Some people died, some were harmed psychologically or physiologically for life, and babies were born deformed, among other results. These same studies would not be approved by institutional review boards today. Instead, to be approved, all experiments on human and animal subjects must have some fact-based logical or theoretical outcomes predicted at the outset.

REFERENCES

Brink, P. J., & Saunders, J. M. (1976). Culture shock: Theoretical and applied. In P. Brink (Ed.), *Transcultural nursing: A book of readings*. Englewood Cliffs, NJ: Prentice Hall.

Brink, P. J., & Wood, M. J. (1978). *Basic steps in planning nursing research: From question to proposal*. North Scituate, MA: Duxbury.

Brink, P. J., & Wood, M. J. (1983). *Basic steps in planning nursing research: From question to proposal* (2nd ed.). Monterey, CA: Wadsworth Health Sciences.

Brink, P. J., & Wood, M. J. (1988). *Basic steps in planning nursing research: From question to proposal* (3rd ed.). Boston: Jones & Bartlett.

Brink, P. J., & Wood, M. J. (1994). *Basic steps in planning nursing research: From question to proposal* (4th ed.). Boston: Jones & Bartlett.

Fawcett, J., & Downs, F. (1986). *The relationship of theory and research*. Norwalk, CT: Appleton-Century-Crofts.

Field, P., & Morse, J. (1985). *Nursing research: The application of qualitative approaches*. Rockville, MD: Aspen.

Foster, G. (1969). *Applied research*. Philadelphia: F. A. Davis.

Glaser, B., & Strauss, A. (1967). *The discovery of grounded theory*. Chicago: Aldine.

Hutchinson, S. (1986). Grounded theory: The method. In P. Munhall & C. Oiler (Eds.), *Nursing research: A qualitative perspective* (pp. 111-129). Norwalk, CT: Appleton-Century-Crofts.

Kus, R. (1985). Stages of coming out: An ethnographic approach. *Western Journal of Nursing Research, 7*(2), 177-193.

Leininger, M. (Ed.). (1985). *Qualitative research methods in nursing*. New York: Grune & Stratton.

Morse, J. (Ed.). (1988). *Qualitative nursing research: A contemporary dialogue*. Rockville, MD: Aspen.

Munhall, P., & Oiler, C. (Eds.). (1986). *Nursing research: A qualitative perspective*. Norwalk, CT: Appleton-Century-Crofts.

Nieswiadomy, R. M. (1987). *Foundations of nursing research*. Norwalk, CT: Appleton & Lange.

Parse, R., Coyne, A., & Smith, M. J. (1985). *Nursing research: Qualitative methods*. Bowie, MD: Brady.

Polit, D. F., & Hungler, B. P. (1987). *Nursing research*. Philadelphia, PA: J. B. Lippincott.

Saunders, J. M. (1983). A study of widow bereavement involving various modes of death. In P. J. Brink & M. J. Wood (Eds.), *Basic steps in planning nursing research: From question to proposal* (2nd ed., pp. 235-260). Monterey, CA: Wadsworth Health Sciences.

Stern, P. (1980). Grounded theory methodology: Its uses and processes. *Image, 12*, 20-23.

Stern, P. (1985). Using grounded theory method in nursing research. In M. Leininger (Ed.), *Qualitative research methods in nursing* (pp. 149-160). New York: Grune & Stratton.

Swanson, J. M., & Chenitz, W. C. (1986). *From practice to grounded theory: Qualitative research*. Menlo Park, CA: Addison-Wesley.

Wilson, H. S. (1985). *Research in nursing*. Menlo Park, CA: Addison-Wesley.

Wilson, H. S. (1986). Presencing: Doing grounded theory. In P. Munhall & C. Oiler (Eds.), *Nursing research: A qualitative perspective* (pp. 131-144). Norwalk, CT: Appleton-Century-Crofts.

Part II

EXPERIMENTAL DESIGNS

The primary purpose of experimental designs is to test theory. The significant difference between experimental designs and all other designs is that in experimental designs the independent variable is manipulated. The research question asks, What is the difference between groups after the independent variable has been altered and why does the alteration produce those differences? The question is answered with "Because . . ." and the explanation provides the theoretical framework for the study. These studies test one portion of a theory rather than the entirety of the theoretical position. Cause and effect is always predicted based on theory. Predictive hypotheses are written at the beginning of the study, stating the precise nature of both the manipulation of the independent variable and its effect on the dependent variable. Manipulation of the independent variable tests theory in a manner not possible with any other design.

The chapters in this section describe types of experimental designs. The single feature that distinguishes these major designs from all other designs is the manipulation of the independent variable. No other designs have this feature. The experiment provides the greatest control over the experimental situation: The experimental variable is manipulated, there is random assignment to groups, and there is at least one control group. *Internal validity* is the key issue in assessing the accuracy of the findings. Other critical features include control and the validity of the measure of the dependent variable. The quasi-experimental design, in contrast to the true experiment, lacks either a control group or random assignment to groups.

The classic work on experimental and quasi-experimental designs by Campbell and Stanley has been used by researchers in many disciplines since it was first published in 1963. Campbell and Stanley developed the concepts of *internal* and *external validity* as they apply to studies with human subjects in natural settings. In the first two chapters that follow, Buckwalter and Maas have used this classic work, adapting the basic principles to make them relevant to nursing studies.

Because of the level of control and the strength of the theoretical base required to support an experimental or quasi-experimental design, these designs will be used as the basis for comparison for the other designs presented in this book.

The third chapter in this section deals with a neglected design in nursing research, the *within-subject* experiment. Here, the task is to randomly assign study participants not to groups but to the treatments they receive. This design is particularly useful when there are a limited number of participants, participants are extremely difficult to recruit, or there are a large number of measurements.

The last chapter in this section deals with the evaluative research design.

2

Classical Experimental Designs

KATHLEEN C. BUCKWALTER
MERIDEAN L. MAAS
BONNIE WAKEFIELD

A number of strategies, blueprints, or research designs can be employed in the systematic study of problems that are of interest to nurses. The experimental design is the appropriate research strategy when the questions to be answered require the testing of theory and causal relationships. Experiments, broadly defined, are tests that involve at least one treatment (independent variable), units (e.g., subjects) to be analyzed by assignment or nonassignment to a treatment, and a comparison for inferring effects that may be attributed to the treatment. Experimental designs are of two major types, true experiments and quasi experiments, although in general, the term *experimental design* is used when referring to true experiments. In addition to the general

AUTHORS' NOTE: We wish to thank Joan Crowe and Nancy Goldsmith for typing the manuscript for this chapter.

characteristics listed above for experiments, *true experiments* include the random assignment of units to comparison groups for inferring a change that has been caused by a treatment. Random assignment is an essential component of true experiments that is designed to achieve comparability of comparison groups. *Quasi experiments* have a treatment (independent variable), outcomes (dependent variable), and units to be analyzed; but random assignment of units to comparison groups is not included for determining the groups of units to be compared. True experiments are described in this chapter. Quasi experiments are discussed in the following chapter. Throughout the remainder of this chapter, the terms *experimental design* and *true experiment* will be used interchangeably, unless otherwise noted.

All experimental designs, true experiments, and quasi experiments are appropriate for answering Level III questions (Brink & Wood, 1983) within a theoretical context and are theory testing in nature. The researcher who appropriately employs experimental designs begins from a position of logical relationships derived from current theory and research findings. All of these designs are powerful methods for testing hypotheses of causal relationships between variables. The emphasis is on four main criteria: (a) establishing causal relationships, (b) manipulating an independent variable, (c) measuring the impact of the independent variable on the dependent variable, and (d) minimizing or accounting for the effects of factors other than the independent variable on the dependent variable.

For these reasons, the true experiment is regarded as the "cornerstone of scientific research" (Ingersoll, 1982, p. 625). It is the *most powerful* strategy for testing causal hypotheses and achieving the above four criteria, because random assignment is used to create the comparison between groups from which a change due to the treatment is inferred.

TYPES OF TRUE EXPERIMENTAL DESIGNS

A number of different experimental designs meet the criteria for true experiments. These include, but are not limited to, the "classical" experimental design, the factorial design, the multiple treatment groups-repeated measures design, and the Solomon four-group design. Although there are a number of additional variations on these designs (see, for example, Pedhazur & Schmelkin, 1991, pp. 265-275), illustration of the use of these four basic experimental designs provides a basis for understanding the strengths and weaknesses of true experiments and for understanding how variations can be structured to maximize strengths to study specific problems. An important assumption underlying all true experimental designs is that equivalence of groups is maintained throughout the course of the experiment and is not compromised by things such as differential attrition—that is, variable dropout rates that may make experimental and control subjects different on critical factors at the time of the analysis. If experimental and control groups become nonequivalent, the design then becomes quasi-experimental.

The "Classical" Experimental Design

All experimental designs are variations on the basic classical experimental design, which consists of two groups, an experimental and a control group, and two variables, an independent and a dependent variable. Units to be analyzed (e.g., subjects) are randomly assigned to each of the experimental and control groups. Units in the experimental group receive the independent variable (the treatment condition) that the investigator has manipulated. Participants in the control group do not receive the independent variable treatment. Pretest and posttest measures are taken on the independent variable(s), and the control group participants are measured at the same time as the experimental group, although no planned change or manipulation has taken place with regard to the independent variable in the control group.

Researchers often use this design when they are interested in assessing change from the pretest to the posttest, as a result of a treatment or intervention. This design is also known as "pretest-posttest" or "before-after" design, to differentiate it from a posttest-only design in which one group receives a treatment, whereas the other group receives no treatment and serves as a control. The key difference in the posttest-only design is that neither group is pretested, and only at the end of the study are both groups measured on the dependent variable. Some researchers favor this latter design over the classic two-group pre- and posttest approach because they are concerned that the pretest measures will sensitize participants or that a learning effect might take place that influences individuals' performance on the posttest.

Factorial Designs

Classical experimental design allows the manipulation of a single variable at a time, holding all other conditions constant. Frequently, problems of interest to nurses are more complex than the classical design permits. Factors (variables) *interact* to produce behaviors of interest to nurse researchers. *Factorial designs* differ from the classical experimental design in that they permit the manipulation of more than one independent variable (or factor) at a time. Furthermore, interaction effects between variables are revealed and the simultaneous testing of multiple hypotheses is thus allowed. In factorial designs, the researcher can study the effects of each of the variables (known as the main effects), and the interactions between them, or their joint effects on the independent variable, making factorial designs an important variation on the classical experimental design.

Although the example used later in this chapter is a 2 × 2 factorial design, factorial experiments can be conducted with any number of categories and independent variables (known as factors). Each factor must have two or more levels; thus, when new factors are added, the analysis becomes more complex. For example, a 4 × 5 factorial design means that one of the factors has four categories and the other has five. These designs can also be extended to have more than two factors, as in a 3 × 2 × 4 factorial design. In this example there are three factors, consisting of three, two, and four categories, respectively.

Factorial designs are also referred to as "levels of treatment" designs. When one of the factors cannot be manipulated, such as sex or race of study participants, it is referred to as a *blocking variable*, and the design that incorporates the blocking variable is known as the *randomized block design*. Stratified randomization is often used in this case to ensure that approximately equal numbers of participants within categories are randomly assigned to the various treatments.

Multiple Treatment Groups—
Repeated Measures Design

This design uses several experimental groups, each of which receives a different treatment. Control is achieved through comparison among groups and from measures taken on the dependent variable for all groups at Time 1 and Time 2. It is not always true that a control group will be used that has no treatment at all. There can also be more than one pretest and posttest measure for the dependent variable for all groups.

Solomon Four-Group Design

This is a rigorous design for controlling effects on the dependent variable that may be due to factors other than the independent variable. It is essentially a combination of the pretest-posttest and posttest-only designs described above. However, it is used less often than other designs because a large group of homogeneous subjects is required to make up the four groups. It is difficult to introduce the treatment simultaneously for all groups in order to avoid extraneous temporal effects, and statistical analysis is complex. These problems will be clarified when they are discussed along with the research example later in the chapter.

Prior to the illustration of these four experimental designs with examples from the nursing research literature, the essential elements that characterize true experiments—their strengths and weaknesses and issues of the research setting, measurement, and analysis—are described. This discussion will make the research examples more understandable and more useful.

ESSENTIAL CHARACTERISTICS OF EXPERIMENTAL DESIGNS

In experimental designs, the investigator predicts an experimental outcome based on theory and previous research findings to explain the results in the context of logical and tested relationships. Basically, the researcher hypothesizes that the dependent variable for the experimental group will be altered in some specific (predicted) way, whereas the same dependent variable for the control group will remain unchanged. To test a relationship and most confidently infer this result, experimental designs must be characterized by three essential elements: randomization, manipulation, and control.

Randomization

In a true experimental design, *randomization* refers to participants being assigned by chance to either receive (the experimental group) or not receive (the control group) the treatment condition or intervention (independent variable). A number of procedures exist for assigning individuals to groups, such as a coin toss, a random numbers table, or computerized random number generators. The key characteristic of all these procedures is that each participant has an *equal* and *known* probability of being assigned to either the control or the experimental group. If any participant has a greater or lesser chance of being assigned to either group, the assignment process is not random, and the assumptions underlying a true experimental design are violated.

The advantage of assigning participants to groups in a random manner is that this should result in the groups' initially being similar to one another prior to the intervention. Basically, randomization helps eliminate bias by spreading variability due to extraneous variables equally across the groups under study (Pedhazur & Schmelkin, 1991). For example, imagine that a nursing intervention for treating depressed patients is being evaluated and a group of persons who have been referred by their family physician to a community mental health center is used as participants in the study. Half of the participants are randomly assigned to participate in the treatment program, and the remaining participants are placed on a waiting list as a control group. On the basis of this method of assigning participants to a condition, the two groups of depressed persons should not differ in their pretreatment level of depression or in other characteristics that may affect the treatment outcome (e.g., levels of social support). Assuming that the group receiving the nursing intervention is significantly less depressed than the control group following completion of the treatment program, it becomes possible to conclude that the nursing intervention was responsible for the improvement in depression that occurred.

Random assignment to condition *does not guarantee* that the two groups will be similar to one another. Based on sampling theory, significant differences ($p < .05$) between the two groups will occur in 1 of 20 cases of assigning participants to groups. If the sample size is not large enough, there is a greater probability that significant variables may not be equally distributed among groups, even with random assignment. In this situation, the researcher may wish to consider some additional methods of distributing important variables, such as matching or use of a more homogeneous population (see also the discussion of control of extraneous variance, below). However, studies have consistently supported the efficacy of random assignment to condition over various ways of matching subjects who are participants in different groups (Sherwood, Morris, & Sherwood, 1975).

In some research, it is necessary to randomly assign treatment conditions to a unit(s) other than the individual participant(s). Take, for example, the study of Abraham, Neundorfer, and Currie (1992) on the effects of group interventions on cognition and depression in nursing home residents. Because of the mix of residents with different physical and mental disabilities, it was necessary for the researchers to recruit participants from seven nursing homes to create three treatment groups. Only one facility yielded enough participants for two groups. Thus, it became necessary to randomly assign treatment conditions (behavioral, visual imagery, and education) to nursing homes. In other studies in which known factors can influence intervention outcomes, modification of the randomization plan, stratified randomization, is recommended. In effect, this controls extraneous variables by inclusion. For example, in one experimental nursing study that examined chest tube stripping in pediatric oncology patients (Oakes et al., 1993), the investigators knew that previous treatment could influence the outcomes of a thoracotomy. They therefore assigned patients to the two groups (chest tube stripping using established-practice methods vs. no chest tube stripping) using a fixed randomization plan with two strata: (a) history of previous thoracotomies or radiation therapy involving the study lung and (b) no such history. Still another variation on randomization that has been used in nursing studies is the cluster-randomized controlled-trial design (Gilliss et al., 1993). In a randomized clinical trial of nursing care for recovery from cardiac surgery, Gilliss and colleagues (1993) used clusters of consecutive groups of patients who were entered conveniently into the trial. This approach was used primarily to avoid contamination between groups of study participants. Size of the clusters, which were stratified by hospital, varied randomly. Clusters were randomized to experimental or control conditions by computer-generated random numbers. Researchers enrolling participants were blind to both cluster size and condition, and random assignment of the cluster was not revealed until a patient had been discharged from the intensive care unit (ICU).

Manipulation

Manipulation is the process of maneuvering the independent variable so that its effect on the dependent variable can be observed (measured). In experimental designs, the causative variable must be amenable to manipulation by the investigator; that is, the researcher "does something" to subjects in the experimental condition. "Manipulation strength" is an assessment of the "likelihood that the treatment could have its intended outcome" (Yeaton & Sechrest, 1981, p. 156), independent of the actual effect of the treatment on the dependent variable. It is also essential that researchers conduct "manipulation checks"— that is, check to see whether the manipulation had its intended effect or perhaps resulted in an unintended effect(s) that could compromise the validity of an experiment (Pedhazur & Schmelkin, 1991). For example, in a caregiver intervention designed to enhance coping ability by providing more information to caregivers, an unintended effect was that some caregivers became depressed when confronted with the reality of the debilitating progression of the disease. In working to avoid unintended effects, researchers should be cautious of the use of reactive measures (those that increase participants' awareness of the experiment), which can influence participants' responses to the dependent variable.

A word of caution is needed regarding the control group. Even though the researcher does not actively manipulate participants in the control group, it is important that he or she be aware of what may be happening to them. Control groups should experience all the same things (including environmental factors and time spent with data collectors) as participants in the experimental group, except, of course, the independent variable. Often, ethical considerations will prohibit manipulation of variables (e.g., introduction of pain or other aversive stimuli to participants). Similarly, some variables that could differentially operate in the groups cannot be manipulated (e.g., attitudes, age, disease, and other such attribution variables). Finally, organizational policy of the research setting may disallow manipulation of variables (such as making dietary changes or altering medication regimens). The ability of the researcher to manipulate the independent variable is a major source of control in experimental studies.

Control

Control is a key concept in experimental designs. Cook and Campbell (1979, p. 8) identify three uses of the term *control* in relation to research designs, all of which involve elimination of threats to valid inference. One type of control refers to the researcher's control over the research environment; a second refers to control over the experimental variable; and the third suggests the ability to identify and rule out threats to internal validity. This last type of control is typically achieved through the use of a comparison or control group and through attention to sources of variance. The control group consists of participants whose scores on the dependent variable are compared to the scores of participants who received the experimental condition. In experimental designs with more than one experimental group, control is present in the sense of a formal comparison between groups. In many nursing studies, control participants receive the usual or traditional methods of care, rather than no treatment, against which the effects of the experimental intervention are measured.

A major strength of experimental designs is their ability to diminish bias, which refers to a misrepresentation of the effect of the independent variable on an outcome(s), because of systematic differences in the way treatment and control participants have been selected or measured or because another variable confounds the estimate of the true relationship between the independent variable and the outcome(s) of interest (Rothman, 1986). Kerlinger (1973) discusses the merit of experimental designs in terms of their ability to *control variance*, or to take into account factors that may contribute to differences in the dependent variable. To provide valid answers to research questions, three kinds of variance must be considered: (a) systematic or experimental variance, (b) extraneous variance, and (c) error variance (Kerlinger, 1973, pp. 306-313).

Systematic or experimental variance refers to the systematic effect of the independent variable(s) on the dependent variable(s) and is a type of variance that should be *enhanced*. That is, experimental conditions should be planned to be as *unlike as possible*. Say an investigator wishes to determine the most effective way to teach psychiatric patients about their psychotropic medication regime by comparing the efficacy of a 1:1, nurse to individual patient, teaching program to that of a group teaching approach. To maximize systematic variance, the two teaching programs (experimental conditions) should be substantially different from each other so that the effects of teaching programs can be separated from the total variance of the dependent variable (in this case, patient knowledge of the medication regime), which is often largely due to chance.

Extraneous variance refers to the effects of extraneous variables (also referred to as "nuisance" or "unwanted" variables) on the dependent variable(s). This source of variance is to be *controlled* by the design, because extraneous variables are factors other than the independent variable that could lead to differences between groups. In addition to randomization, which is the most ideal way to control all possible extraneous variables simultaneously, Isaac and Michael (1971, p. 54) list four ways the researcher can control extraneous variance. All of these techniques require that the researcher know in advance which extraneous variables need to be controlled:

1. *Building the extraneous variable into the design,* as an independent variable (e.g., if sex of participants is considered an important variable in determining response to an intervention, a randomized block design with sex [male/female] as one of the factors may be used).

2. *Eliminating or holding constant* an extraneous variable by selecting participants as homogeneous as possible on that variable (e.g., all elderly female participants).

3. *Matching* participants on one or more extraneous variables, as long as those variables are highly correlated with the dependent variable(s) (e.g., matching participants for rural/urban residency or type of disease). It should be noted that matching is *never* an adequate substitution for randomization and should be used only when other techniques are not feasible. Furthermore, if matching is required on three or more variables, this method becomes too complex and impractical to implement. For example, if participants are matched on two categories of three variables, they must be matched on six combinations. If matching is desired for more categories or more variables, the difficulty in accomplishing all of the matches becomes more obvious.

4. *Statistical* control of variance, such as analysis of covariance (ANCOVA). This procedure is explained more fully in the section on data analysis.

Error variance refers to the variability of measures due to random fluctuations, including errors of measurement. Control of error variance is achieved principally by standardizing the measurement (experimental) conditions, by increasing the sensitivity of measurement instruments, and by increasing reliability of measurement instruments.

1. *Control of experimental conditions* can be enhanced by keeping factors such as place, time of day, instructions to participants, and experimental

personnel constant. Otherwise, factors such as noise, hunger, fatigue, or anxiety may create errors of measurement.

2. *The reliability of measurement instruments* (e.g., their accuracy) can be increased by writing items clearly, adding more similar items, and providing clear, consistent instructions (Kerlinger, 1973, p. 454). Unreliable instruments increase error variance, and this in turn compromises the effects of systematic variance. Furthermore, unreliable human measurements can affect study outcomes. For example, a nursing study of the accuracy of apical pulse rate measurements in young children (Margolius, Sneed, & Hollerbach, 1991) compared the measurements made by a variety of health care providers with ratings made by a Hewlett-Packard electrocardiographic monitor and found an average error rate of 8 bpm, although errors as high as 58 bpm were found in the sample.

Experimental designs are considered the most powerful research approach because they permit the researcher to maximize systematic variance and to control for extraneous and error variance. This is principally a problem of establishing internal validity of the experiment. Experiments, however, are often limited in generalizability because they intrude on natural settings and participants are not randomly selected from a target population. They are powerful designs for controlling threats to external validity, which are an important aspect of generalizability. Experimental designs also best control threats to internal validity and thus are the most powerful for testing causal relationships.

Internal validity is the primary objective of experimental methodology. The researcher essentially asks the question, Was the effect observed on the dependent variable actually due to the action of the independent variable? Egan, Snyder, and Burns (1992) argue for the need for clarity in describing the intervention, noting that the validity of a study may be compromised by the researcher's failure to thoroughly describe the independent variable. These authors also stress the need for what has been called "treatment integrity"—that is, for researchers to question whether each protocol was executed in exactly the same manner for each treatment session, as a means to control variance, both for repeated uses of the intervention with the same subject and across subjects. Because nurses study complex treatments and diverse participants in a variety of settings, differences in implementing intervention protocols may account for inconsistencies in outcomes related to the effectiveness of a particular intervention (Egan et al., 1992).

Essentially, this is a design issue related to how to obtain and maintain high compliance (Hennekens & Buring, 1989). Two strategies to accumulate sufficient outcome measures are to select a high-risk study population and to extend the duration of the study. With regard to the latter strategy, researchers have postulated that their interventions may have had the desired impact if they had lasted longer (De Berry, Davies, & Reinhard, 1989). However, there should be clinical and empirical support for long protocols, and researchers must weigh extension of the study against the likelihood of increased participant attrition, especially in populations such as the frail elderly (Abraham et al., 1992, p. 201).

When a high proportion of participants are noncompliant, the treatment and control groups become increasingly alike with respect to exposure to the variables of interest, and this in turn may obscure any true effects of the treatment. If a substantial number of participants become noncompliant, say, because of the adverse side effects of an experimental drug, their experience must still be "counted" to allow for a fair and valid trial of the intervention. One method to enhance compliance is the run-in or "washout" period prior to randomization. That is, potential study participants are given practice with all or part of the study protocol prior to randomization, and those who experience difficulty complying with the protocol are then excluded from the study (Lang, 1990). This allows for an increase in the power of the study by yielding a committed group of participants, especially for long-term follow-up studies, and because the observed effects of the difference between the groups will show less of the diluting effects of noncompliance (Hennekens & Buring, 1989; Lang, 1990). Although the use of a run-in may enhance the validity of the study, external validity may be limited, particularly if compliance is in some way related to the outcome of interest.

Thus, the nurse who is critiquing a proposal or published report using an experimental design will want to evaluate the study in terms of its treatment integrity and how well it controls for extraneous variables that might invalidate the results of the experiment by introducing rival and plausible hypotheses. Cook and Campbell (1979) identified 12 types of extraneous variables that, if left uncontrolled, may produce effects that the researcher could mistake for the effect of the independent variable. These threats to internal validity—history, maturation, testing, instrumentation, statistical regression, selection, experimental mortality, selection/maturation interaction, diffusion or imitation of treatments, selection/history interaction, compensatory equalization of treatments, and compensatory rivalry by respondents receiving less desirable treatments—are explained briefly below and are discussed in relation to quasi-experimental designs in the next chapter.

- *History* refers to the events or circumstances other than the introduction of the treatment variable that occur coincident with the time interval between the pretest and posttest measurements. For example, history could have compromised the results of a (hypothetical) experiment to determine the best educational method to increase AIDS awareness among black teenage males, if the study was being conducted at the same time that Magic Johnson announced he was HIV positive—an event that received much media coverage and attention and that may have influenced responses in the target population. In this era of health care reform and rapid technological developments, clinical researchers must be attuned to changes at one study site (such as new staffing patterns in a hospital) that could make comparison of outcome variables (such as staff satisfaction) across several hospitals biased.

- *Maturation* refers to changes within the study participants themselves that occur over time and that are not related to any specific event, such as tiring, gaining weight, or becoming more knowledgeable. Thus, it becomes difficult for the researcher to determine whether changes observed over time can be attributed to the independent variable (or treatment), to maturational changes in the participants, or perhaps to an interaction effect between the treatment and maturational changes. Maturational threats to internal validity are a particular issue in longitudinal studies and in research using people with chronic, degenerative diseases such as Alzheimer's disease.

- *Testing* refers to the learning that results from being tested at Time 1 that affects responses to the test at Time 2, regardless of the introduction of the treatment variable. Thus, the process of measuring itself can introduce a threat to internal validity, especially when reactive measures (see discussion under Manipulation) are used. Participants may recall information on the pretest or be sensitized to aspects of the experiment, especially when the tests are unusual or memorable.

- *Experimental mortality (attrition)* refers to nonequivalent (or differential) attrition of study participants from the experimental and comparison groups that renders meaningful comparisons between the groups difficult. Random attrition is a far less serious threat than when participants are systematically dropping out of one treatment condition more than another. When the latter occurs, researchers should attempt to evaluate a small random sample of dropouts to determine why they left the study. As with maturational changes discussed above, experimental mortality is a particular threat in longitudinal studies.

The nursing study described earlier in the section on randomization (Oakes et al., 1993) that examined the effects of chest tube stripping in pediatric oncology patients illustrates several of the potential threats to validity that were addressed by the researchers, including history, adaptation, testing, and attrition. One of the important outcome variables in this study was self-reported pain. The authors note that history could influence pain scores if other painful events unrelated to the intervention (chest tube stripping) or thoracotomy occurred at the same time as the stripping. They controlled for this possibility by adding a checklist that included a place for noting other painful events that were then transferred to the data collection sheet and considered in interpretation of pain scores. In addition, participants could have become so accustomed to pain that they adapted to it and therefore failed to report it. This threat to validity was reduced by the design of the study that included random assignment of participants to groups, thereby making it more likely that adaptation to pain would occur equally across both groups. The researchers also noted that repeated testing of participants might result in a memory effect that could influence their responses. To decrease this threat, the investigators used two instruments to measure pain, and the sequence of their administration was randomized. Unequal attrition did not occur in the two groups over the course of the study, but the researchers kept careful notes regarding attrition nonetheless (Oakes et al., 1993).

- *Instrumentation* refers to changes that occur in the measurement instruments, observers, or raters that potentially produce changes in the dependent variable measurements. For example, batteries that power a scale may run down, or interviewers may become fatigued or bored over time, such that measurements taken later in the course of the study are different from those at baseline. This threat to validity is most pronounced in studies using repeated measures designs (see discussion of multiple treatment—repeated measures designs elsewhere in this chapter).

■ *Statistical regression* refers to the movement of mean scores from Time 1 to Time 2 that most often results when study participants are selected on the basis of scores that are at the extremes of the distribution. For example, a multigenerational study of persons with unusually high IQ scores (greater than 140) might reveal that the IQ scores of their children and grandchildren were closer to the average distribution (e.g., 100) on this variable.

■ *Selection bias* refers to the selection of participants on a nonrandom basis that may produce differences in the experimental and comparison group participants with regard to the criterion measurement irrespective of the differential exposure to the treatment. This threat occurs, for example, when an investigator (consciously or unconsciously) assigns all the smarter, sicker, or wealthier individuals to one treatment condition and not the other or when participants are pregrouped in a long-term care facility according to acuity levels or stage of disease. Thus, if only residents in the less severely ill group are exposed to the intervention, outcomes will be biased in terms of the effectiveness of the treatment.

■ *Interactions with selection* means that a number of the previously described threats to internal validity can interact with selection, causing spurious treatment effects. The combined effects of nonrandom selection of participants and differential changes that occur within the participants on dependent variable measurements between Time 1 and Time 2 may be interpreted as changes that are due to the treatment when in fact they result from selection and maturation interaction. Selection-history and selection-instrumentation are among the additional interaction effects that can be erroneously interpreted as treatment effects. Because of these types of interaction effects, participants that are in any way self-selected should be scrutinized carefully for differential treatment effects at Time 2 even though the groups demonstrated equivalence on the dependent variable measurements at Time 1. Selection maturation interaction occurs when some process within the participants is changing at a differential rate regardless of the introduction of the treatment. Selection-history results when participants are drawn from different unique settings that have exposed the participants to variable local historical events that may influence the outcome measure. Selection-instrumentation can result when participants achieve different mean scores on an instrument that is not constructed with equal intervals, producing "ceiling" and "floor" effects on the measurement. When a ceiling effect occurs, a larger number of participants in one group will be unable to achieve more true change in the measurement score. Conversely, when more individuals in one group are clustered at the lower end of a scale, it may be because the instrument is not capable of measuring true scores below a certain point (floor effects). An example of a ceiling effect with the Family Perceptions of Care tool used in the Maas and Buckwalter (1990) study of special care units is described in the next chapter on quasi-experimental designs. Floor effects, on the other hand, occur in instruments such as mental status tests when they are used to measure cognitive impairment in the later stages of dementia, when participants' scores tend to cluster around zero.

■ *Diffusion or imitation of treatments* refers to the introduction of a treatment that involves information when the experimental and control group participants may be able to interact with one another, directly or indirectly, and learn about information intended for others. This threat to internal validity may be a particularly salient contaminating effect for many nursing research studies in which study participants are physically proximal to one another and likely to communicate, as in a hospital ward area. A community-based example of this threat to validity occurred in a nursing study in which rural caregivers of persons with Alzheimer's Disease (AD) were randomly assigned to either an experimental strategy teaching them to manage behavioral problems associated with AD or to a control group in which they received routine referrals and a copy of the book, *The 36-Hour Day*. Midway through the 1-year study, in one of the rural communities where the study took place, caregivers from both the experimental and control groups ended up joining the same newly formed AD caregivers' support group. At one of the support group meetings, a participant from the experimental group brought his research notebook and shared behavioral management information from the experimental protocol with a participant from the control group—thus contaminating the design.

■ *Compensatory equalization of treatments* refers to the use of an experimental treatment that has actual or potential value to participants in cases in which authorities or participants may be unwilling to tolerate an imposed inequity in the distribution of the treatment. The result may be that the treatment is obtained by participants making up the control group so that the planned experimental contrast is compromised. For example, in recent Phase III randomized, double-blind, controlled trials of a drug to manage symptoms associated with AIDS, compelling evidence emerged during the course of the study that the experimental agent drastically decreased the likelihood that a pregnant woman would pass the HIV virus on to her unborn child. Midway through the study, federal authorities mandated that participants in the control group have access to the potentially life-saving (in the case of the fetus) agent.

- *Compensatory rivalry by respondents receiving less desirable treatments* refers to the assignment of study participants to experimental and control groups in which control group participants are disadvantaged by the absence of the treatment in contrast to experimental participants and thus are motivated to compete for equity. Like compensatory equalization, compensatory rivalry is a response to the inequity of benefits imposed by the presence of an experimental condition. However, compensatory equalization is mainly a response by administrators, and compensatory rivalry is a response by participants in a disadvantaged no-treatment group. For example, in the AD caregiver example noted above under diffusion of treatments, once the control group participant became aware of the training her counterpart in the experimental group had received as part or the experimental protocol, she contacted the investigator and "demanded" to be given a copy of the research notebook and to learn about the behavioral management strategies that were being taught only to caregivers in the experimental group.

In general, experimenters are primarily concerned with the internal validity of their design. However, they are also interested in the *external validity,* or generalizability, of their findings with respect to other participants, settings, and variables. The researcher and those critiquing a proposal or study may ask, "Are the findings relevant beyond the experimental condition?" Both the representativeness of the participants and the experimental settings must be considered when judging whether the findings can be applied elsewhere. Cook and Campbell (1979) identified six main factors that may jeopardize the external validity of a design: interaction effects of selection biases and the independent variable, the reactive effect of pretesting, the reactive effect of experimental procedures, multiple treatment interferences, interaction of history and treatment, and interaction of setting and treatment. When they are controlled, the researcher can achieve generalizability by replicating the study with different participants, in different settings, and at different times. These six threats to external validity are briefly described below:

- *Interaction of selection and treatment* refers to the effects obtained that are applicable only to the specific individuals who participated in the study.

This threat to external validity is especially apt to occur the more unusual the requirements for participation. If participation is made as convenient and unextraordinary as possible, there is less likelihood of systematic recruitment factors operating that lead to results that apply only to the "very special people" who agree to participate and are able to comply with protocol.

- *Interaction of setting and treatment* refers to the effects obtained that are applicable only to the specific setting in which the experiment is conducted. This threat also contains an element of selection bias because persons from some settings are more apt to agree to participate than those from others. The milieus of settings vary widely, with some being more innovative, more pleasant, and more competitive. The question is whether or not results obtained in one setting can be generalized to other settings that, because of their particular environments, would be different from the original setting. For example, a study of the effects of a series of geriatric mental health training programs on the behavior, knowledge, and attitudes of nursing home staff in rural long-term care facilities was developed and evaluated in nursing homes in Iowa (Smith et al., 1994). When the same training series was implemented and tested in nursing homes in the Appalachian region of rural Virginia, the findings were very different because some of the training content was culturally "irrelevant" and insensitive and the literacy level of the predominantly minority nursing home staff conducting the training was considerably different from that of staff members in the Midwest.

- *Interaction of history and treatment* refers to the effects obtained that are applicable only to the specific time period within which the study is conducted. Unusual occurrences that coincide with a study period can make the extrapolation of results to other periods of time questionable. Although the researcher can attempt to plan in a way that avoids obvious unusual occurrences, it is often impossible to avoid happenings that could make the findings unique to the study time period. Also, the generalization of findings to future time periods is always questionable. Replication of studies at different times is the logical approach to counteracting the interaction effect of history.

Cook and Campbell (1979) refer to additional threats to external validity that have been described by Campbell and Stanley (1963) as "threats to construct validity." Because most research texts continue to subsume "threats to construct validity" under "threats to external validity," these threats are listed and described below:

- *Reaction or interaction effect of pretesting* means that following exposure to the pretest, the participants no longer remain representative of the target population, which has not been pretested. Thus, the findings cannot be generalized to the target population. This effect occurs because the nature of the pretest makes participants aware of certain issues or events of which they would not otherwise be aware, causing them to respond to the treatment in a unique way. For example, in an experimental study of the effects of a family-staff partnership intervention on selected resident, staff, and family outcomes in a nursing home setting, staff participants in both experimental and control nursing homes were pretested at base- line using several instruments that evaluated staff member perceptions of family involvement in care. As a result of sensitization to family-related issues due to pretesting, there is potential that staff members in one of the control settings could initiate a family support group soon after the research was begun.

- *Reactive effect of experimental procedures* is the effect produced by the procedures of the experiment that make the participants who are exposed to these procedures no longer representative of the target population, this is commonly known as the "Hawthorne effect."

- *Multiple treatment interference* refers to effects produced by multiple expo- sures of participants to a treatment so that the results may be gener- alizable only to individuals who also receive the same multiple exposures to the treatment in the same sequence.

Causality. Experimental designs are used to test hypotheses of cause- and-effect relationships between variables; that is, when X occurs, it is likely that Y will result. Although causal laws can never be proved, researchers proposing or critiquing experimental designs should be aware of the three criteria for causality (Selltiz, Wrightsman, & Cook, 1976, p. 115): (a) a temporal relationship—that is, the cause must pre- cede the effect in time; (b) an empirical relationship—that is, there must be evidence that the independent variable and the dependent variable are associated; and (c) the relationship cannot be explained by the influence of a third variable (or spurious relationship). Some examples may serve to clarify these criteria: A correlational study in which the researcher proposes that X, decreased nurse responsiveness (as mea- sured by amount of time taken to answer call lights) causes Y, increased number of patient complaints, fails to meet the criterion of a temporal relationship because it is *equally* possible that the effect (Y) may precede the cause (X). That is, increased complaining on the part of patients may lead nurses to stop responding efficiently, because they dread dealing with patient complaints and therefore delay unpleasant encounters by failing to respond to call lights.

A study suggesting that excessive trace elements such as aluminum (X) causes Alzheimer's disease (Y) would have to meet the criterion of an empirical relationship by demonstrating an association between the ingestion of aluminum and the presence of Alzheimer's disease using, for example, specimens from the hippocampus region of the brain on autopsy.

Finally, a nurse researcher who has observed a relationship between number of ice cream cones consumed (X) and number of drownings (Y) cannot conclude there is a causal relationship between eating ice cream and drowning without taking into consideration a third spurious variable, Z (season of the year), that influences both X and Y. That is, there are more ice cream cones consumed in the warm summer months, and there are more drownings also, because more people go to the beach in the summer months as well. This somewhat humorous example illustrates an important point—that correlation is a necessary but insufficient condition for causality. However, knowledge gained about the relationship between variables using correlational designs can serve as the basis for the testing of causal relationships using experimental designs.

Only in true experimental designs can plausible alternative explanations for observed relationships be eliminated or discredited. This is because experimental designs have the highest internal validity and thus the greatest control over factors other than those advanced by the research hypotheses that might explain the findings. When a smaller number of plausible interpretations are available to account for the data, a theory is confirmed to a greater degree (Campbell & Stanley, 1963).

SUMMARY OF STRENGTHS AND WEAKNESSES

A major advantage of experimental designs is the degree of confidence they allow the researcher in inferring causal relationships. This is the case because true experiments have greater internal validity than other methodological approaches. A high degree of internal validity enables the researcher to rule out rival or alternative explanations to a causal interpretation. Establishing causal relationships is important to researchers because it enhances their ability to predict and therefore control phenomena. Despite these advantages, the proportion of experimental studies reported in the nursing literature remains relatively small, although experimental research conducted by nurses is increasing. For example, Abraham, Chalifoux, and Evers (1992) reviewed 2,746 articles from six scholarly journals over the period from 1981 to 1990. Of those, only 293 (10.7%) were reports of nursing intervention studies, both experimental and quasi-experimental.

Experimental designs are not perfect. Among the limitations already noted are the number of potentially interesting research variables that are not within the researcher's purview to manipulate. Ethical concerns, organizational prohibitions, and human characteristics often interfere with the researcher's ability to control a number of variables experimentally. Moreover, the sample is usually not representative. To increase control of extraneous variables, the sample is often quite homogeneous prior to random assignment, and therefore, many replications may be required to achieve any generalizability.

Another design limitation, apparent in laboratory experiments especially, is their artificiality and, thus, diminished external validity. Yet another compromise to generalizability is the "Hawthorne effect," or the reactive effects created by individuals' knowledge that they are participating in an experiment. Finally, many of the phenomena of interest to nursing are simply not yet well described and do not have an adequate theoretical base to be tested appropriately in an experimental mode. Rather, these phenomena are best approached in exploratory and/or descriptive studies that will generate hypotheses for experimental testing at a later stage in the development of nursing knowledge.

Research Settings. Researchers frequently distinguish between "field experiments" and "laboratory experiments" based on the setting in which the research is conducted. Field experiments are conducted in real-life settings, such as hospitals, that are particularly well suited to the study's external validity, but field experiments often lack control of variance, because it is difficult to control extraneous environmental variables in real-life settings. Conversely, laboratory experiments are conducted in highly controlled, artificial settings in which the investigator has great control over all experimental conditions. Because of these characteristics, laboratory experiments usually contain less error variance and are more easily replicated than field studies. The artificiality of the research setting, although boosting the internal validity of the experiment, diminishes its generalizability and occasionally the impact of the experimental treatment as well. Both types of experiments are crucial to the generation of nursing knowledge. Both have inherent strengths and weaknesses that the researcher should consider when choosing a research setting. As with the choice of design, the choice of research setting (e.g., field or laboratory) should be determined by the nature of the research questions under consideration, the culture in which they are studied, and the historical context.

Sampling Issues. In many experimental situations, study participants cannot be randomly selected from a defined population. In other words, a complete list of all persons in a population (the sampling frame) cannot be obtained from which a random sample can be drawn. Although probability sampling of participants is ideal, and the best way to generalize research findings beyond the sample, the realities of clinical research, in particular, often prohibit random sampling. In experimental designs, the use of random assignment provides control of sample variables by the random distribution of important characteristics to both experimental and control groups.

In many clinical experiments, participants are selected on the basis of variables such as presence of a given disease or syndrome at a given point in time. All persons who meet selected inclusion criteria and who consent to participate are thus enrolled in the study. More often than not, participants are selected sequentially as they arrive for a particular treatment. In these field settings, it is frequently infeasible to locate and list the population in advance of participant selection. Moreover, in many cases, the population is unknown.

Lack of probability sampling poses several methodological disadvantages. First, without random sampling, it is difficult to generalize research findings beyond the sample. In addition, experimental designs employ rigorous control over many variables, making the sample unrepresentative of real-world cohorts and thus generalizations to the population questionable. Second, inferential statistics should be applied only to data obtained from probability samples. Parametric statistical procedures commonly used to analyze experimental results, such as analysis of variance, have a number of underlying assumptions that are best met through random sampling.

Third, only with probability sampling are researchers able to determine sample size according to how much sampling error (the differences between population values and sample values) they are willing to accept. In experimental designs without probability sampling, the desired sample size depends on the number and type of variables under study. If subgroups within the sample are to be analyzed, the sample size often must be increased. Ns of 20 to 30 participants per subdivision of the data (or each cell of a factorial design) are recommended, with the minimum being 10 per group.

The researcher must ensure the generation of sufficient data for purposes of analysis through the testing of an adequate number of participants. Power is defined as the probability that a statistical test will support a research hypothesis when it should be supported or the probability that it will reject the null hypothesis when it should be rejected. Analysis of the power of the statistical tests to be used in an experiment is a function of effect size, power, and significance level. Formulas are available that permit investigators to calculate the necessary sample size to detect a statistically significant effect if one exists. Discussion of these formulas is beyond the scope of this chapter, and the interested reader is referred to additional references on this topic (Cohen, 1988; Hennekens & Buring, 1989; Kraemer & Thiemann, 1987; Rudy & Kerr, 1991; Shott, 1990; Slakter, Wu, & Suzuki-Slakter, 1991; Yarandi, 1991). In general, and when economically feasible, large samples are preferable to small samples. Data from larger samples usually are more reliable, are more representative of the population of interest, have fewer sampling errors, and provide more statistical power for purposes of analysis. Increased sample size also decreases the probability of Type I (alpha) and Type II (beta) errors in hypothesis testing. (See the discussion of hypothesis testing, below.)

Finally, larger samples permit the principle of randomization to function better in the distribution of sample characteristics between groups.

Measurement of Outcomes in Experimental Design. Selection of poor or insensitive outcome measures (dependent variables) can seriously undermine a nursing research project. Insensitive measure bias occurs, for example, when dependent measures are inadequate to differentiate among subgroups of patients and to detect a clinically meaningful change. In an excellent two-part series, Stewart and Archbold (1992, 1993) have outlined seven questions that should be addressed when choosing an outcome measure:

1. *Is the conceptual link between the intervention and the outcome variable logical?* The investigator must be able to logically define the expected relationship between the intervention and outcome. In addition, the outcome measure should not be so global in nature that factors other than the treatment could be causing the change. To rule out other causes, specific outcome measures should be used.

2. *To what extent is the outcome variable amenable to change?* When considering the ability of the outcome measure to change, the investigator must also define whether the change is expected to be short- or long-term (e.g., measures to stabilize blood glucose immediately vs. long-term control).

3. *Is the content validity of the outcome measure adequate for detecting the effect of the proposed intervention?* The investigator should consider whether items on the outcome measure adequately capture the specific effects of the treatment.

4. *Does evidence for the construct validity of the outcome measure argue for its potential to detect change as a result of the proposed intervention?* Because one of the primary purposes of experimental studies is to detect change, an important consideration for the outcome measure is its validity sensitivity to change and ability to detect differences between the experimental and control groups. The investigator should consider whether the outcome measure has been used in previous intervention studies and how well it was able to detect change.

5. *Does the instrument used to measure the attribute have a potential distribution of scores that will allow detection of change?* Researchers should examine the potential range of scores to determine whether there is room for change and whether the measurement units are sufficiently fine-tuned to detect differences. Measures with a floor or ceiling effect should be evaluated to make sure there is room for change in the desired direction within those limits.

6. *What type of reliability assessment is appropriate to consider for this outcome measure?* Reliability estimates must reflect a small degree of measurement error. The focus is on within-subject changes that occur as a result of treatment, as opposed to between-subjects differences. If feasible, parallel forms for the outcome measure can be used; reliability will be

reflected in the agreement between the two forms on changes in the dependent variable. Empirical evidence of construct validity may be an indirect measure of reliability.

7. *How should the level of correlational stability over time be interpreted?* High test-retest correlation over long periods of time may indicate that the outcome measure is stable and unlikely to change. High correlations may also mean that the participant has not yet received the intervention or an adequate "dose" of the intervention. Low test-retest correlations over time may indicate that the measure is sensitive to change.

The four main issues related to outcome measurement—relevant outcome variables, validity, reliability, and systematic biases—are discussed in more depth in the following section.

Relevant outcome variables are crucial for answering causal research questions. In the example of depressed patients randomly assigned to an experimental nursing intervention designed to treat depression, one obvious criterion measure of effectiveness of the intervention is whether treated patients improve on measures of depression. There are a number of ways to measure depression, ranging from indirect physiological parameters such as MHPG levels in urine to self-report instruments such as the Beck Depression Inventory. Which outcome variables are most relevant depends on the study's theoretical framework, the objectives of the intervention, and the research questions addressed. In this example, the nurse researcher might also be interested in recidivism and/or suicide rates, vocational adjustment following the intervention, and family attitudes toward the patient. To measure these diverse aftercare variables the nurse researcher might use structured observations or interviews and archival data. The point is that whether and how these variables are measured depends on the objectives of the particular intervention. The independent variable and its outcome criteria must be correlated in the theoretical framework. For example, if the nursing intervention to alleviate depression is cognitive restructuring, a dependent variable that captures cognitive changes is most appropriate. Similarly, if an intervention is psychopharmacological in nature for purposes of altering selected catacholamines, a physiological measure of those catacholamines or their breakdown products is most relevant.

Often, a variety of data collection methods is required to assess all the relevant outcome measures. If the intervention is truly effective, and the theoretical framework sound, differences should be found on all reliable and valid outcome measures. Furthermore, because these measures often involve different methods of assessment (see the discussion of triangulation, below), the nurse researcher can have increased confidence in the findings. This is because the more numerous and independent the ways in which the experimental effect is shown, the less plausible alternative explanations or rival hypotheses become (Campbell & Stanley, 1963).

The employment of measures that have demonstrated reliability and validity is critical to the success of any experiment. For an in-depth discussion of these issues, see Chapter 10 of this volume, "Methodological Studies: Instrument Development," by Merle Mishel.

Validity refers to whether a particular instrument actually measures the construct it is designed to assess (Carmines & Zeller, 1979). In the example of an experimental nursing intervention to treat depression, if an *invalid* measure of depression is used to assess patient outcome, the researcher might falsely conclude that the intervention is effective or ineffective. Because of the instrument's lack of validity, scores would not be indicative of any true changes in depression that occurred due to the intervention. An invalid measure could be measuring some other property, such as powerlessness.

In selecting measures to use in any experiment, the researcher should carefully review the validity evidence for the measure. Mishel's chapter provides an excellent description of the different forms of validity employed in evaluating measurement instruments, including self-evident measures such as face and content validity, pragmatic measures or criterion-related validity (both concurrent and predictive), and construct validity. Construct validity deals with validation of the theory or construct underlying an experimental study. Ideally, experimental designs should use instruments with established construct validity. However, the multitrait, multimethod techniques used to establish construct validity are complex, and more often than not, experiments are conducted using tools that have not yet achieved this highest level of validation.

Certain instruments may be valid only for selected populations or age groups. For example, if our nursing intervention was for treatment of the depressed *elderly*, then standard measures of depression widely used with younger age groups might not be valid for this study (Kane & Kane, 1981). Failure to use age-validated criteria could result in changes in cognitive abilities and physiological processes being labeled as pathological when in fact they are normal consequences of aging. Thus, it is critical that measures of depression be validated for the elderly before they are used in this study.

Reliability is concerned with the accuracy (consistency, stability, and repeatability) of a measure in representing the true score of the participant being assessed on a particular dimension. Mishel's chapter presents an in-depth discussion of the ways to conceptualize and evaluate a measure's reliability, including tests of stability, such as test-retest; tests for equivalence, such as alternate forms; and tests of internal consistency, which ensure that the concept is measured consistently throughout the instrument.

It is important to employ reliable measures in any experimental study, because unreliable measures may not be sensitive or accurate enough to detect differences in the experimental versus the control group. That is, the effect of measurement error (discussed earlier in this chapter in the section on *control of variance*) is to attenuate or reduce the differences between groups, which can undermine efforts to demonstrate the effectiveness of a particular intervention. In general, reliability coefficients should be at least 0.70. The reliability coefficient is determined by what proportion of the test variance is *nonerror* variance.

Biases in measurement can be minimized by using more than one method of measurement. The use of multiple methods of data collection and sources (*triangulation* of the measurement process) is recommended to ensure assessing the range of relevant outcome measures for a particular experiment. This approach, using multiple methods of assessment, also helps to counteract systematic biases that may be present in some measures. Often, patients or staff may be biased in their assessments, out of a desire to see a particular intervention succeed. These biases can lead to false conclusions of effectiveness on the part of the researcher. Employing a variety of data collection methods will help to counteract this type of bias.

It is important to use data collectors who are "blind" to (that is, unknowledgeable about) which participants received the experimental condition and which are controls. This means that the same research assistant who delivers the nursing intervention should not collect the outcome data related to that intervention. Additional personnel who do *not* hold preconceptions should be employed to collect the outcome data. An experimental ideal in terms of decreasing bias is the *double blind* procedure, in which neither the participant nor the observer knows the group to which the participant is assigned (see discussion of the Physician's Health Study under 2 × 2 factorial designs as an example of a double-blind study). Randomized, double-blind crossover studies have also been used in nursing research. For example, Simms, Rhodes, and Madsen (1993) used this design strategy to compare the antiemetic effectiveness of intravenous Compazine and Ativan in the management of postchemotherapy symptoms during two initial cycles of therapy. Only the staff pharmacist who randomized participants into one of the two antiemetic regimen groups knew the regimen for a particular patient. Yet another approach to decreasing bias is to assign more than one data collector for each participant and then calculate interrater agreements. It is often sufficient to check interrater reliability on only a random 10% of all data sets.

In experimental designs, the data collection methods are highly structured, the approach to data collection is deductive and theory testing, and the researcher controls the variables and the experimental conditions. A wide variety of data collection methods are acceptable, and multiple methods of assessment are encouraged, as long as the conditions and measurements are identical for all participants. This high degree of structure is usually an asset when it comes to data preparation and analysis.

Hypothesis Testing. Experimental research is theory-testing research, and whereas experimental findings can never be used to "prove" a theory, successful theories avoid disconfirmation. A useful tool for both designing and interpreting the results of a study is *substruction*. This is a process by which both the conceptual and operational indicators assessed in the study and their relationships are diagrammed. This diagram more clearly portrays the relationships between the variables and hypotheses in a study and is a valuable aid in specifying appropriate hypotheses and interpreting data in the context of the theoretical framework (Hinshaw, 1979; Phillips, 1986).

Hypotheses are statements concerning predicted relationships between the variables under study that link a study's theoretical framework to experimental realities. Hypotheses provide overall direction to any experiment and guide every aspect of the research process, including sampling, data collection, and analysis. The components of a hypothesis are examined in detail in Brink and Wood (1983, pp. 67-73). In general, a well-written hypothesis (a) is neutral in tone rather than value-laden, (b) precisely and parsimoniously identifies the independent and dependent variables, and (c) identifies how the dependent variable is measured. The research hypothesis in experimental designs should be derived from a theory, must specify the predicted relationship between two or more variables, and must be testable; that is, the variables specified must be measurable.

The *null hypothesis* is set up for purposes of possible rejection. It is an arbitrary convention and the hypothesis that is tested statistically. The null hypothesis postulates that any differences found between the experimental and control groups would be due to chance alone or to sampling errors. The *research* (or working) *hypothesis* states the researcher's expectations, identifying the factors in a causal relationship that are believed to account for the findings. Rejecting the null hypothesis suggests support for the research hypothesis. Researchers can commit two types of errors in accepting or rejecting the null hypothesis. *Type I error* (alpha) occurs when the null hypothesis is rejected and it is true; that is, no differences actually exist in the data. Alpha errors are best avoided by choosing a conservative (alpha = .05) level of significance. *Type II error* (beta) occurs when the null hypothesis is accepted falsely; that is, the researcher concludes that no difference exists when it actually does. There is no established beta error level; rather, Type II error is addressed through its relationship to power (Rudy & Kerr, 1991), defined earlier in this chapter.

Data Analysis. Tests of hypotheses are one form of analysis that experimenters engage in. Which statistical test is selected depends on what the hypothesis predicts, the level of measurement, and assumptions related to the data. In the classic experimental design, a comparison of two sample means (the posttest data for the control and experimental groups) is made to determine whether or not the independent variable "made a difference." The null hypothesis under test is that the two means are the same (H_0: $X_1 = X_2$), and the alternative or research hypothesis is that the two means differ (H_1: $X_1 > X_2$, $X_1 < X_2$, or $X_1 \neq X_2$). Statistical procedures such as a t test for differences between two groups or analysis of variance (ANOVA) for differences among multiple groups can be used to test these hypotheses. A significant F statistic using the ANOVA procedure indicates that the "among-group" variance is larger than the "within-group" variance. Because these tests are based on comparisons of sample means, the level of measurement must be at least interval level. These parametric tests assume (1) that the data are normally distributed and (2) that the variances of the data are similar. Both the t test and ANOVA have nonparametric or "distribution-free" counterparts, including the Mann Whitney U test and the Kruskall-Wallis one-way ANOVA for ordinal data, respectively. Siegel and Castellan (1988) provide an excellent reference on nonparametric procedures.

It can be misleading to compare t tests on a before-and-after basis without first comparing initial differences between the control and experimental groups. If the researcher has collected pretreatment data on both the experimental and control group using the same outcome measure, these pretest measures can be employed as covariates in an ANCOVA procedure. The effect of this procedure is blocking or "leveling out" of the pretest scores and the adjustment of posttest scores to compensate for initial lack of equivalence between groups. Thus, AN-COVA adjusts for initial differences between groups and for the correlation between means. A more complete discussion of ANCOVA appears in Chapter 3 of this volume, on quasi-experimental designs. On occasion, problems may arise in experimental studies that employ random assignment that result in the randomly assigned groups becoming nonequivalent over the course of the study. As discussed earlier in this chapter, this may be due to differential attrition, noncompliance with the study protocol, or crossover between groups. It is tempting in these cases to analyze only data from participants who actually receive treatment as indicated in the initial assignment to treatment and control groups. However, analyzing only those participants who fully comply with the study protocol may actually introduce bias. For example, if participants who did not comply with the study protocol are removed from the analysis, the findings of an effect for the intervention are confounded by compliance, because noncompliant participants are excluded. Therefore, it is important to analyze *all* randomized participants, because comparisons of any subgroups that are defined after randomization are no longer valid. Known as "intention-to-treat" analysis (Newell, 1992), the concept implies that all patients randomly allocated to a treatment group should be analyzed together as representing that treatment, whether or not they completed or even received the treatment at all; that is, "once randomized always analyzed." Indeed, one important purpose of randomization is to decrease selection bias and to generate comparable groups. Any changes to these groups destroys that comparability. In sum, intention-to-treat analysis is critical, especially in randomized clinical trials, because the prognostic balance brought about by randomization will be disturbed, the sample size will be reduced, and the validity of the statistical tests used will be undermined (Lee, Ellenberg, Hirtz, & Nelson, 1991).

PILOT STUDY

A pilot study is strongly recommended before the conduct of any major experiment. This preliminary investigation or "trial run," using a limited number of participants permits the researcher to test and possibly reshape or add hypotheses. The pilot study is an ideal time to conduct manipulation checks, enabling the researcher to determine whether or not the desired level of strength has been achieved through manipulation of the independent variable(s) (Pedhazur & Schmelkin, 1991). The proposed data collection and analysis procedure can also be evaluated and changed as needed. Unanticipated problems arise during the course of almost any study, and a pilot study enables the researcher to identify and deal with these before the major study is sabotaged. In addition, pilot studies can indicate the proportion of respondents likely to return mailed follow-up questionnaires, for example, so that the researcher can address issues related to obtaining complete follow-up data on all participants, if the design calls for multiple data collection points (Hennekens & Buring, 1989). The value of pilot studies is emphasized by the fact that grants submitted to the National Institutes of Health are rarely awarded without evidence of pilot data.

ETHICAL CONSIDERATIONS

The protection of the rights of all human and animal subjects is the obligation of every researcher, and these rights are protected by federal law. Perhaps the most important concern for human subjects comes in the area of informed consent. All people who participate in an experimental study must clearly understand its purpose, procedures, the researcher's expectations of them as study participants, the length of the experiment, and projected use of the data. Researchers must further provide adequate treatment and referral mechanisms for participants should injury or other untoward complications develop during the course of the experiment. Participation must be voluntary, and participants must be assured of their right to withdraw from the study at any time without prejudice. True informed consent means that the researcher cannot withhold information or deceive participants in any way, even if knowledge of the research purpose or methods might affect their response. Nor can participants be coerced in any way to participate—for example, by intimating that needed treatment might be withheld.

Of particular concern in experimental designs, which typically employ a control or comparison group, is the notion that the research approach should not deprive control participants of necessary care or information. Experimental studies that employ a placebo drug or effect must therefore be carefully scrutinized. As in other methodologies, the researcher using an experimental design must avoid an invasion of participants' privacy, assure participants of anonymity or confidentiality, and inform them of plans for publishing findings of the study without identification of individual participants (Silva, 1995; Armiger, 1977; Jacobsen, 1973).

CRITIQUING EXPERIMENTS

Although experimental designs provide for the most rigorous tests of hypotheses, no one design is perfect, and many experiments reported in the literature are flawed and subject to question. Perhaps the experiment was not well-conceptualized to begin with, or perhaps the experimental conditions were not carefully controlled, the analyses imprecise, or interpretations rendered that went beyond the scope of the data. Especially in field settings, adequate control over all variables is extremely difficult to achieve.

Batey (1971) has classified experimental pitfalls into three major areas: conceptual, empirical, and interpretive. Conceptual problems most frequently encountered have to do with poorly defined or inconsequential research problems and with a lack of congruence between study variables and the theoretical "roots" of the study. Hypotheses may be poorly stated, or it may be inappropriate to be testing the hypotheses altogether. That is, perhaps exploratory (Level I) or descriptive (Level II) questions (Brink & Wood, 1983) are better suited to the phenomena under study, and it is premature to test hypotheses and attempt to establish cause-and-effect relationships between the variables.

Empirical problems center largely on control-of-variance issues, discussed earlier in this chapter. Without adequate control over extraneous variables, the researcher cannot be confident that it was the independent variable(s) that was (were) responsible for any observed changes in the dependent variable(s), an issue of the internal validity of the study. The external validity, or generalizability of findings, is also subject to criticism. For example, if characteristics of either the sample or population are unknown, inferences from one to the other may not be valid.

Problems of interpretation of the data may arise from a variety of sources, including inappropriate analysis procedures and lack of congruence with the study's theoretical framework. It is not uncommon for beginning researchers, in particular, to make assertions that have no basis in the research findings (that is, that go beyond the data) or to fail to consider adequately the study's limitations (e.g., small sample size or measurement errors) when developing inferences from results. In experimental designs, which are theory testing in nature, the supporting theoretical framework should guide all interpretations of the data. It is essential to report data that support, as well as disconfirm, the null hypotheses. Reviewers may also question whether human subjects' rights were adequately protected in the experiment and whether the merit of the study was proportionate to the risks incurred.

Although a number of approaches to critiquing experimental studies are available, Binder (1981, pp. 158-159) has developed a comprehensive criterion checklist for critiquing nursing research using experimental designs. The checklist is based on Batey's (1971) three-part classification scheme. Many of the pitfalls and issues related to the conduct and analysis of experimental studies discussed thus far will become clearer in this final section, in which three designs are examined in relation to actual nursing studies.

USE OF EXPERIMENTAL DESIGNS IN NURSING RESEARCH

In reviewing the classic experimental design (pretest, posttest, control group), subjects are randomly assigned to the experimental and control groups.

$$RA \ \frac{O_1 \ X \ O_2 \ (Ex)}{O_3 \quad O_4 \ (Con)}$$

where RA = random assignment, O = observations, Ex = experimental group, and Con = control group.

Participants are pretested on the dependent variable (O_1, O_2) before participants in the experimental group receive the experimental manipulation (X). Both groups are subsequently posttested (O_2, O_4) and the differences between their scores on the dependent variable are analyzed using a t test or F test. This design has many advantages. First, it is simple, and random assignment of participants helps to ensure that the groups are equivalent at the beginning of the study. The comparison group controls for threats to internal validity such as history (the influence of events that might occur during the study and that could affect the dependent variable) and maturation (processes occurring within the participants themselves as a function of the passage of time). As both groups are pretested, any sensitizing effects of the pretest should be equally distributed (controlling for the effects of testing). However, results can be generalized only to similarly pretested groups, which decreases the study's external validity.

A number of variations on the classic experimental design exist. This design can be extended to more than one independent variable, as in the Eland (1982) example below, and to more than one measurement of the dependent variable(s), as noted in the Layton (1979) example that follows.

Factorial Designs

Classical experimental design allows the manipulation of a single independent variable at a time, holding all other conditions constant. Frequently, phenomena of interest to nurses are more complex than the classical design permits, and factors may *interact* to produce behaviors of interest to nurse researchers. As noted earlier, *factorial designs* permit more than one independent variable to be manipulated at a time and thus allow the testing of multiple hypotheses simultaneously. Furthermore, interaction effects between variables are revealed, making factorial designs an important variation on the classical experimental design.

Although the example used in this chapter is a 2 × 2 factorial design, factorial experiments can be conducted with three or more independent variables (known as factors). Each factor must have two or more levels. Thus, when new factors are added, more hypotheses can be tested simultaneously. Concurrently, the interpretation of main effects and interaction effects becomes more complex with the addition of new factors. Factorial designs are also referred to as "levels by treatment" designs. When one of the factors cannot be manipulated, such as sex of participants, it is referred to as a *blocking variable*. The design that incorporates the blocking variable is known as a *randomized block design*.

Design 1: 2 × 2 Factorial

The purpose of this study was to investigate the effects of two separate nursing interventions on the amount of pain experienced by prekindergarten children undergoing a routine DPT immunization (Eland, 1982). A 2 × 2 factorial design was used to test the two nursing interventions. Intervention 1 altered the transmission of pain messages from the skin surface by spraying a skin coolant, Frigiderm, on the injection site immediately prior to the injection. One half of the partici-pants had Frigiderm sprayed on the injection site prior to the injection, and the other half had aerosol air sprayed on their legs prior to injection. Intervention 2 altered the processing and interpretation of injection pain by giving cognitive information. One-half of the participants were told by the nurse prior to injection, "I'm going to spray something on your leg before your shot that will not hurt, that will make your leg feel cool, and the spray will make this shot hurt less than other shots you've had." The other half of the participants were told only that the nurse was "going to spray something on their leg before their shot." The sample consisted of 20 male and 20 female prekindergarteners. There were 5 males and 5 females included in each of the two levels of the two treatment groups. Children scheduled for physical exams during a 1-month period were stratified by the variables of sex and nurse who would give the injection. Each child was then *randomly assigned* to one of the treatment groups. The dependent variable, amount of pain expe-rienced with the injection, was assessed using the Eland color tool, with its 4-point pain scale (0 = *no pain* to 3 = *severe pain*). Participants in Group A received Frigiderm and cognitive information, those in Group B received air and cognitive information, those in Group C received Frigiderm but no cognitive information, and those in Group D received air and no cognitive information (see Figure 2.1).

A two-factor analysis of variance was used to answer the research question. The ANOVA test dimensions consisted of (a) a *main effect* for type of spray, (b) a *main effect* for type of cognitive information, and (c) the *interaction effects* of spray and cognitive information. The main effect for type of spray was significant ($p = .029$). The main effect for cognitive information and the interaction effects of spray and cognitive information did not reach significance ($p = .521$ and $p = .337$, respectively), suggesting that Frigiderm used before the injection resulted in significant pain reduction regardless of the type of information given to the child about the spray.

This same design (2×2 factorial) was used in the Physician's Health Study, a randomized, double-blind, placebo-controlled trial of aspirin and beta-carotene in the reduction of cardiovascular mortality and cancer incidence (Steering Committee of the Physician's Health Study Research Group, 1988). In this large-scale study, the 22,071 participants were randomly assigned first to two groups, one taking aspirin and the other an aspirin placebo. Each of these two groups was then subdivided into groups taking either beta-carotene or a beta-carotene placebo. Thus, this study employed four treatment groups: (a) aspirin only, (b) beta-carotene only, (c) both aspirin and beta-carotene, and (d) both placebos (Hennekens & Buring, 1989).

Design 2: Multiple Treatment Groups— Repeated Measures Design

This experiment tested various combinations of modeling, labeling, and videotaped rehearsal to teach empathy to upper-division baccalaureate nursing students (Layton, 1979). There were four experimental groups: (a) modeling alone (X_1), (b) modeling and labeling (X_2), (c) modeling and rehearsal (X_3), and (d) modeling and labeling and rehearsal (X_4). A fifth group served as a no-treatment control (C). This design incorporates multiple experimental groups that receive different treatments. Control is present in two ways: (a) in the sense of a formal comparison and (b) in the notion that it is not always true that a control group is always the "no-treatment" group.

	Frigiderm	Aerosol Air	
Cognitive Information	$X = 1.90$ $N = 10$	$X = 2.30$ $N = 10$	$X = 2.10$
	A	B	
	C	D	
No Cognitive Information	$X = 1.80$ $N = 10$	$X = 2.80$ $N = 10$	$X = 2.30$
	$X = 1.85$	$X = 2.55$	

Figure 2.1. Amount of Pain Experienced by Prekindergarten Children During Routine DPT Immunizations

	Time 1	Time 2
X_1	O_1	O_2
X_2	O_3	O_4
X_3	O_5	O_6
X_4	O_7	O_8
C	O_9	O_{10}

Each participant was posttested on two occasions, immediately after treatment and 3 weeks later. A repeated measures design with time as a variable was employed, using student volunteers from the six junior and senior courses ($N = 56$). Assignment was randomized within the courses rather than within the total group of participants to equalize systematic differences because of class level and prior learning experiences. Empathy, the dependent variable, was measured in three ways: (1) empathy test completed by participants, (2) evaluation of a student-client interview using (a) the Barrett-Lennard Relationships Inventory and (b) the Carkhuff Empathetic Understanding in Interpersonal Processes Scale. On the second posttest, an alternate form of the empathy test was used; otherwise all measurements were the same. Data were analyzed using multivariate analyses of variance. First, a repeated measures analysis of treatment by time was conducted, followed by separate analysis of the two posttest sessions. Findings for the total group of participants were not significant, but when results of junior nursing students were analyzed separately, they were significant for treatment and interaction effects, especially on the Carkhuff scale.

Thus, the modeling intervention appeared to produce a change in junior, but not senior, students. Regarding treatment effects, Scheffe post hoc procedures indicated that only the groups receiving modeling and rehearsal (X_3) performed better than the no-treatment control group. Modeling alone (X_1) and modeling and labeling (X_2) were not effective treatments—rehearsal was the only effective condition in this study.

Design 3: Solomon Four-Group Design

One of the most rigorous designs in terms of control of threats to both internal and external validity is the Solomon four-group design (Campbell & Stanley, 1963, p. 24). Study participants are randomly assigned to one of the four groups to promote statistical equivalence at the outset of the experiment. Lines 1 and 2 (pretested experimental and pretested control groups) control for the effects of history and maturation. Line 3 (unpretested experimental group) controls for the effects of pretesting, and the fourth line (unpretested control) controls for contemporaneous effects occurring between pre- and posttesting periods. Although it is a rigorous design, the Solomon four-group design is seldom employed in nursing research for a number of reasons. First, the four groups require a large number of homogeneous participants. Second, conducting the four groups concurrently to avoid temporal extraneous variables is demanding and usually requires multiple investigators and a great deal of coordination of research activities. Third, the four groups do not produce four complete sets of data, leading to a more complex statistical analysis, as illustrated in the research example below:

$$
\begin{array}{cccc}
 & O_1 & X & O_2 \\
RA & O_3 & & O_4 \\
 & & X & O_5 \\
 & & & O_6 \\
\end{array}
$$

Silva (1979) used the Solomon four-group design to test the effects of orientation information on spouses' anxieties and attitudes toward hospitalization and surgery. The theoretical base for her study was cognitive dissonance theory. A total of 48 participants (spouses of patients, $N = 12$ per group) were randomly assigned to one of four groups: (a) orientation information, pretest and posttest (Line 1), (b) no orientation information, pretest and posttest (Line 2), (c) orientation information, posttest only (Line 3), and (d) no orientation information, posttest only (Line 4). The two dependent variables of anxiety and attitudes toward hospitalization and surgery were measured using a standardized anxiety inventory and a scale measuring spousal perception, developed by the researcher. Data analysis involved three tests. A 2×2 factorial analysis of variance tested the presence or absence of pretesting and orientation information. Pretest scores were additionally used as the covariate in a one-dimensional analysis of covariance with homogeneity of regression test. Finally, chi-square tests were performed on 2×3 frequency contingency tables (pretest groups × anxiety × attitude).

Data supported the hypothesis that spouses given orientation information would experience less anxiety than those not receiving information for the Spouse Questionnaire, but *not* for the State Anxiety Inventory. Spouses who received orientation information did exhibit better attitudes toward hospitalization and surgery than did spouses in the control group. It is interesting to note that both the main and interactive effects of pretesting were insignificant.

CONCLUSION

The purposes of research designs are to answer research questions in a valid manner and to control sources of variance. Experimental designs are the most precise method researchers can employ to generate evidence in support of postulated causal relationships between variables. Experimental research should be well-grounded theoretically and based on cumulative research findings. In experimental studies, three elements are essential: randomization, control, and manipulation of the independent variable(s) by the investigator. Within these criteria, a number of variations on the classic experimental design permit use of multiple groups, multiple independent variables, and multiple measurements of the dependent variable over time. Although experimental designs offer the most rigorous control over extraneous variables and therefore have strong internal validity, they are by no means always the ideal choice for answering a research question. Pragmatic considerations such as cost, time, generalizability, and factors associated with the research setting must also be evaluated when one is choosing a research strategy. In general, however, experimental designs are considered to be the most powerful approach available to nurse researchers in that they maximize the effect of the independent variable, minimize error, and control extraneous variables better than any other research mode.

REFERENCES

Abraham, I. L., Chalifoux, I. L., & Evers, G. C. M. (1992). Conditions, interventions, and outcomes: A quantitative analysis of nursing research (1981-1990). In *Patient outcomes research: Examining the effectiveness of nursing practice* (Proceedings of the State of the Science Conference; NIH Publication No. 93-3411). Rockville, MD: NIH National Center for Nursing Research.

Abraham, I. L., Neundorfer, M. M., & Currie, L. J. (1992). Effects of group interventions on cognition and depression in nursing home residents. *Nursing Research, 41*(4), 196-202.

Armiger, Sister B. (1977). Ethics of nursing research: Profile, principles, perspectives. *Nursing Research, 26*, 330-336.

Batey, M. W. (1971). Conceptualizing the research process. *Nursing Research, 20*, 296.

Binder, D. M. (1981). Critique: Experimental study. In S. D. Krampitz & N. Pavlovich (Eds.), *Readings for nursing research*. Chicago: Rand McNally.

Brink, P. J., & Wood, M. J. (1983). *Basic steps in planning nursing research: From question to proposal* (2nd ed.). Monterey, CA: Wadsworth Health Sciences.

Campbell, D. T., & Stanley, J. (1963). *Experimental and quasi-experimental designs for research*. Chicago: Rand McNally.

Carmines, E. G., & Zeller, R. A. (1979). *Reliability and validity assessment*. Beverly Hills, CA: Sage.

Cohen, J. (1988). *Statistical power analysis for the behavioral sciences* (2nd ed.). Hillsdale, NJ: Lawrence Erlbaum.

Cook, T. D., & Campbell D. T. (Eds.). (1979). *Quasi-experimentation: Design and analysis issues for field settings*. Chicago: University of Chicago Press.

De Berry, S., Davis, S., & Reinhard, K. E. (1989). A comparison of medication-relaxation and cognitive/behavioral techniques for reducing anxiety and depression in a geriatric population. *Journal of Geriatric Psychology, 22*, 231-247.

Egan, E. C., Snyder, M., & Burns, K. R. (1992). Intervention studies in nursing: Is the effect due to the independent variable? *Nursing Outlook, 40*(4), 187-190.

Eland, J. M. (1982). Minimizing injection pain associated with prekindergarten immunization. *Issues in Comprehensive Pediatric Nursing, 5*(5/6), 361-372.

Gilliss, C. L., Gortner, S. R., Hauck, W. W., Shinn, J. A., Sparacino, P. A., & Tompkins, C. (1993). A randomized clinical trial of nursing care for recovery from cardiac surgery. *Heart & Lung, 22*(2), 125-133.

Hennekens, C. H., & Buring, J. E. (1989). Methodologic considerations in the design and conduct of randomized trials: The U.S. Physician's Health Study. *Controlled Clinical Trials, 10,* 142S-150S.

Hinshaw, A. S. (1979). Theoretical substruction: An assessment approach. *Western Journal of Nursing Research, 1*(3), 317-324.

Ingersoll, G. M. (1982). Experimental methods. In H. E. Mitzel (Ed.), *Encyclopedia of educational research* (5th ed.). New York: Free Press.

Isaac, S., & Michael, W. B. (1971). *Handbook of research and evaluation.* San Diego, CA: EDITS.

Jacobsen, S. F. (1973). Ethical issues on experimentation with human subjects. *Nursing Forum, 12,* 58-71.

Kane, R. A., & Kane, R. L. (1981). *Assessing the elderly: A practical guide to measurement.* Lexington, MA: Lexington Books.

Kerlinger, F. N. (1973). *Foundations of behavioral research* (2nd ed.). New York: Holt, Rinehart & Winston.

Kraemer, H. C., & Thiemann, S. (1987). *How many subjects? Statistical power analysis in research.* Newbury Park, CA: Sage.

Lang, J. M. (1990). The use of a run-in to enhance compliance. *Statistics in Medicine, 9,* 87-95.

Layton, J. M. (1979). The use of modeling to teach empathy to nursing students. *Research in Nursing and Health, 2,* 163-176.

Lee, Y. J., Ellenberg, J. H., Hirtz, D. G., & Nelson, K. B. (1991). Analysis of clinical trials by treatment actually received: Is it really an option? *Statistics in Medicine, 10,* 1595-1605.

Maas, M. L., & Buckwalter, K. C. (1990). *Nursing evaluation research: A special Alzheimer's unit* (Final report). Rockville, MD: NIH National Center for Nursing Research.

Margolius, F. R., Sneed, N. V., & Hollerbach, A. D. (1991). Accuracy of apical pulse rate measurements in young children. *Nursing Research, 40*(6), 378-380.

Newell, D. J. (1992). Intention-to-treat analysis: Implications for quantitative and qualitative research. *International Journal of Epidemiology, 21*(5), 837-841.

Oakes, L. L., Hinds, P., Rao, B., Bozeman, P., Taylor, B., Stokes, D., & Fairclough, D. (1993). Chest tube stripping in pediatric oncology patients: An experimental study. *American Journal of Critical Care, 2*(4), 293-301.

Pedhazur, E. J., & Schmelkin, L. P. (1991). *Measurement, design, and analysis: An integrated approach.* Hillsdale, NJ: Lawrence Erlbaum.

Phillips, L. R. (1986). *A clinician's guide to the critique and utilization of nursing research.* Norwalk, CT: Appleton-Century-Crofts.

Rothman, K. J. (1986). *Modern epidemiology.* Boston: Little, Brown.

Rudy, E. B., & Kerr, M. (1991). Unraveling the mystique of power analysis. *Heart & Lung, 20*(5, Part 1), 517-522.

Selltiz, C., Wrightsman, L. S., & Cook, S. W. (1976). *Research model in social relations* (3rd ed.). New York: Holt, Rinehart & Winston.

Sherwood, C. D., Morris, J. N., & Sherwood, S. (1975). A multivariate, nonrandomized matching technique for studying the impact of social interventions.

In E. L. Struening & M. Guttentag (Eds.), *Handbook of evaluation research* (Vol. 1, pp. 183-224). Beverly Hills, CA: Sage.

Shott, S. (1990). *Statistics for health professionals.* Philadelphia: W. B. Saunders.

Siegel, S., & Castellan, N. J. (1988). *Nonparametric statistics for the behavioral sciences* (2nd ed.). New York: McGraw-Hill.

Silva, M. C. (1979). Effects of orientation information on spouses' anxieties and attitudes toward hospitalization and surgery. *Research in Nursing and Health, 2,* 127-136.

Silva, M. C. (1995). *Ethical guidelines in the conduct, dissemination, and implementation of nursing research.* Washington, DC: American Nurses Publishing.

Simms, S. G., Rhodes, V. A., & Madsen, R. W. (1993). Comparison of prochlorperazine and lorazepam antiemetic regimens in the control of postchemotherapy symptoms. *Nursing Research, 42,* 232-239.

Slakter, M. J., Wu, Y., & Suzuki-Slakter, N. S. (1991). *, **, and ***: Statistical nonsense at the .00000 level. *Nursing Research, 40*(4), 248-249.

Smith, M., Buckwalter, K. C., Garand, L., Mitchell, S., Albanese, M., & Kreiter, C. (1994). Evaluation of a geriatric mental health training program for nursing personnel in rural long-term care facilities. *Issues in Mental Health Nursing, 15*(2), 149-169.

Stewart, B. J., & Archbold, P. G. (1992). Nursing intervention studies require outcome measure that are sensitive to change: Part one. *Research in Nursing and Health, 15,* 447-481.

Stewart, B. J., & Archbold, P. G. (1993). Nursing intervention studies require outcome measure that are sensitive to change: Part two. *Research in Nursing and Health, 16,* 77-81.

Yarandi, H. N. (1991). Planning sample sizes: Comparison of factor level means. *Nursing Research, 40*(1), 57-58.

Yeaton, W. H., & Sechrest, L. (1981). Critical dimensions in the choice and maintenance of successful treatments: Strength, integrity, and effectiveness. *Journal of Consulting and Clinical Psychology, 49,* 156-167.

3

Quasi-Experimental Designs

MERIDEAN L. MAAS
KATHLEEN C. BUCKWALTER
DAVID REED
JANET K. PRINGLE SPECHT

Very often in the "real world" of nursing research the use of the true experiment is not a viable option. Much of the research that is relevant for nursing practice and for the development of nursing science must be conducted in natural settings. The researcher is often not allowed control of the treatment variable and cannot achieve randomization because of ethical considerations, institutional policies, or other situational factors. When these circumstances are present, the nurse researcher can look to quasi experiments for alternative research strategies rather than forgo the systematic study of many phenomena for which the use of an experimental design is not possible. Quasi experiments are sufficiently probing to be worth employing, especially when more efficient probes are not possible (Campbell & Stanley, 1963). They are appropriate for Level III questions (Brink & Wood, 1994), which aim to explain why a relationship exists, and are very often the strategy that the nurse in the clinical field setting will use to test theories of causal relationships. In a review of 720 nursing research articles, Moody et al. (1988) found that quasi-experimental designs were used more frequently than true experimental designs. Similarly, Abraham, Chalifoux, and Evers (1992), found that quasi experiments were more prevalent than experiments in their review of 2,746 published nursing research articles.

In some circumstances, randomization may be the source of problems that the researcher would not want to introduce into the study. For example, the nursing administration of a hospital may want to study the effects of flextime on staff nurses' job performance. Staff nurse participants are drawn from two different patient care units and randomly assigned to experimental and control groups. A problem that can arise when this method is used is referred to by Cook and Campbell (1979) as "resentful demoralization." Because the experimental and control participants work daily in close proximity, nurses in the control group who are not allowed flextime may become resentful of the nurses in the experimental group and experience demoralization. In this situation, the objectives of the investigation would be better served by selecting nurses from one unit for the experimental group and nurses from another unit for the control group. This is so even though there may be a number of differences between the two groups of nurses and the patient care units that will introduce sources of variance in job performance.

QUASI-EXPERIMENTAL DESIGNS

Quasi experiments, as the name implies, are designs that resemble true experiments. Quasi-experimental designs partially employ the control over threats to internal validity that are provided by true experimental designs. The inability to achieve experimental controls in field experiments led to the development of quasi-experimental designs and to special controls if random assignment was not possible (Cook & Campbell, 1979). Quasi experiments are experiments that do not have equivalence created by random assignment or that do not have control groups for comparison so that the researcher can infer change due to a treatment effect. Rather, comparisons must be made with nonequivalent groups or with periodic measurement on the same group that may be different due to a number of variables extraneous to the causal variable of interest. Thus, the major problem facing the researcher who uses quasi-experimental designs is in distinguishing the effects that are due to the treatment from those that are due to uncontrolled extraneous variables.

Quasi-experimental designs can be described in two general categories (Cook & Campbell, 1979). *Nonequivalent group designs* are those in which dependent variable measures are obtained for an experimental and a comparison group (nonrandomly assigned) before and after introduction of the independent variable to the experimental group. *Interrupted time-series designs* are those in which the independent variable effects are inferred by comparing measures of the dependent variable obtained at multiple time intervals with multiple dependent variable measures obtained after introduction of the independent variable. The basic time-series design uses a single group of participants. There are several, if not an unlimited number of, variations of each of these two basic experimental designs. Campbell and Stanley (1963) and Cook and Campbell (1979) are the seminal works that contain the numerous variations of these basic designs that are available to the field researcher.

For whatever reason(s) that the rigorous criteria of true experiments cannot be met, quasi-experimentation represents a logical and useful framework for research to answer causal questions. Since introduced by Campbell and Stanley (1963), quasi-experimental designs have been described as a taxonomy of strategies that compromise as minimally as possible the internal validity achieved by the true experiment. More recently, an integrated and synthesized view of quasi-experimental and experimental research has been advanced (Trochim, 1986). This view emphasizes the advantages of different combinations of design features and principles that cut across traditional design distinctions and de-emphasizes the taxonomic smorgasbord approach to quasi-experimental design selection (Trochim, 1986). Thus, the narrowness and passivity of earlier quasi-experimentation approaches have begun to be replaced by more comprehensive and active processes. Cordray (1986) discusses structural models and "patched up quasi-experiments" as two types of quasi experiments that represent the increasingly comprehensive and active approaches.

ADVANTAGES AND DISADVANTAGES
OF QUASI-EXPERIMENTAL DESIGNS

Strengths

The major advantage of quasi-experimental designs is their useful-ness as strategies for testing causal hypotheses field settings. Many research questions of interest to nurse investigators are not amenable to random assignment of participants to experimental and control conditions. Quasi-experimental designs are not only practical and fea-sible, they are directly relevant to the "real nursing world." Quasi experiments represent essential alternative strategies to extend the scope of nursing research and to prevent the loss of causal tests due to the deterioration of true experiments in field settings. Quasi experi-ments provide a systematic framework for answering questions that might otherwise be left to subjective analysis, trial and error, or conclu-sions drawn from compromised experiments in which rival causal hypotheses have not been explicitly evaluated. Furthermore, quasi experiments enhance generalizability over true experiments. Although replication is needed for maximum generalizability, quasi experiments are ordinarily less intrusive on conditions in natural settings, less arti-ficial, and more apt to be representative of the real world of nursing practice. Finally, through the active use of mediating explanatory mod-els, contextual factors, and multiple methodologies to probe and search causal linkages, quasi experiments offer useful strategies to test and build nursing practice theory.

Weaknesses

Quasi-experimental designs, by definition, lack the controls inherent in experimental designs, such as variance in the dependent variable from sources other than the treatment variable. The principal purposes of designs for testing causal relationships are to provide controls to maximize the effect of the independent variable on the dependent variable, to minimize the effects of extraneous variables on the depen-dent variable, and to minimize measurement error. The major short-coming of the quasi-experimental design is its lack of control over extraneous sources of variance that threaten the conclusion that the treatment variable produced the measured changes in the criterion variable (Campbell & Stanley, 1963). Because of the lack of random assignment, the experimental and comparison participants may be different in some systematic way. These differences may then be the reason for any measured differences in the criterion variable that are obtained. It is essential, therefore, to analyze actively and attempt to rule out other causal explanations for the findings before concluding that the treatment variable produced the measured differences in the criterion variable.

Rather than foregoing randomization or chancing gross imbalances in group assignments, investigators may consider use of an alternative to complete randomization, such as use of a permuted block design and assigning participants by blocking them into groups (Rudy, Vaska, Daly, Happ, & Shiao, 1993). In the Rudy et al. (1993) study comparing patient outcomes for patients cared for on a special unit (SU) for chronically, critically ill patients with outcomes for patients on a traditional intensive care unit, study participants were randomized in blocks of three with two of the three always assigned to the SU. This procedure was used to ensure an adequate number of patients so that the SU was financially feasible and could be studied, a circumstance that might not result if complete randomization were employed. Thus, a coin was always flipped for the first participant assignment of each block of three. If that participant was randomly assigned to the experimental group, the coin was flipped again for the second participant. However, if the first coin flip resulted in assignment to the control group, the next two patients were automatically assigned to the SU. Although this permuted block design ensured balance in the assignments made to the experimental and control groups, a major disadvantage of the approach is that at times researchers are aware of the group assignment of particular individuals, which has potential for selection bias. To avoid selection bias, Rudy et al. (1993) used a process for determining who was next in line for assignment in the study that was not under the investigator's control, and the nursing and medical personnel in the two units were not involved in determining patient eligibility or assignment to the units.

Despite repeated warnings of the need to actively shore up inferential weaknesses, quasi experiments have too often been treated as second-best substitutes for true experiments with the only difference being a lack of random assignment to treatment conditions. This limited and passive use of quasi experiments results in underdeveloped explanations of treatment effects and of understandings of why treatments have specific effects.

The rival variables that may cause the group differences on the criterion variable are described as "threats to internal validity" and "threats to external validity" or generalizability of results (Campbell & Stanley, 1963; Cook & Campbell, 1979). In addition, Cordray (1986) argues that the credibility of evidence for causal connections bears greatly on the internal validity in practice and policy applications.

CRITERIA FOR EVALUATING DESIGNS

Threats to Internal Validity

Campbell and Stanley (1963) present eight types of extraneous variables that potentially jeopardize internal validity. Cook and Campbell (1979) describe 12 threats to internal validity that need to be considered for different types of designs. The sources of extraneous variance that can confound the effects of the treatment on the criterion, if not controlled, that are especially critical for the evaluation of the adequacy of quasi-experimental designs are history, maturation, testing, experimental mortality, instrumentation, statistical regression, selection bias, selection/maturation interaction, selection/history interaction, diffusion or imitation of treatments, compensatory equalization of treatments, and compensatory rivalry by respondents receiving less desirable treatments. Finally, an important threat to internal validity of any study, regardless of the design, is the underspecification of the causal linkages. This is especially a serious threat when the treatment being tested is complex, requiring a process of change for implementation. (See Chapter 2 for a description of these variables.)

Threats to External Validity

Cook and Campbell (1979) assert that the external validity of a design is reflected in the design's ability to produce outcomes that can be generalized to particular target persons, settings, and times and that can be generalized across types of persons, settings, and times. Thus, they emphasize the need to distinguish clearly between generalizing to a specific target population and generalizing across populations in evaluating the external validity of an experimental design.

In other words, research results obtained with a randomly selected representative sample could be generalized to the target population, but not necessarily to specific subgroups of the population. Although both aspects of generalizability are relevant to assessing external validity, Cook and Campbell (1979) focus more on generalizing across subpopulations. This is because random sampling for representativeness that would allow generalization to a target population is not often done in field research. In addition, experiments that employ representative sampling with random assignment invariably experience attrition, so that when the research is completed the sample no longer represents the same population. For these reasons, external validity is considered to be strengthened more by multiple small studies with nonrandom samples even if a single study could be implemented with a representative sample.

Thus, the analyses of the ability to generalize across various subpopulations are basically tests of statistical interactions (Cook & Campbell, 1979). The different magnitudes of effects across types of participants, settings, and other subpopulations must be specified to explain these different effects. The threats to external validity are expressed as the following statistical interaction effects: (a) interaction of selection and treatment, (b) interaction of setting and treatment, (c) interaction of history and treatment, (d) reaction or interaction effect of pretesting, (e) reactive effects of experimental procedures, and (f) multiple treatment interference. See Chapter 2, on experimental design, for a description of these effects.

Knowledge of these basic designs and the assumptions underlying them is critical to the effective use of the variations of quasi-experimental designs. Discussion of these variations will be limited to those most likely to be employed by nurse researchers.

A NURSING RESEARCH EXAMPLE

Maas and Buckwalter (1990) designed a study to evaluate experimentally the effects of a special Alzheimer's care unit. The study assessed the effects of the therapeutically structured unit environment on Alz-

heimer's patient functioning, selected staff responses, and family attitudes toward care, as well as the cost-effectiveness of the unit (Maas,
Buckwalter, Kelley, & Stolley, 1991; Maas, Buckwalter, Swanson, &
Mobily, 1994; Mobily, Maas, Buckwalter, & Kelley, 1992; Swanson, Maas,
& Buckwalter, 1993, 1994). Patients with AD who met specific inclusion
criteria were initially randomly assigned either to the special care unit
group or to the group whose care was provided on traditional, integrated nursing home units. Mostly due to attrition by death, randomization could not be maintained. Patients were followed for 12 months
before and after implementation of the special care unit to gather
baseline and within- and between-group comparison data. The specific
aim of the study is to answer the following questions:

1. Are there slower rates of deterioration in terms of functional and cognitive abilities for patients with Alzheimer's disease (AD) on the special
   care unit?
2. Are there fewer falls for the patients on the special care unit?
3. Are fewer medications used for patients on the special care unit?
4. Is it more cost-effective to care for patients with AD on a specialized care
   unit as opposed to the traditional approach of caring for them on
   integrated long-term care units?
5. Do staff members report more satisfaction with their jobs, less burnout,
   and less stress when they care for patients with AD on a special care
   unit?
6. Are family members' perceptions of the care of the patient with AD more
   positive if patients are cared for on the special care unit?

Measures of each of the effect variables were collected every other
month throughout the study period. The design for this research is
illustrated in Figure 3.1. There is no symbol R that indicates random
assignment to the comparison groups. Rather, the dashed line separating the parallel rows indicates comparison groups that are not equated
by random assignment. The X notation indicates introduction of the
treatment variable and O indicates measurements of the dependent
variable(s) (Campbell & Stanley, 1963). Both of the basic nonequivalent
groups and time-series designs are embedded in Figure 3.1.

$$O_1 \quad O_2 \quad O_3 \quad O_4 \quad X \quad O_5 \quad O_6 \quad O_7 \quad O_8$$
- -
$$O_1 \quad O_2 \quad O_3 \quad O_4 \qquad O_5 \quad O_6 \quad O_7 \quad O_8$$

Figure 3.1. Design to Evaluate the Effects of a Special Alzheimer's Unit
SOURCE: Cook and Campbell (1979). Reprinted by permission.
NOTE: X = introduction of the treatment (independent variable); O = Observations or measures; dashed line = nonrandom assignment to groups/nonequivalent groups; numerical subscripts = same measures at different times.

NONEQUIVALENT GROUPS DESIGNS

In the basic nonequivalent groups design, one group of individuals is designated to receive a program, service or treatment (experimental group) and a second group of individuals is designated as a control group. This design is called the *untreated control group design with pretest and posttest* (Cook & Campbell, 1979). Figure 3.2. presents the schematic of the basic nonequivalent groups design, using the codes defined in Chapter 2.

$$O_1 \quad X \quad O_2$$
- - - - - - - - - - - - - -
$$O_1 \qquad O_2$$

Figure 3.2. The Nonequivalent Groups Design
SOURCE Cook and Campbell (1979). Reprinted by permission.
NOTE: See note to Figure 3.1. for explanation of figure elements.

This design is often used in field research in which variable relationships characterizing human subjects are tested. The design is identical to the classical experimental pretest-posttest control group design except that participants are *not* randomly assigned to the experimental and control groups. Because it is frequently an interpretable design (effects on the outcome variable that are due to the treatment variable can be separated from effects due to extraneous variables), it is recommended when a true experimental design cannot be achieved (Cook & Campbell, 1979).

When the nonequivalent groups design is employed, the control group may also receive a treatment. The control group of patients might receive the traditional nursing intervention, whereas the experimental group would receive the innovative intervention being tested. This is true in the example of AD patient research. The two groups of participants represent preexisting groups of patients who are separated from one another either temporally or spatially. With temporal separation, the two groups may represent different cohorts of patients who have received care at a single nursing service site. The control group could be patients who received care during the year prior to the institution of the innovative nursing intervention, whereas the treatment or experimental group could consist of patients who received care in the year following use of the innovative intervention. Nicholson et al. (1993) used temporal separation of experimental and control groups in their pilot study of the effects of child visitation on surgical intensive care unit (SICU) patients' emotional and behavioral outcomes and on family functioning. First, a convenience sample of 10 patients was designated as the control group (no child visitation on the SICU) and outcome measures were taken. After a 2-week waiting period, another 10 SICU patients and families were enrolled in the experimental group with the child visitation intervention. Outcome measures were taken for the experimental group within 48 hours of the child's visit. The authors note that the 2-week interval between groups with the intervention implementation with the second group was selected to avoid carryover and other contaminating effects on the control participants.

In evaluating an elderly outreach project (EOP) designed to identify and provide mental health services to rural elderly, Buckwalter, Smith, Zevenbergen, and Russell (1991) matched the two experimental counties where the EOP was carried out with two control counties in Iowa. This illustrates use of spatial separation of experimental and control groups, with little chance of contamination of control participants by the experimental condition. However, the equivalence of spatially separated groups is still an issue. In the Buckwalter et al. (1991) study, significant differences were found in the need for mental health services at baseline between the experimental and control counties with greater need found in the experimental counties. After implementation of the EOP for a 2-year period, no differences were found in the need for care. Analysis of changes over time indicated no differences in need for care in the experimental counties and a significant increase in need for care in the control counties, suggesting that the EOP may have been effective in preventing an increase in need for mental health care in residents in the experimental counties.

A study by Nath and Rinehart (1979) employed the nonequivalent group design to compare the effects of individual and group relaxation therapy on blood pressure of essential hypertensives. Fifteen hypertensives were taught progressive muscle relaxation. Nine were taught individually and six were taught as a group. The choice of individual or group instruction was made by the participants. The relaxation teaching sessions were held once weekly for 4 weeks. Blood pressure measurements were taken at the beginning and end of each session and at the beginning of the first and last sessions. No differences were found between the two methods of instruction. Decreases in both systolic and diastolic blood pressures from the beginning to the end of each session were found, as well as decreases in systolic pressure from the first session to the fourth. It was concluded (a) that group instruction and individual instruction are equally effective, (b) that progressive muscle relaxation is effective in reducing blood pressure, and (c) that 4 weeks is inadequate for reducing diastolic blood pressure.

Several threats to internal and external validity are associated with the basic nonequivalent group design. *Selection bias* is an especially relevant threat. It is important to distinguish two versions of the nonequivalent control group design. In one, two natural groups are available and the experimenter has free choice of who receives the treatment. In the other, the experimental group is self-selected and participants deliberately seek out the treatment. This was the case in the Nath and Rinehart (1979) study described earlier in which participants selected the type of progressive muscle relaxation instruction. In this case, no control group is available from the same population, so selection interactions become more likely in the latter version.

The basic nonequivalent groups design is clearly superior, however, to the nonequivalent groups, posttest-only design, with data collected at two different points in time, used by Williams, Campbell, Raynor, Mlynarczyk, and Ward (1985), to test the effects of interventions to reduce acute confusional states in elderly patients with hip fractures. In the Williams et al. research, the design does not allow assessment of the effects of history as well as being subject to systematic selection differences in the two groups.

In the Maas and Buckwalter research it was not possible to assign patients, staff, or family members randomly to experimental and control groups. Patients were originally randomized, but their assignment

eroded because of attrition, mostly due to death, and subsequent relo-
cations by clinicians and families. Staff members were assigned to the
special care unit or traditional units according to agency personnel
procedures. The two groups of AD patients were likely not to be
comparable at baseline, making it more difficult to rule out competing
explanations for results obtained. To help rule out such explanations,
the two groups were compared on their demographics, mental status,
and functional status. Although there were no statistically significant
differences between the two groups on any of the variables, statistical
procedures such as analysis of covariance (ANCOVA) could have been
employed to evaluate the viability of these alternative explanations.

The nonequivalent groups design is particularly vulnerable to the
threat of *selection-maturation*. This occurs where one group has a pre-
ponderance of participants who tire more easily or experience some
other internal change that influences the criterion variable irrespective
of the treatment effect. In the case of the evaluation of the special unit
for AD patients, this type of threat is present if the two groups differ in
the natural course of the Alzheimer's disease process. In this situation,
effects attributed to the special unit may actually result from different
patterns of naturally occurring changes in the disease over time for the
two groups. One method that can be used to assist with the interpretation of this source of variation involves adding another measure of the
criterion variable prior to exposure to the treatment being tested. Group
mean differences can also be inspected to assess whether groups are
maturing at different rates. If mean difference is due to selection only,
the difference in growth between groups should also be occurring
within groups. Thus, one would expect an increase in within-group
variances at posttest when compared to pretest (Cook & Campbell,
1979). Second, selection-maturation can be inferred from the regression
of the maturation variable on the pretest outcome scores for both
groups. Different linear slopes of the two regression lines indicate that
there is a difference in the average change in the outcome scores in the
two groups.

A problem may also arise due to the interaction of selection and
history. Cook and Campbell (1979) refer to this threat to internal validity
as *selection-history* or *local history*. These effects result from the combined
influence of nonrandom selection of participants and events that affect
the groups differentially. *History* in this sense refers to any events
occurring between the assessment periods that have an influence on the

outcome variable(s). Events that affect one group more than the other are of particular concern. Therefore, the researcher carefully scrutinizes any events that may occur during the course of the study. An example of the threat of selection-history to the internal validity of the Alzheimer's study could have been the exposure of participants in one group and not the other to programs, such as a friendly visitor program, that were extraneous to the study. If special care unit participants were exposed to the program and participants on traditional units were not, the effects could have served to make the special care unit program appear more or less effective than it was.

The remaining threats to internal validity that are relevant to the basic nonequivalent groups design have to do with measurement of the outcome variable(s). The first threat is *instrumentation*. This occurs when there are floor or ceiling effects or when the units of measurement on a scale are not uniform. In other words, some scales are more or less sensitive to change at certain points on the scale than at other points. Inspection of the distribution of scores on the measure may indicate the presence of instrumentation problems. If so, the distributions will be skewed, the group means and variances will be correlated, or both will happen (Cook & Campbell, 1979). A potential instrumentation bias was discovered during pretest of the Family Perceptions Tool (Maas & Buckwalter, 1985) that was developed to measure the attitudes of family members regarding the care of their AD relatives. A possible ceiling effect occurred. The mean score of family members was 6.4 on a 7-point Likert-type scale, where 7 indicated the most positive attitude toward care the AD patient was receiving. This indicated that the instrument was likely not sensitive to variation in the attitudes of family members and that scores could not go above a certain level of positive attitude. Thus, the instrument was revised by adding additional items designed to elicit more discriminating information about the care of their relatives from family members (Maas et al., 1991).

Regression is the final threat to internal validity that is relevant to the nonequivalent groups design. In this case, if the experimental AD group had much lower cognitive and functional abilities than did the control group prior to the special unit intervention, the special unit would appear to be effective in that the two groups do not appear to differ on the posttest measures. The change in cognitive and functional abilities scores could, however, be due to the measurement problem termed *regression toward the mean*. Due to errors in measurement, individuals who received extreme scores on an instrument at a first measurement are likely to receive scores closer to the population mean on that instrument at the second assessment. As a result, a group of individuals who receive extreme scores on a measure will tend to show a significant change on the measure at retesting toward the population mean in the absence of any real change in true scores. Thus, the change in the experimental AD group could simply reflect regression toward the mean and not indicate that the special unit program caused a significant change in an outcome measure.

To obtain groups whose scores are as equivalent as possible on pretest measures, researchers sometimes misguidedly match controls with experimental participants known to have extreme scores. This results in the control group's mean regressing to its population mean and the experimental group's mean not regressing when the experimental participants are not selected on the basis of their extreme scores. Obviously, true score comparisons are obscured in this circumstance.

One way of assessing the presence of regression artifacts is to employ multiple assessments prior to the intervention. This permits an evaluation of whether the differences reflect regression toward the mean or real treatment effects. The design for this Alzheimer's research project (Figure 3.1) contained multiple pretest measures and thus allowed assessment of possible bias in the results due to statistical regression. The *untreated control group design with pretest measures at more than one time interval* is the variation of the untreated control group design most commonly used (Cook & Campbell, 1979). This design is presented in Figure 3.3. There are advantages to administering pretests at more than one time that strengthen the basic nonequivalent groups design. Multiple pretests permit assessment of whether the groups are becoming disparate at different rates from O_1 to O_2, when the effect could not be due to the treatment (selection-maturation threat). Multiple pretests also allow assessment of spurious treatment effects due to statistical regression.

$$O_1 \quad O_2 \quad X \quad O_3$$
$$\text{-----------------------}$$
$$O_1 \quad O_2 \qquad\quad O_3$$

Figure 3.3. The Untreated Control Group Design With Pretest Measures at More Than One Time Interval
SOURCE: Cook and Campbell (1979). Reprinted by permission.
NOTE: See note to Figure 3.1 for explanation of figure elements.

Because the untreated control group with multiple pretests variation of the basic nonequivalent group design considerably strengthens the interpretation of results, it would seem that this quasi-experimental approach could be used more than it is. However, it is often problematic to obtain pretest measures when the field researcher is unable to delay implementation of the treatment. Furthermore, funding sources are often unwilling to expend monies for pretests, preferring instead to commit resources only for posttest measures. However, researchers should try to achieve the addition of at least one more pretest measure to the basic nonequivalent groups design and should attempt to convince funding agencies of its merit for conducting quality studies.

Three additional variations of nonequivalent group designs are worthy of discussion because they can often be used by nurse researchers in field settings. These designs are useful when a nonequivalent control group cannot be obtained and are applicable when the researcher must create circumstances that are conceptually similar to the no-treatment control group, or in other words, when only a single group of participants is available for the research. The first of these designs, illustrated in Figure 3.4, is the *removed-treatment design with pretest and posttest*.

$$O_1 \quad X \quad O_2 \quad O_3 \quad X \quad O_4$$

Figure 3.4. The Removed Treatment Design With Pretest and Posttest
SOURCE: Cook and Campbell (1979). Reprinted by permission.
NOTE: X = treatment removed; see note to Figure 3.1 for explanation of other elements.

Removed-Treatment Design
With Pretest and Posttest

This design can be advantageous when participants self-select out of a treatment. When the effects of interventions such as reminiscence therapy or exercise are being evaluated, patients often remove themselves from the intervention or are removed by factors that cannot be controlled. A single group pretest-posttest is fundamental. However, a third posttest is added, which is followed by removal of the treatment (X) and one more posttest. The O_3-O_4 data collections serve as the no-treatment control for the O_1-O_2 data collections. One group of individuals participates throughout the course of the study. When a treatment is effective, there are expected differences between O_1 and O_2 and between O_3 and O_4. These differences must be in opposite directions, with a clear change following removal of the treatment variable. This latter result is needed to distinguish differences between the experimental and control conditions that are due to removal of the treatment rather than to the treatment simply having no long-term effect.

One difficulty with this design is that in using it, it may be hard to demonstrate a pattern of effects on which a valid statistical conclusion can be based. That is, the difference between O_1, O_2, and O_3, O_4, must not be equal, and the difference between O_2, O_3, and O_3, O_4, must also not be equal. Furthermore, the researcher must be aware that maturation effects could explain any differences that occur. Another difficulty can arise with this design if the treatment has to be removed deliberately. Because the treatment was likely introduced because of its positive benefits, participants may become frustrated and agitated when it is removed. These responses may correlate with the outcome measures and obscure the effect of the removed treatment. Thus, the design may not be a good choice when the researcher must deliberately remove the treatment. Finally, it is important that observations be made at equal time intervals, to assess any spontaneous changes that may be occurring with the passage of time, irrespective of the introduction and removal of the treatment.

The Repeated-Treatment Design

Figure 3.5 depicts the repeated-treatment design, in which the researcher uses a single group of study participants because he or she has access to only one population. Participants are exposed to the treatment, removed from treatment, and then exposed again to the treatment. This design is best employed when the treatment effects are expected to dissipate rapidly or when the effects are expected to be cumulative. To interpret the effects of the treatment, the O_3, O_4, difference must be in the same direction as the O_1, O_2, difference. This design is vulnerable to regularly occurring extraneous sources of variance due to participant maturation or history. Furthermore, there is potential for participant resentment or frustration when a treatment is removed, just as in the removed-treatment design with pretest and posttest, described above. This frustration can confound the O_3, O_4, difference, which could be inferred to be due to replication of the treatments when in fact it was due to a reduction in frustration when the treatment was again introduced. To enhance the external validity and statistical validity of the

$$O_1 \quad X \quad O_2 \quad X \quad O_3 \quad X \quad O_4$$

Figure 3.5. The Repeated-Treatment Design
SOURCE: Cook and Campbell (1979). Reprinted by permission.
NOTE: See note to Figure 3.1 for explanation of figure elements.

design, large samples of participants should be used. The design is particularly vulnerable to the reactive effects of experimental procedures. Thus, the design is best when the treatment being tested is unobtrusive and there is a long time interval before reintroduction of the treatment. To prevent the effects of extraneous cyclic rival causes (e.g., seasonal influences, budget cycles), it is best to distribute reintroductions of the treatment randomly.

The repeated-treatment design could be useful for testing many nursing interventions that are not especially conspicuous or invasive to the patient, such as interaction or psychosocial modalities or touch or reflective techniques. This design is embedded in the Buckwalter, Cusack, Sidles, Wadle, and Beaver (1989) study described in the section on interrupted time-series design.

The Reversed-Treatment Nonequivalent Control Group Design With Pretest and Posttest

This design is diagrammed in Figure 3.6, where X+ represents an expected effect in one direction and X– represents an expected effect in the opposite direction (Cook & Campbell, 1979). The reversed-treatment design is resistant to selection-maturation threats because maturation rarely occurs at the same time in opposite directions in the two groups. It is also stronger than basic nonequivalent group designs in terms of construct validity because it necessitates a carefully specified causal theory to hypothesize an effect in one direction in one group and an opposite effect in the other group. Reactive effects of the experimental procedures are less likely to explain hypothesized effects that are obtained in many types of studies, because social desirability would be expected to ameliorate effects of the conceptually opposite treatment. However, this should not be taken to mean that the design is totally resistant to the Hawthorne effect. Cook and Campbell (1979) emphasize that to be maximally interpretable the reversed-treatment design requires (a) a placebo control group that receives a treatment not expected

O_1	$X+$	O_2
O_1	$X-$	O_2

Figure 3.6. The Reversed-Treatment Nonequivalent Control Group Design With Pretest and Posttest
SOURCE: Cook and Campbell (1979). Reprinted by permission.
NOTE: X+ and X– = reversed treatments; see note to Figure 3.1 for explanation of other elements.

to influence the outcome measure except through a reactive effect of experimental procedures and (b) a control group that receives no treatment for a baseline of no cause.

The reversed-treatment design is often difficult to implement in social and clinical settings. Treatments that produce negative effects are considered unethical. Thus, the deliberate design of these experimental conditions is questionable. It may be possible, however, for nurse researchers to capture the reversed-treatment experimental conditions as natural, unplanned occurrences that result from changes in the availability of resources or differing philosophies regarding nursing administration, education, and practice.

The Cohort Design
With Cyclical Turnover

The cohort design, Figure 3.7, can be useful for studies in which (a) some participants (cohorts) are exposed to a treatment, because they cycle through an organization, but other participants (cohorts) are not; (b) it can be assumed that the cohorts differ only minimally; and (c) archival records can be used to compare cohorts on specific characteristics. The extent to which groups can be assumed to be comparable depends on the researcher's ability to examine background characteristics.

Hamera and O'Connell (1981) used this design to study the effects of primary and team nursing on patient-centered variables such as nurturance received, patient involvement, and frequency of nurse-patient contacts. Baseline observational data were collected on 12 randomly selected adult medical patients experiencing team nursing care. A primary nursing care approach was then implemented on the same nursing unit. Six months later, 12 randomly selected medical patients

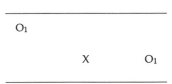

Figure 3.7. The Cohort Design With Cyclical Turnover
SOURCE: Cook and Campbell (1979). Reprinted by permission.
NOTE: See note to Figure 3.1 for explanation of figure elements.

were observed under this system. Patients were observed 24 hours a day for 5 days of hospitalization. Results showed that there were no differences between primary and team nursing care groups in the number of contacts, nurturance, or patient involvement with all nursing personnel or with professional nurses. However, when the primary group was adjusted to include only those patients for whom primary nursing care was fully implemented, the primary group received more nurturance and tended to be more actively involved than did the team group. *t* tests indicated no statistically significant differences between the groups on age, number of days hospitalized, or number of patients observed over weekends, providing some check on selection bias. However, history could have differentially affected the groups during the 18-month span of the study. Furthermore, the nursing personnel who implemented the two types of care may have been an extraneous source of variance due to characteristics and behavior that were not necessarily a function of the system of care. Unfortunately, the investigators did not report data for the nursing personnel who implemented team nursing and primary nursing.

INTERRUPTED TIME-SERIES DESIGNS

The basic interrupted time-series design involves multiple observations over time, usually with a single group of participants. However, the time-series design can also use different but similar units of analysis (Cook & Campbell, 1979). Figure 3.8 depicts the basic interrupted time-series design. For nursing research, the design has particular relevance whenever a program or intervention is hypothesized to affect variables that are regularly measured and contained in archival sources.

$$O_1 \quad O_2 \quad O_3 \quad O_4 \quad O_5 \quad X \quad O_6 \quad O_7 \quad O_8 \quad O_9 \quad O_{10}$$

Figure 3.8. Interrupted Time-Series Design
SOURCE: Cook and Campbell (1979). Reprinted by permission.
NOTE: See note to Figure 3.1 for explanation of figure elements.

It is especially relevant for many quality assurance studies and also can be convenient for conducting "pure" research. Time-series analyses can supplement information gathered using nonequivalent group designs. This combination of methodologies represents a rigorous form of evaluation, even in the context of quasi-experimental design.

Tilden and Shepherd (1987) used a simple interrupted time-series design to examine the effects of an educational intervention on nurse's identification of battered women in a large urban hospital emergency department. They looked at records of all adult, female trauma patients ($N = 447$) for a 4-month period, followed by an education program and a new interview protocol for staff. Following the education program and new interview protocol, data were again collected from records of all adult, female trauma patients ($N = 445$) for another 4 months to identify those women who were battered. Data from the two, 4-month data collection periods were compared, and it was found that statistically significantly more battered women were identified in the second 4-month period after the introduction of the intervention. As expected for optimum interpretation of results, the graphic presentation of the data showed a sharp increase in the percentage of patients who were identified as battered women by the emergency department nurses following the education and change in interview. The design, however, does not control well for influences of history (e.g., hospitalwide encouragement to improve charting after the education and change in interview were introduced was mentioned by the researchers as a possible threat) or for the potential halo effects of the focus on the staff members by the researchers. The investigators did try to control some seasonal effects of history by comparing the same 4-month periods in two successive years. The investigators also noted the potential bias of selection due to turnover attrition of staff nurses during the period between the two data collection periods, which could have added records from nurses who were more skilled with conducting and documenting the interviews to the second 4-month data collection period.

When the interrupted time-series design is used, the researcher must know exactly when the participants were exposed to the treatment variable in order to infer its effects. If a treatment effect occurs, the outcome measures taken after exposure to the treatment should be different from those taken before exposure to the treatment. Hence, the time-series measures are "interrupted."

At least 30 time periods should be available when the researcher considers using the interrupted time-series design without a comparison group. This allows sufficient data to be gathered for an evaluation of a trend over time following the intervention. Cook and Campbell (1979) describe several types of interruption effects that can occur. The first is a sharp change in mean scores when the interruption occurs, indicating different levels or intercepts of the slopes of pre- and post-treatment scores. The second interruption effect that can be observed is a change in the slope of the mean scores before and after treatment. The change observed in the Tilden and Shepherd (1987) study illustrates both a sharp change in mean scores and a change in the slope of the scores. In addition to changes in slope and intercept of mean scores, the interruption effect can also be characterized as continuous or discontinuous and as instantaneous or delayed. Note, however, that the different effects can occur simultaneously in various combinations.

A major strength of the basic time-series design is that it allows the assessment of outcome effects that are due to maturation prior to the introduction of a treatment. Multiple observations also make it possible to examine the trend of pretest scores for an effect that is due to statistical regression. Furthermore, with a large number of time period observations, extraneous effects due to history or cyclic influences can also be evaluated. However, history remains the main threat to internal validity of the design. Data collections at frequent intervals (weekly versus monthly or yearly) and the careful recording of all possible events or circumstances that could reasonably influence outcomes should make it possible for the researcher to determine whether any event that occurred between the last pretest and the first posttest may have caused the interruption effect.

Instrumentation and selection bias are additional threats to the internal validity of the basic time-series design. Instrumentation can produce spurious effects due to differences in the way data are recorded or maintained over time. Changes can also come about in the way variables are conceptually and operationally defined. These sources of extraneous variance are most likely to result from changes in personnel or philosophy within an organization. However, they can also be the result of changes in the knowledge and motivation of key persons involved in the study. Selection effects threaten the validity of interpretation when changes in the experimental groups occur simultaneously with the introduction of the treatment. Often, this occurs because the treatment itself causes participant attrition from the study. This problem can be resolved by restricting either all or part of the data analysis to a subset of the participants from whom data on reliable and relevant background characteristics, such as age, education, occupation, show a distinct change when the treatment is introduced. Selection is apt to be a problem if a distinct change is found.

Reactive effects of experimental procedures threaten the external validity of any study that uses a time-series design if the same participants are aware of treatment exposure. These conditions are not likely to occur with archival studies, but they often exist with clinical nursing research, particularly when the time intervals are sufficiently short to make the recall of responses probable. The lack of availability of multiple measures of variables may also be a constraint when the researcher depends on archival sources of data. Nurse administrators, researchers, nurses responsible for quality assurance studies, and clinical practitioners are advised to consider this potential constraint on the conduct of research prior to the collection of archival data.

Certainly, the time-series design that has an adequate number of time period observations has a distinct advantage for generalization of results over a variety of time periods. A final advantage of the basic time-series design is the opportunity that is often present to examine results within subgroups of participants. When this is possible, the external validity of the design is strengthened. Study participants can be stratified according to individual and setting characteristics to determine if effects hold across subgroups. Of course, the researcher who uses archival data is limited to the variables measured in the setting and to the ranges of values recorded.

Interrupted Time-Series Designs With a Nonequivalent No-Treatment Group Time Series

Time-series design variations become more complicated and combine a number of the nonequivalent group design variations. Combinations of variations provide the means whereby researchers can enhance their ability to interpret both of the basic quasi-experimental designs.

The first variation on the basic interrupted time-series design results when a nonequivalent no-treatment group time series is added. This design is illustrated in Figure 3.9 and is the design used by Maas and Buckwalter (1990). In the Maas and Buckwalter (1990) Alzheimer's unit research example, two basic quasi-experimental designs (nonequivalent groups and time series or repeated measures) were combined. The combined design increased the probability that the investigators could better interpret results that could potentially be confounded by threats to internal validity that would be present if either of the two basic designs was used alone. Multiple measurement points before and after introduction of the special Alzheimer's unit intervention permitted the analysis of baseline patterns and thus more accurate assessment of treatment-related changes. Multiple observations after the treatment decreases the potential for measurement error and thus reduces the risk of Type I (alpha) errors (Abraham & Neundorfer, 1990).

$$O_1 \quad O_2 \quad O_3 \quad O_4 \quad O_5 \quad X \quad O_6 \quad O_7 \quad O_8 \quad O_9 \quad O_{10}$$
$$\text{---}$$
$$O_1 \quad O_2 \quad O_3 \quad O_4 \quad O_5 \quad\quad\quad O_6 \quad O_7 \quad O_8 \quad O_9 \quad O_{10}$$

Figure 3.9. Interrupted Time-Series Design With a Nonequivalent No-Treatment Group Time Series
SOURCE: Cook and Campbell (1979). Reprinted by permission.
NOTE: See note to Figure 3.1 for explanation of figure elements.

The addition of a no-treatment control group time series to the basic time-series design makes it strong in terms of the threat of history to internal validity because the effects of history can be tested. This design can still be subject to the threat of selection-history interaction, however, if one group is exposed to a unique event and the other is not. The threat can occur only if one group is influenced by an event *at the time that it is also exposed to the treatment.* The threat is enhanced by the addition of factors that increase the nonequivalence of the groups. These are viable threats for the Alzheimer's research example because one of the groups of participants was housed on a unit that was isolated to some extent from the rest of the agency and because participants might have been selected for admission to the special care unit based on factors that made them noncomparable to control group participants (e.g., more problem behaviors). Isolation from the other agency units could make the differential exposure of each of the groups to a unique situation even more likely.

The more comparable the groups are, the stronger this design is for testing other factors threatening the internal validity of the basic time-series design. Matching is not a solution for noncomparability. Rather, matching can produce the same distortion in the outcome due to regression effects as was described for the nonequivalent control group design. In general, the threats to external validity are the same as those described for the basic time-series design.

The Interrupted Time-Series Design
With Nonequivalent Dependent Variables

This design, depicted in Figure 3.10, is included because of its value for testing the effects of history and for the advantage it has for enhancing construct validity. The effects of history can be assessed and the construct validity strengthened by collecting data for some variables that should show treatment effects and for others that should not.

$$O_{A1} \quad O_{A2} \quad O_{A3} \quad O_{A4} \quad O_{A5} \quad X \quad O_{A6} \quad O_{A7} \quad O_{A8} \quad O_{A9} \quad O_{A10}$$

$$O_{B1} \quad O_{B2} \quad O_{B3} \quad O_{B4} \quad O_{B5} \quad \quad O_{B6} \quad O_{B7} \quad O_{B8} \quad O_{B9} \quad O_{B10}$$

Figure 3.10. Interrupted Time-Series Design With Nonequivalent Dependent Variables
SOURCE: Cook and Campbell (1979). Reprinted by permission.
NOTE: Letter subscripts = different measures; see note to Figure 3.1 for explanation of other elements.

For the nonequivalent dependent variables design, as well as for the interrupted time-series design with nonequivalent dependent variables, sufficient theory must exist to establish the conceptual relationship of the dependent variables with the treatment. For example, based on the theoretical framework of person-environment fit and the PLST model (Hall & Buckwalter, 1987; Lawton, 1972), we can expect the special Alzheimer's unit and program to have a positive impact on the behaviors (number of catastrophic behaviors; social interactions) of residents with Alzheimer's but little if any effect on standardized measures of their functional abilities. As with other designs, questions arise as to whether or not the relationships will hold for other populations and across subgroups of the target population.

Interrupted Time-Series Design With Removed Treatment

Figure 3.11 illustrates this design, which is actually two interrupted time series joined together: O_1 to O_9 represents one time series that allows assessment of a treatment effect; O_5 to O_{13} allows assessment of the removal of the treatment.

$$O_1 \quad O_2 \quad O_3 \quad O_4 \quad X \quad O_5 \quad O_6 \quad O_7 \quad O_8 \quad O_9 \quad \overline{X} \quad O_{10} \quad O_{11} \quad O_{12} \quad O_{13}$$

Figure 3.11. Interrupted Time-Series Design With Removed Treatment
SOURCE: Cook and Campbell (1979). Reprinted by permission.
NOTE: X = treatment; $\overline{X}$ = treatment removed.

For maximum inference of effect, the researcher would expect one form of change between O_4 and O_5 and an opposing change between O_9 and O_{10}. Certainly, the design has all of the strengths characteristic of the simple time series. However, the second time series adds protection from the threat of history to internal validity. This is because any historical event that could pose a threat would have to operate in opposite directions at different times, or two events would have to operate in different directions at different times. Of course, the resentful demoralization described earlier in designs that remove participants from treatment can also occur with this design. Thus, the designs are best interpreted when the treatment is not perceived as particularly important to the participants. Regardless of the effects of resentful demoralization, the design is quite strong because two alternative explanations are required to negate results that occur in a different direction after removal of a treatment.

Buckwalter et al. (1989) used a variation of the interrupted time-series design with removed treatment and multiple replications to test the effects of an individualized speech therapy enhancement program

(STEP) for brain-damaged patients with diagnoses of aphasia and or dysarthria. Phases of the study were in the following sequence: (a) a 3-month baseline phase; (b) implementation of the STEP intervention for 3 months; (c) a 3-month control period during which STEP was withdrawn and only usual treatment was provided; (d) a 3-month alternative intervention (systematic attention); (e) 3 months of the STEP intervention; and (f) a second and final 3-month control period with the STEP intervention withdrawn. Measures of dependent variables were collected at regular intervals (speech tasks weekly and speech battery every 3 months) throughout the study period. Results showed improvement in speech tasks over baseline, and the participants scored better during STEP segments than during the alternative systematic attention intervention period or during control phases. The study illustrates how the creative use of combinations of time-series design variations can be useful strategies to test important clinical nursing interventions.

Interrupted Time-Series Design With Switching Replications

In this design (Figure 3.12), two nonequivalent groups are exposed to a treatment and serve as control groups for each other. There are two important reasons for including this design in a discussion of quasi experimentation. First, the design has strong internal and external validity. Second, it is a practical design that nurse researchers should consider whenever a nonequivalent control group is available. The advantage of replication built into the design makes it possible to extend the findings beyond a single population. In view of the considerable costs of conducting research studies, this efficiency should be most attractive. Furthermore, one should expect that cooperating settings, from which nonequivalent control groups are obtained, would find the demonstration of treatment effects in these groups beneficial. An additional advantage for nursing is the potential for greater use of findings by settings where effects of a treatment have been demonstrated, causing them to acquire a more vested interest in the research. One additional benefit of the switching replications time-series design is that it makes it possible to assess delayed effects. If the effect is delayed equally in each group, it should be observed in an earlier discontinuity in one group. Maas and Swanson (1994) used a variation

$$O_1 \ O_2 \ O_3 \qquad O_4 \ O_5 \ O_6 \ O_7 \ O_8 \ X \ O_9 \ O_{10} \ O_{11}$$

- -

$$O_1 \ O_2 \ O_3 \ X \ O_4 \ O_5 \ O_6 \ O_7 \ O_8 \qquad O_9 \ O_{10} \ O_{11}$$

Figure 3.12. Interrupted Time Series With Switching Replications
SOURCE: Cook and Campbell (1979). Reprinted by permission.
NOTE: See note to Figure 3.1 for explanation of figure elements.

of this design in a study designed to test the effects of a family involvement in care (FIC) intervention on family members of institutionalized Alzheimer's residents and staff caregivers' stress and satisfaction. Using a repeated measures, nonequivalent groups design, the FIC intervention was introduced with the comparison group family members and staff following the completion of the intervention trial with the experimental participants. Thus, the intervention was switched and replicated with the comparison participants with these participants used as their own controls.

Interrupted Time-Series Design With Multiple Replications

The interrupted time-series design is presented in Figure 3.13. The design is very powerful for testing causal hypotheses and has the added advantage of modifications that allow the testing of more than one treatment in a single study, as well as testing interaction effects of treatments. Two treatments can be tested by substituting X_1 for X and X_2 for $\overline{X}$.

$$O_1 \ O_2 \ X \ O_3 \ O_4 \ \overline{X} \ O_5 \ O_6 \ X \ O_7 \ O_8 \ \overline{X} \ O_9 \ O_{10} \ X \ O_{11} \ O_{12} \ \overline{X} \ O_{13} \ O_{14}$$

Figure 3.13. Interrupted Time Series With Multiple Replications
SOURCE: Cook and Campbell (1979). Reprinted by permission.
NOTE: $\overline{X}$ = treatment removed; see note to Figure 3.1 for explanation of other elements.

Parsons, Smith-Peard, and Page (1985) used the interrupted time-series design with multiple replications to assess the effects of oral, body, and catheter care on the cerebrovascular status of 19 severe closed-head-injured patients. Measures of heart rate, arterial blood pressures, intracranial pressures, and cerebral perfusion pressures were taken at baseline, peak nursing intervention, and 1-minute recovery times for each patient. Statistically significant increases in the dependent variables were observed at peak intervention. By recovery time, these values had returned to baseline levels. Because cerebral perfusion pressures never fell below 50 mm Hg, the three hygiene interventions were considered safe for the patient with closed-head injury.

Martinson and Anderson (1983) used another variation of the interrupted time-series design with multiple replications to study the effects of thermal applications to the abdomens of four dogs. A silicone rubber envelope through which water circulated at 0, 10, 20, 30, 40, or 50 degrees centigrade was applied. Skin surface, subcutaneous, intraperitoneal, intestinal, and colonic temperatures were measured at baseline (10 minutes after starting the procedure) and 90 minutes after application of the thermal pad. For the control conditions (no pad), measurements were taken at 10 minutes and 100 minutes after initiating the procedure. The first 100-minute procedure for each dog was a no-pad treatment. Then, the 6 applications were chosen at random with replacement. The eighth 100-minute procedure was another no-pad treatment. This was followed by 6 additional random thermal applications, 1 no-pad treatment, 6 thermal applications, 1 no pad treatment, 6 thermal, and 1 final no-pad treatment. Each dog had 24 sessions of temperature application and 6 sessions of no-pad application. Results of the study showed that both cutaneous and subcutaneous temperatures were affected by surface application of heat and cold to the area, but core temperature remained unaffected.

As with the removed-treatment design (Figure 3.11), the direction of treatment and removal of treatment must be opposite. Furthermore, a treatment effect can be inferred if the same pattern of effects for both the treatment and its removal occurs throughout the data collection. The design is vulnerable to the extraneous effects of cyclical maturation, so random scheduling of treatments and their removal is suggested, while preserving the alternating treatment and removal, unless cyclic effects can be ruled out by a strong theoretical base.

Practicality is, however, a weakness of this design. The design is possible only when the effects of a treatment are expected to extinguish rapidly. Also, the design ordinarily requires that the researcher have the ability to control the circumstances of the experiment. This is usually not possible with nursing phenomena, although educational and mental health settings may be exceptions. For example, it may be a useful design for testing forms of behavior modification interventions.

In conclusion, a number of problems may arise with time-series designs that have not been included in the discussion thus far. First, some treatments cannot be introduced quickly; rather, their impact on participants evolves over time. Second, treatment effects may have a variety of periods of delay that differ among specific populations and from one time to another. Third, although an abundance of archival data exist that theoretically could be used for time-series analysis, they are often difficult to locate and the researcher may have problems obtaining their release. The time intervals of archival data may also be inappropriate for the research. Data may be missing or unreliable. Fourth, it is often problematic to obtain the 30 or more observations recommended for data analysis. Because of the advantages of these designs for nursing research and the problems that have just been listed, nurse administrators, educators, researchers, and clinicians are encouraged to consider their potential applications and to anticipate their use when data are routinely gathered and stored. Many of these designs could be employed with relative ease to answer nursing questions if these recommendations are followed. Most important, standardized classifications of nursing phenomena (nursing diagnoses, interventions, and outcomes) must be developed and used in computerized nursing databases to take maximum advantage of these designs for nursing research.

Patched-Up Designs and Structural Modeling

As stated earlier, researchers are often flexible in their use of quasi-experimental strategies, which results in designs that do not necessarily neatly fit the typology of designs presented in this chapter. The notion of "patched-up" designs allows the researcher to mix and match strategies to best achieve practicality, feasibility, and research rigor. These designs are often difficult to label because they are not like the designs ordinarily described in texts. One example of the patched-up design is the study by Williams et al. (1985). In Phase I of the Williams et al. study, one group of study participants was used to develop a method of assessing risk for confusion, and in Phase II the same participants were used as a comparison group for participants who received a confusion reduction intervention. The object is to present a plausible pattern of evidence while controlling threats to validity. The switching of the test of the FIC intervention to the control group using participants as their own controls by Maas and Swanson (1994) following testing the intervention with the experimental participants is another example of "patching up" a design. Some general techniques for building additional evidence for valid findings and patterns of findings with quasi-experimental approaches include multiple measures, multiple research designs, multiple analyses, and supplemental data collection (Lipsey, Cordray, & Berger, 1981).

Structural modeling depends on strong theory to specify the relevant variables influencing specific hypothesized outcomes. The focus is on comprehensive identification and measurement of all input, process, and outcome variables. Structural modeling entails specifying the true pretreatment assignment processes, theory-based specification of outcomes, and modeling of extraneous factors that influence the outcomes beyond the intervention, including treatment and mediating subject and treatment system variables (Cordray, 1986). A more detailed discussion of structural modeling with examples can be read in Chapter 8 of this volume.

ISSUES OF DATA ANALYSIS FOR NONEQUIVALENT GROUP DESIGNS

Data analysis for quasi-experimental designs presents a number of complex problems. With nonequivalent group designs, it is likely that pretreatment differences on the outcome variable(s) exist between the experimental and control groups as a result of the nonrandom selection process and other sources of extraneous variability discussed above. Because these pretest differences may be reflected in posttest differences even without a treatment effect, an objective of the analysis should be to correct for the effects of initial differences when estimating the effect of treatment. In general, this objective has been pursued by employing statistical means to fashion a pretreatment equivalence between the two groups of participants. How effectively this objective is achieved depends on the statistical procedures employed, the kind of data available for the analysis, and the actual causal relationships that determine both selection and outcome.

Because of the complexity of the issues that arise in the analysis of quasi-experimental data, only a general introduction to those issues and the methods that can be employed to resolve them can be provided here. Greater detail can be found in the sources cited in this section. Several statistical procedures have traditionally been used for the analysis of quasi experiments. Analysis of variance (ANOVA), ANCOVA, ANOVA with blocking or matching, and ANOVA with gain scores are four of the more common procedures (Reichardt, 1979). Repeated measures analysis of variance is also a possibility when repeated measures have been taken on nonequivalent groups.

These procedures vary in the manner and extent to which they control for pretreatment differences. Thus, the procedures should not be viewed as interchangeable. Which will be employed will be determined by the particular circumstances of the quasi experiment.

Analysis of Variance

ANOVA is the least elaborate of the five procedures. ANOVA provides three components: (a) the grand mean of the posttest scores; (b) the treatment effect, the average value that the treatment adds to or subtracts from the posttest scores in the treatment group; and (c) the error (residual), which represents the effect of all extraneous factors on the scores. Pretest scores are not assessed in this model, nor are interaction treatment effects. In essence, the treatment is assumed to be the only factor producing posttest differences, and there is no control for initial differences on outcome or other variables. Because this assumption is unlikely to be valid, simple ANOVA has generally been seen as the least satisfactory of the approaches. However, under certain circumstances (see Achen, 1986), it may be preferable to more elaborate analyses.

The use of ANOVA is based on certain assumptions. One is that the dependent variable is at least at the interval level of measurement. A second is that the dependent variable is normally distributed. A third is that variance in the dependent variable is homogeneous across groups, and a fourth is that the observations are independent of one another. In general, moderate violations of the normal distribution assumption will not invalidate significance tests.

Even if a separate ANOVA is used to find "no significant difference" between the groups in pretest scores, it is not possible to unequivocally attribute posttest differences to the treatment. This is because differences may have emerged over time due to other factors, such as selection-maturation interaction.

Analysis of Covariance

ANCOVA has been the most widely used alternative to the simple ANOVA analysis described above. ANCOVA adds one or more covariates as predictors of outcome. Most commonly, the covariate added is a pretest measure of the outcome variable, but ANCOVA also may be used to adjust for pretreatment differences on other variables believed to be related to outcome. The effect is a statistical adjustment to equate the experimental and control groups on pretest measures as the estimate of the effect of treatment is obtained. Interaction terms may also be introduced to determine if the relationship of pretest measures to outcome are the same within experimental and control groups.

It is not often noted, but ANCOVA can be useful in an analysis even if the experimental and control groups do not differ on pretreatment measures. This is so because the use of covariates that are related to the outcome measure will reduce the error term, making for a more powerful test of the treatment effect. Including covariates that are not related to outcome yields no benefits, but including those that are could be the difference between establishing a treatment effect and not doing so.

When ANCOVA is used, an additional assumption beyond those required for ANOVA must be met: The correlation between the covariate(s) and the outcome measure (dependent variable) must be the same across all treatment groups. The standard statistical programs offer a test for this assumption.

Analysis of Variance With Blocking or Matching

Another approach to fashioning an equivalence between groups that differ on pretest measures is the use of blocking or matching. Matching involves pairing a participant in one group with a participant in the other group who has the same, or more likely nearly the same, value on a pretest measure. Participants without a match in the other group are not used in the analysis. Blocking involves dividing each group into subgroups (blocks) based on a *range* of the pretest measure. In non-equivalent group designs, participants have been selected for experimental and control groups before they are blocked or matched on the pretest scores.

The exclusion of participants from one group because they have no match or comparable block in the other group(s) can lead to erroneous conclusions about the impact of treatment. If the participants remaining are ones with more extreme values for the group, then posttest measures will reflect regression toward the mean, as discussed earlier. This will give the appearance of a treatment effect even when there is none. This is a serious cause for caution in the use of matching or blocking.

As a control for pretest differences, the effect of matching or blocking is much the same as the use of ANCOVA. In fact, if the relationship of pretest scores to outcome is perfectly linear and the pairs are matched perfectly, the effect is exactly the same as using ANCOVA with the pretest measure as a covariate. If matching is not perfect, which is likely, but the relationship is linear, the estimate of treatment effect by the use of matching will be less satisfactory than that derived from ANCOVA. The estimate should, however, be superior to that derived from the simple ANOVA, given that causal relationships are correctly specified.

With blocking, again assuming a strictly linear effect for the pretest measure, effectiveness increases and approaches that of ANCOVA the greater the number of blocks that are used. In the instance that the effect of the pretest measure is not linear, blocking may produce a better estimate of treatment effect. Consequently, it cannot be assumed that ANCOVA is always preferable to blocking or matching.

Analysis of Variance With Gain Scores

An ANOVA using gain scores examines the change that occurs from pretest to posttest scores (Reichardt, 1979). The gain scores (posttest minus pretest) are used as the dependent variable for the ANOVA procedure. This approach assumes that a treatment effect would result in more or less change in the experimental group than in the control group. The ANOVA with gain scores does not allow an assessment of interaction of the treatment with pretest. As with the ANCOVA procedure, additional variables can be added to the gain score analysis. However, gain score analysis cannot assess selection-maturation interaction, instrumentation (floor and ceiling effects), or statistical regression effects.

The fundamental problem with the use of gain scores is that they will be generally less reliable than the pre- and posttreatment scores on which they are based. Thus, although it has been widely used in many fields of research, the use of gain score analysis is not recommended (Burckhardt, Goodwin, & Prescott, 1982; Russell & Buckwalter, 1992).

Repeated Measures Analysis of Variance

For nonequivalent group designs involving a small number of pretest and posttest measures, time-series analysis is not appropriate. To take advantage of the additional information provided by pretest and/or posttest measurements, repeated measures ANOVA may be used to test for the effect of treatment. This is preferable to a series of ANOVAs repeated for each time period. There are univariate and multivariate approaches to repeated measures ANOVAs. The univariate approach treats the time dimension as an additional independent variable, and there is only a single dependent variable. The multivariate approach includes the time dimension through multiple dependent variables, one for each time period, which are subjected to a transformation that reduces their number by one.

Of the two, the univariate approach requires stricter conditions for use but is more powerful if those conditions are met. However, conditions for the multivariate approach are more likely to be met, and this approach permits easy testing of a variety of hypotheses about the pattern of values for the multiple measures. This is accomplished by using transformations for the dependent variables. For example, each measure might be compared to the mean of the succeeding measures to test at what point in the sequence mean values shift. A transformation equivalent to difference scores between measures for adjacent time periods could be used to see if there were significant pretest changes in scores indicative of regression toward the mean.

Advances in Quasi-Experimental
Analysis Measurement Error

In recent years, developments in approaches to analyzing quasi-experimental data have focused on two concerns. The first of these is the effect of error in the measurement of control variables employed as covariates. What one wants to adjust for are the true differences between the groups, but this is not what happens if one uses a measure that includes error. Adjustment with such a measure includes the error in the adjustment. To equate the treatment and control groups on true values for the covariate, the covariate must have a reliability of 1.00 (i.e., must be error free) (Reichardt, 1979). Error in the covariate results in an underadjustment for group differences on the pretreatment measure. The same principle applies when variables other than outcome variables are used in an attempt to equate groups with pretest differences. The procedure will correctly adjust for differences only when the pretest measure is error free.

One solution to this problem is use of the LISREL program developed by Jöreskog and Sörbom (1989). The program was designed to permit testing of theoretical models involving relationships between latent or unobserved variables. Scores on these latent variables are estimated by employing several measured variables as indicators for each latent variable in the theoretical model. For example, a latent variable representing the functional ability of Alzheimer's patients would be estimated in the LISREL procedure by employing a number of different indicators (preferably three or more) (Bentler, 1980). The procedure is designed to derive a true score for participants on the constructs being assessed—that is, a score uncontaminated by measurement error. Therefore, LISREL could be used to conduct an ANCOVA in which the biasing effects of measurement error in the covariate are eliminated. The limitations are that LISREL requires the use of multiple measures of each construct and requires a larger sample size than simple ANCOVA because of the large number of parameters estimated. Both multiple measures and larger sample sizes may be difficult to obtain in practice.

Causal Modeling

A second concern emphasized in recent years is the need for adequate modeling of the causal process involved in producing both selection to groups and outcome. This concern arose from the recognition that the best application of the traditional procedures to control for pretest differences may not at all improve the estimate of the effect of the treatment variable. In fact, under certain conditions, *the use of ANCOVA or matching may even worsen the estimate of the treatment effect* (Achen,

1986). This is a separate problem from that created by regression toward the mean. This is a problem created by failure to specify causal relationships fully.

To be certain that ANCOVA or matching will properly control for initial differences between the experimental and control groups, *all* variables affecting both assignment and outcome must be included in the analysis. The omission of any variable affecting both selection and outcome will result in biased estimates of the treatment effect. One approach to dealing with this problem has been to focus on selection modeling, or identifying the determinants of selection to the experimental or control group. If selection can be completely predicted, then a completely unbiased estimate of treatment effect can be obtained. If prediction is less than perfect, but more than 75% successful, the bias will still not be large (Rindskopf, 1986). The difficulty is that in many, perhaps most, quasi-experiments, it will not be possible to identify the determinants of selection that well. Quite frequently, the researcher will not be able to specify with confidence all the variables that affect selection, and even if the researcher could do so, he or she still would probably not have data for all those variables.

Achen (1986) suggests an approach to this concern that does not require full specification of the determinants of selection. This is an instrumental variable approach using two-stage least squares. To implement this approach, the researcher must be able to use at least one variable that reasonably can be said to affect assignment, but *not* to affect outcome. The selection of this variable must be made on sound theoretical grounds, because there is no way statistically to verify that the causal relationships are as assumed. If the assumptions about the causal effects of this variable be true, then unbiased estimates of the treatment effect can be obtained. Reichardt and Gollob (1986), on the other hand, suggest approaches that are not intended to eliminate bias in the estimate of treatment effects but, rather, to provide estimates for the upper and lower bounds of the treatment effect.

To summarize, statistical procedures such as ANOVA and ANCOVA are appropriate for randomized designs. However, for quasi-experimental designs, there are problems associated with employing ANOVA, ANCOVA, or other traditional approaches. These problems have been the focus of recent developments in the analysis of quasi-experimental data. The LISREL procedure has promise for overcoming the biasing effects of measurement error in covariance analysis and in permitting a more appropriate and powerful analysis of data from quasi-experimental designs. Several approaches have been devised to deal with omitted variable bias, and more will likely be proposed in the future. What is most important is that the statistical procedure used must be carefully selected to fit the particular characteristics of the data to be analyzed.

ISSUES OF DATA ANALYSIS
WITH TIME-SERIES DESIGNS

Although time-series analysis (TSA) has been in the nursing literature for more than a decade, it is underused in nursing research (Abraham, Nadzam, & Fitzpatrick, 1989). Statistical procedures based on ordinary least squares (OLS) analysis are not appropriate for time-series data analysis, principally because OLS assumes independent error and, with any time-series design, the errors will almost certainly be serially related (autocorrelated). Although the estimates of the parameters obtained by OLS will not themselves be biased, the significance tests will be biased, most often overestimating the significance level of parameters (McCain & McCleary, 1979). Conceptually, time-series analysis is very similar to OLS regression models $(Y = b_0 + b_1x + e)$ but does not make the assumption that the errors are independent. One reason why TSA may be underused is that a minimum of 30 observation or data points (rather than participants) are needed for analysis. Chatfield (1980) maintains that a minimum of 50 observation points are needed. However, many physiological variables that nurses measure, such as vital signs, are taken frequently, and large numbers of observations will often be available. The rapid development of standardized and computerized nursing databases should yield more than sufficient numbers of observations to lend themselves to TSA. When a sufficient number of observations are not available for TSA, the use of repeated measures multivariate analysis of variance (MANOVA) should be considered (see discussion above).

Time-series data lend themselves well to graphical presentation. In fact, time-series analysis has generally been seen as a means to provide a statistical significance test for effects observed by visual inspection of graphed time series. Ideally, the researcher should develop, through experience, skill in visual interpretation of time-series data according to specific principles, with statistical tests used to corroborate visual analysis.

Autoregressive integrated moving average (ARIMA) models and the modeling techniques developed by Box and Jenkins (1976) are recommended for obtaining unbiased estimates of the error component in time-series data (McCain & McCleary, 1979). These procedures estimate the systematic portion of the error component, that portion that produces autocorrelation among time-series scores so that unbiased estimates of the standard deviations of parameters can be calculated for statistical tests.

An ARIMA model is developed to fit a particular time series by an iterative, that is, repetitive process. An initial model is identified by inspection of what are called the autocorrelation function (ACF) and the partial autocorrelation function (PACF). Particular patterns in these indicators correspond to ARIMA models with a particular structure. Once an initial model is identified, estimates of model parameters are obtained that permit calculation of the residual errors. If statistical tests indicate that these errors are not serially related, the model is accepted. If the tests indicate that there remains a systematic component in the error, the process is repeated. Although model identification is developed with the aid of statistical tests, the analyst must depend on skill developed through experience to conclude that the model finally accepted is the "true" model.

With the ARIMA model developed, it is then possible to estimate the effect of the treatment. The time series is said to be "interrupted" because the intervention is expected to alter the pretreatment pattern of the series in some way. As discussed earlier, the treatment effect may take three basic forms: (a) abrupt, constant change; (b) gradual constant change; and (c) abrupt, temporary change.

If the researcher wishes to rule out history as an alternative explanation of an apparent treatment effect, a parallel TSA may be done with a control group. Repeated measures MANOVA also could be considered for this purpose, because it permits simultaneous analysis of data from both experimental and control groups.

In summary, time-series analysis is an underused technique that could be applied to many research questions in nursing. Only with the accumulation of experience can the researcher become confident in the interpretation of a time-series analysis, but this should not be a deterrent to its use; TSA is superior to OLS regression when data represent sequential measurements over time. Readers are therefore encouraged to seek information beyond the scope of this chapter about time-series analysis in several excellent nursing sources (Abraham & Neundorfer, 1990; Clinton, 1986; Jensen, 1990; Jirovec, 1986; Lentz, 1990a, 1990b; Lentz & Woods, 1989; Metzger & Schultz, 1982; Taylor, 1990; Thomas, 1990).

SUMMARY

Quasi-experimental designs offer a variety of alternative strategies for the conduct of nursing field research. They are especially important for assessing causal relationships between nursing interventions and desired patient outcomes when the researcher is unable to implement all of the characteristics of a true experimental design. Although quasi-experimental designs are not as elegant for the control of threats to internal validity and therefore are not as rigorous as true experimental designs for testing causal relationships, the nurse researcher who is knowledgeable about the variety of quasi-experimental designs can often combine the strengths of nonequivalent groups and time-series designs to optimize controls on internal validity. In addition, the use of structural modeling and "patched up" designs further extends the nurse researcher's strategies for assessing linkages without the benefit of a true experimental design. A substantial increase in the number of clinical nursing field studies conducted with many different populations could result, which would have the additional advantage of improving generalizability of findings.

REFERENCES

Abraham, I. L., Chalifoux, Z. L., & Evers, G. C. M. (1992). Conditions, interventions, and outcomes: A quantitative analysis of nursing research (1981-1990). In *Patient outcomes research: Examining the effectiveness of nursing practice* (Proceedings of the State of the Science Conference; NIH Publication No. 93-3411). Rockville, MD: NIH National Center for Nursing Research.

Abraham, I. L., Nadzam, D. M., & Fitzpatrick, J. J. (1989). *Statistics and quantitative methods in nursing: Issues and strategies for research and education*. Philadelphia: W. B. Saunders.

Abraham, I. L., & Neundorfer, M. (1990). The design and analysis of time series studies. In L. Moody (Ed.), *Advancing nursing science through research* (Vol. 2, pp. 143-176). Newbury Park, CA: Sage.

Achen, C. (1986). *Statistical analysis of quasi-experiments.* Berkeley: University of California Press.

Bentler, P. M. (1980). Multivariate analysis with latent variables: Causal modeling. *Annual Review of Psychology, 31,* 419-456.

Box, G. E. P., & Jenkins, G. M. (1976). *Time series analysis: Forecasting and control.* San Francisco: Holden Day.

Brink, P. J., & Wood, M. J. (1994). *Basic steps in planning nursing research: From question to proposal* (4th ed.). Boston: Jones & Bartlett.

Buckwalter, K. C., Cusack, D., Sidles, E., Wadle, K., & Beaver, M. (1989). Increasing communication ability in aphasic/dysarthric patients. *Western Journal of Nursing Research, 11*(6), 736-747.

Buckwalter, K. C., Smith, M., Zevenbergen, P., & Russell, D. (1991). Mental health services of the rural elderly outreach program. *The Gerontologist, 31*(3), 408-412.

Burckhardt, C. S., Goodwin, L. D., & Prescott, P. A. (1982). The measurement of change in nursing research: Statistical considerations. *Nursing Research, 31,* 53-55.

Campbell, D. T., & Stanley, J. C. (1963). *Experimental and quasi-experimental designs for research.* Chicago: Rand McNally.

Chatfield, C. (1980). *The analysis of time series: An introduction.* London: Chapman & Hall.

Clinton, J. (1986). Conceptual and technical issues in using time-series methodology in clinical nursing research. In P. L. Chinn (Ed.), *Nursing research methodology: Issues and implementation.* Rockville, MD: Aspen.

Cook, T. D., & Campbell, D. T. (Eds.). (1979). *Quasi-experimentation: Design and analysis issues for field settings.* Chicago: Rand McNally.

Cordray, D. S. (1986). Quasi-experimental analysis: A mixture of methods and judgment. In W. M. K. Trochim (Ed.), *Advances in quasi-experimental design and analysis* (pp. 9-28). San Francisco: Jossey-Bass.

Hall, G. R., & Buckwalter, K. C. (1987). Progressively lowered stress threshold: A conceptual model for care of adults with Alzheimer's disease. *Archives of Psychiatric Nursing, 1*(6), 399-406.

Hamera, E., & O'Connell, K. A. (1981). Patient-centered variables in primary and team nursing. *Research in Nursing and Health, 4*(1), 183-192.

Jensen, L. (1990). Guidelines for the application of ARIMA models in time series. *Research in Nursing & Health, 13,* 429-435.

Jirovec, M. M. (1986). Time series analysis in nursing research: ARIMA modeling. *Nursing Research, 35,* 315-319.

Jöreskog, K. G., & Sörbom, D. (1989). *LISREL VII: User's Reference Guide.* Mooresville, IN: Scientific Software.

Lawton, M. P. (1972). Assessing the competence of older people. In D. Kent, P. Kastenbaum, & S. Sherwood (Eds.), *Research planning and action for the elderly.* New York: Behavioral Publications.

Lentz, M. J. (1990a). Time series—Issues in sampling. *Western Journal of Nursing Research, 12,* 123-127.

Lentz, M. J. (1990b). Time series analysis—Cosinor analysis: A special case. *Western Journal of Nursing Research, 12,* 408-412.

Lentz, M. J., & Woods, N. F. (1989). Women's health research: Implications for design, measurement, and analysis. In I. L. Abraham, D. M. Nadzam, & J. J. Fitzpatrick (Eds.), *Statistics and quantitative methods in nursing: Issues and strategies for research and education.* Philadelphia, PA: W. B. Saunders.

Lipsey, M. L., Cordray, D. S., & Berger, D. E. (1981). Evaluation of a juvenile diversion program: Using multiple lines of evidence. *Evaluation Review, 5,* 283-306.

Maas, M. L., & Buckwalter, K. C. (1990). *Nursing evaluation research: A special Alzheimer's unit* (Final report). Rockville, MD: NIH National Center for Nursing Research.

Maas, M., Buckwalter, K., Kelley, L., & Stolley, J. (1991). Family members' perceptions: How they view care of Alzheimer's patients in a nursing home. *Journal of Long Term Care Administration, 19*(1), 21-25.

Maas, M., Buckwalter, K., Swanson, E., & Mobily, P. (1994). Staff knowledge, satisfaction, and absenteeism on a special Alzheimer's care unit. *Journal of Long Term Care Administration, 22*(1), 23-26.

Maas, M., & Swanson, E. (1994). *Nursing Interventions for Alzheimer's: Family Role Trials* (Progress report; Grant #R01 NR01689). Rockville, MD: NIH National Institute of Nursing Research.

Martinson, I. M., & Anderson, S. E. (1983). Effects of thermal applications on the abdominal temperature of dogs. *Research in Nursing and Health, 6*(2), 89-94.

McCain, L. J., & McCleary, R. (1979). The statistical analysis of the simple interrupted time-series quasi-experiment. In T. D. Cook & D. T. Campbell (Eds.), *Quasi-experimentation: Design and analysis issues for field settings.* Chicago: Rand McNally.

Metzger, B. L., & Schultz, S. (1982). Time series analysis: An alternative for nursing. *Nursing Research, 31,* 375-378.

Mobily, P., Maas, M., Buckwalter, K., & Kelley, L. (1992). Taking care of the caregivers: Staff stress and burnout on a special Alzheimer's unit. *Journal of Psychosocial Nursing, 30*(9), 25-31.

Moody, L., Wilson, M., Smyth, K., Schwartz, R., Tittle, M., & Van Cott, M. (1988). Analysis of a decade in nursing practice research. *Nursing Research, 37,* 374-379.

Nath, C., & Rinehart, J. (1979). Effects of individual and group relaxation therapy on blood pressure in essential hypertensives. *Research in Nursing and Health, 2*(3), 119-126.

Nicholson, A. C., Titler, M., Montgomery, L. A., Kleiber, C., Craft, M. J., Halm, M., Buckwalter, K., & Johnson, S. (1993). Effects of child visitation in adult critical care units: A pilot study. *Heart & Lung, 22*(1), 36-45.

Parsons, L. C., Smith-Peard, A. L., & Page, M. C. (1985). The effects of hygiene interventions on the cerebrovascular status of severe closed head injured persons. *Research in Nursing and Health, 8*(2), 173-182.

Reichardt, C. S. (1979). The statistical analysis of data from nonequivalent group designs. In T. D. Cook & D. T. Campbell (Eds.), *Quasi-experimentation: Design and analysis issues for field settings.* Chicago: Rand McNally.

Reichardt, C. S., & Gollob, H. F. (1986) Satisfying the constraints of causal modeling. In W. M. K. Trochim (Ed.), *Advances in quasi-experimental design and analysis.* San Francisco: Jossey-Bass.

Rindskopf, D. (1986). New developments in selection modeling for quasi-experimentation. In W. M. K. Trochim (Ed.), *Advances in quasi-experimental design and analysis.* San Francisco: Jossey-Bass.

Rudy, E. B., Vaska, P. L., Daly, B. J., Happ, M. B., & Shiao, P. (1993). Permuted block design for randomization in a nursing clinical trial. *Nursing Research, 42*(5), 287-289.

Russell, D. W., & Buckwalter, K. C. (1992). Researching and evaluating model geriatric mental health programs Part III: Statistical analysis issues. *Archives of Psychiatric Nursing, 5*(3), 151-162.

Swanson, E., Maas, M., & Buckwalter, K. (1993). Catastrophic reactions and other behaviors of Alzheimer's residents: Special unit compared with traditional units. *Archives of Psychiatric Nursing, 7*(5), 292-299.

Swanson, E., Maas, M., & Buckwalter, K. (1994). Alzheimer's residents cognitive and functional measures. *Clinical Nursing Research, 3*(1), 27-41.

Taylor, D. (1990). Time series analysis: Use of autocorrelation as an analytic strategy for describing pattern and change. *Western Journal of Nursing Research, 12,* 254-261.

Thomas, K. A. (1990). Time series analysis: Spectral analysis and the search for cycles. *Western Journal of Nursing Research, 12,* 558-562.

Tilden, V. P., & Shepherd, P. (1987). Increasing the rate of identification of battered women in an emergency department: Use of a nursing protocol. *Research in Nursing and Health, 10*(4), 209-215.

Trochim, W. M. K. (1986). *Advances in quasi-experimental design and analysis.* San Francisco: Jossey-Bass.

Williams, M. A., Campbell, E. B., Raynor, W. J., Mlynarczyk, S. M., & Ward, S. E. (1985). Reducing acute confusional states in elderly patients with hip fractures. *Research in Nursing and Health, 8,* 329-337.

4

Within-Subject Designs

JANICE LANDER

How researchers view or frame their research problem determines the procedures that will be undertaken during an investigation. Research designs lay down a blueprint that guides the investigator. Fortunately, the many research designs that exist have been categorized into families of designs. One classification scheme consists of true experiments, quasi experiments, and descriptive designs. Each category of designs has unique features as well as some that are shared.

True experiments, quasi experiments, and descriptive studies have in common within-subject and between-subjects designs. The names *within* subject and *between* subjects derive from the distinctive methods of each design.

HOW DO BETWEEN-SUBJECTS AND WITHIN-SUBJECT DESIGNS DIFFER?

Between-Subjects Designs

- Subjects are assigned to groups, either randomly or because they possess a particular attribute or experience.

- Subjects may be enrolled in only one group.
- Each group is exposed to, or represents, different values of the independent variable (examples are control and treatment groups or females and males).
- Responses of all members of one group are compared with those of another group. The groups are expected to differ.

An example of a between-subjects design is the classical posttest-only control group experimental design in which subjects are randomly assigned to either a treatment or a control group.

Within-Subject Designs

- Subjects are handled in one of the following ways:
  — Subjects are observed or assessed repeatedly.
  — Subjects are exposed to *all* interventions associated with the investigation.
  — Related subjects, those who have been *matched* on important attributes or experiences, are delegated to different groups or are taken to be representatives of different groups. Matching approaches include *matching by mutual selection* (Kirk, 1982). Those who are matched in this way include people who have paired off (without the assistance of researchers), such as husbands and wives. A pair may be considered as matched by mutual selection when it is reasonable to presume that the pair is more similar on the outcome measure than those who have not been matched.
- Responses of individual subjects (or related subjects) are expected to differ; the researcher begins by comparing the responses of the subject (or related subjects)—that is, by making within-subject comparisons. These comparisons are aggregated for all subjects.

An illustration is the comparison of measures obtained from a subject before-and-after treatment. This comparison is repeated for all subjects.

You may find the following terms used when researchers are referring to use of within-subject strategies: *repeated measures, using subjects as their own control, crossover, correlated groups, split plots,* and *randomized block designs.* Some of these terms have different meanings for researchers of various disciplines.

Choice of Design: Between-Subjects or Within-Subject?

Some research questions may be answered with *either* a between-subjects or within-subject design. For various reasons, however, only one approach will be possible for other questions. As researchers begin to plan the study, they will discard some potential designs on the grounds that the designs are not practical or feasible. The choice of strategy, ultimately, will be based on pragmatic issues:

- Is it possible to assess the subject repeatedly?
- Is it possible to administer all interventions to subjects?
- Are good matches available so that related pairs of subjects can be formed?
- What resources are available for the study?
- What time constraints do the investigators face?

Each research problem (including the context in which the problem will be addressed) requires an appraisal of the relative merits of between-subjects and within-subject designs. Whenever a choice can be made, it is prudent to choose the within-subject approach to achieve a powerful test of the hypothesis (Christensen, 1991).

Strengths and weaknesses associated with within-subject designs will be discussed later in the chapter. Before undertaking a description of within-subject designs, we will define several terms: *conditions, sessions,* and *trials* (see Table 4.1).

CONTROLLING THREATS TO INTERNAL VALIDITY

To accomplish excellent within-subject research, investigators must diligently attend to internal validity. They do this by employing familiar control strategies as well as those devised especially for within-subject designs.

Random Assignment

As mentioned by Buckwalter and Maas in Chapter 2, between-subjects true experimental designs require random assignment of sub-

Table 4.1   Conditions, Sessions, and Trials

Term	Definition
Condition	Refers to specific treatment interventions or independent variable values (denoted as $X_1, X_2, \ldots X_n$)
Sessions	Denotes the succession of various conditions; for example, Session 1 for a particular subject involves exposure to one treatment condition, and Session 2 involves exposure to the other condition
Trials	Refers to a series of observations or measures of the dependent variable. A pretest is Trial 1, and ensuing posttests become consecutively numbered trials.

jects; this creates an equal probability of any subject's being assigned to any group. Hence, for a two-group between-subjects study, the probability must be 0.5 that any subject will be assigned to treatment X_1 or X_2.

The purpose of using random assignment is to create *equivalent* groups that will have identical exposure to extraneous variables, thus ruling out rival hypotheses. In particular, random assignment will equalize the groups with respect to subject (or individual) differences. This ensures that any group differences on the outcome measure(s) cannot be attributed to preexisting differences in groups.

An alternative strategy is to use a within-subject approach. By exposing the same subjects to all conditions or treatments, there can be no preexisting differences that can be attributed to the individual in the sample.

Random assignment can also be found in conjunction with a control technique that is unique to within-subject designs: *counterbalancing.*

Counterbalancing

Although within-subject designs offer maximum control over individual differences, they can potentially fail to control other extraneous variables such as history, maturation, and instrumentation. Accordingly, use of a counterbalancing strategy (which is a technique for control of *sequencing effects*) is an added requirement of within-subject true experiments in which all subjects are to be exposed to all conditions.

Without counterbalancing, uncontrolled extraneous variables will originate from sequencing effects. Christensen (1991) defines two types of sequencing effects: *order* and *carryover.* Order effects are sometimes called practice or fatigue effects. If subjects have been exposed first to treatment X_1 then to treatment X_2, order effects may arise from a number of sources. Subjects may learn or become fatigued, bored, or distracted from one treatment assessment (that is, session) to the next. Instruments or observers may vary in accuracy. When order effects occur, they may positively or negatively influence performance, producing an unfounded or exaggerated effect for treatment X_1 or X_2.

These performance increases and decreases occur as a backdrop to the study, coinciding with the introduction of the experimental interventions and masking the true effects of interventions. It should be emphasized that order effects do not originate from the treatment but from environmental, intrasubject, or instrument factors.

Order effects can be illustrated by the comparison of two sleeping environments (Deiriggi, 1990). The two interventions consisted of having preterm infants spend 3 days on a standard mattress and 3 days on a waterbed. Assume, for now, that the mattress sequence was the same for each infant—first standard, then waterbed. The primary outcome measure was time spent in various sleep-wake states. It is conceivable that during the 6 days of the study, changes may have occurred in infant sleep-wake state that could be attributed to infant maturation or to environment (such as from variations in noise or light level). Changes may also have occurred in rater assessment skill. These changes could coincide with the introduction of one of the mattresses, spuriously inflating or deflating the outcome measure. Any significant difference between mattresses, or lack thereof, could be due to order effects.

Carryover effects, another sequencing effect, are permanent or transient changes occurring in the subject as the result of a prior treatment condition in the study. These can be obvious or subtle. Consider, for example, a within-subject design to compare motor skills with and without alcohol. Each subject will be exposed to both conditions. Motor skills in the no-alcohol condition could be good or poor depending on whether the alcohol condition occurred before or afterward.

A more subtle carryover effect may be observed in a within-subject comparison of two strategies for managing anticipatory anxiety about invasive procedures. Behavior observed during Session 2 (following the second anxiety management treatment) may be influenced by the first treatment provided in Session 1. The second treatment may be more or less effective when preceded by the first treatment. If, for example, the first treatment is beneficial, it could reduce anxiety and provide subjects with a sense of accomplishment, resulting in a change of view about invasive procedures. Indeed, the first treatment may have a very different effect if positioned as the second treatment rather than the first. Some carryover effects therefore may preclude use of the within-subject design.

There are several strategies for controlling or minimizing carryover effects. One strategy to minimize temporary carryover effects is to allow sufficient time to elapse between treatments, permitting the first treatment effect to disappear. That solution will not resolve permanent carryover effects. Furthermore, allowing time to elapse may be an unacceptable solution for researchers if carryover effects resolve slowly.

Because sequencing effects can be subtle, appropriate controls must be employed to eliminate rival hypotheses. Counterbalancing strategies are therefore mandatory for many within-subject designs. The cornerstone of all counterbalancing strategies is the control of sequence of treatments.

The first step in planning counterbalancing is the enumeration of all possible sequences of treatments. This can be determined by computing the factorial of the number of treatments. There are only two possible sequences for two treatments, whereas there are six unique sequences for three treatments (see Table 4.2).

Likewise, for four treatments, there are 24 sequences ($4! = 4 \times 3 \times 2 \times 1$). Once the sequences are enumerated, subjects are randomly assigned to one of the possible sequences. Every sequence must be represented in the study, preferably with equal numbers of subjects in each sequence. When these requirements are met, complete counterbalancing has been used.

The sample size will be a multiple of the number of sequences. Assume that power analysis has indicated that 50 subjects are required for a study with three treatment conditions. The subjects must be randomly assigned, in equal numbers, to the six sequences. Therefore, 54 subjects will be enrolled and assigned randomly with 9 subjects per sequence.

The number of sessions will be equal to the number of treatments or conditions. What happens in each session depends on a subject's as-

Table 4.2   Sequences of Treatments

	Number of Treatment Conditions	
	Two	*Three*
Factorial of number of conditions	$2! = 2 \times 1 = 2$	$3! = 3 \times 2 \times 1 = 6$
Enumeration of all possible sequences	1. X_1 X_2 2. X_2 X_1	1. X_1 X_2 X_3 2. X_1 X_3 X_2 3. X_2 X_1 X_3 4. X_2 X_3 X_1 5. X_3 X_1 X_2 6. X_3 X_2 X_1

signed sequence. In a three-treatments example, subjects in Sequences 1 and 2 will have X_1 at Session 1 and X_2 or X_3 at Session 2 (see Table 4.2).

Another counterbalancing strategy is incomplete counterbalancing. This is an enticing alternative when there are many treatments because fewer subjects will be required. For example, with five conditions, multiples of 120 subjects would be required for complete counterbalancing, whereas multiples of 10 would satisfy incomplete counterbalancing.

Incomplete counterbalancing requires that each treatment condition appear once in each position (first session, second, third, and so on) and precede and follow every other condition. This results in a reduction of the number of required sequences. Odd numbers of treatments require careful planning to achieve the requirement that every condition or treatment appear once before and after each other condition. Christensen (1991) can be consulted for further details about procedures.

Incomplete counterbalancing of four treatments would consist of four sequences instead of the 24 required for complete counterbalancing. Table 4.3 displays sequences and sessions for four conditions.

How does counterbalancing control sequencing effects? The assumption is made that if intrasubject or environmental or instrument confounders occur at any time, they will equally affect all conditions. For example, if some environmental factors influence behavior of subjects during Session 1 in the preceding counterbalancing arrangement, they will influence each treatment condition equally because X_1, X_2, X_3, and

Table 4.3   An Illustration of Sessions and Sequences for Four
                  Incompletely Counterbalanced Treatment Conditions

	Sessions			
Sequences	1	2	3	4
First	X_1	X_2	X_4	X_3
Second	X_2	X_3	X_1	X_4
Third	X_3	X_4	X_2	X_1
Fourth	X_4	X_1	X_3	X_2

X_4 all have been presented in Session 1. This meets the important experimental control requirement of equally distributing extraneous variables over all treatments.

Of the two approaches, complete counterbalancing is more efficient at resolving carryover effects because it will resolve linear and nonlinear carryover effects. By contrast, incomplete counterbalancing is unable to resolve nonlinear carryover effects and can handle only linear carryover effects—that is, those in which the sequencing effect is constant for each treatment position (Christensen, 1991).

Matching

A matching strategy may be undertaken in the quest to construct equivalent groups. The researcher is most likely to decide to match groups when random assignment is not possible or feasible. Matching can, however, also be done in combination with random assignment in true experiments.

As mentioned, matching will create correlated groups because, by definition, subjects who are most alike on the matching variable will be paired. The simplest level consists of a matched pair. The following discussion about matching refers to a matched pair, although three or more individuals may be matched. The complexity and difficulty of the matching procedure increases with the number of matches to be made.

One or more matching variables may be identified. Usually, these are extraneous variables that are to be controlled because they potentially influence the outcome variable. Health status, age, or socioeconomic status are familiar matching variables in health research because these variables are frequently related to outcome measures.

Matching is often undertaken with existing groups consisting of members who have chosen to belong or whose lot in life has earned them membership. The groups are often referred to as *self-selected*. The groups represent values of independent variables that cannot be randomly allocated. These variables include individual characteristics (e.g., gender or age) and diseases or unhealthy behaviors (e.g., smoking). A subject from one group will be paired with a subject from the second group, because they are most alike on important extraneous variables. Consequently, each pair consists of subjects who differ maximally on the study independent variable and minimally on the matching variable. This strategy is employed to minimize differences among groups on key extraneous variables when random assignment is not possible.

Matching may also occur in combination with random assignment. Once pairs are formed, one member may be randomly assigned to one of the intervention groups and the other automatically will be allocated to the second.

Several obstacles may hinder researchers who wish to employ a matching procedure. Use of matched groups requires that researchers know what variables should be matched. This is not always the case. A second obstacle to matching is that a large population may be required if there are many variables on which subjects are to be matched. As a general rule, matching becomes more complex as the number of variables increases and, as mentioned earlier, when matching goes beyond pairs. Another obstacle stems from the nature of some variables. Even though levels of a variable may appear similar, they may be qualitatively different. For example, subjects matched on number of years of education may not be equivalent because of qualitative differences in type of education.

Use of random assignment will control many threats to internal validity, thus allowing an unambiguous test of the hypothesis. When used as a replacement for random assignment, matching leads to a situation in which there may be several explanations for the results. Any differences found between matched groups may be attributed to the independent variable as well as to an extraneous variable, such as selection.

Table 4.4   An Illustration of Sessions and Sequences for a Basic
Within-Subject Design

Sequences	1		2	
First	X_1	O_1	X_2	O_2
Second	X_2	O_1	X_1	O_2

MODELS OF WITHIN-SUBJECT
TRUE EXPERIMENTS

In the nursing literature, the within-subject true experiment is frequently and incorrectly labeled as a quasi experiment. Designs discussed in this section entail (a) taking repeated measures on subjects, (b) exposing subjects to all levels of the independent variable, or (c) both.

Basic Within-Subject True Experiment

The sequences and sessions of the design are illustrated in Table 4.4. The two unique sequences include both of the interventions set up in reverse orders. Subjects are exposed to both treatment X_1 and X_2, with half of the subjects randomly assigned to be treated with one order of treatments and half assigned to the other order. Every condition or intervention is followed by a measure taken on the dependent variable. For this basic design, complete and incomplete counterbalancing are equivalent. Both order and carryover effects are controlled. The exemplar case, presented at the end of this chapter, is a basic within-subject true experiment.

Completely Within-Subject Factorial Design

As Buckwalter and Maas indicated (in Chapter 2), a factorial design includes more than one independent variable. Therefore, a completely within-subject factorial design contains at least two independent variables, each with a minimum of two values, with each subject exposed to all values of all independent variables.

The simplest case consists of two independent variables, A and B, each with two values. Every subject must be exposed to four conditions: A_1, A_2, B_1, and B_2, and the order of presentation must be counterbalanced.

Complete counterbalancing for this simple within-subject factorial design requires arranging 24 sequences and using a minimum of 24 subjects (or multiples of 24). Four sequences will be required for incomplete counterbalancing, as illustrated in Table 4.3. Additional values of independent variables or additional variables can be included; however, the complexity of the design and the counterbalancing scheme will increase with each addition.

A simple modification of the basic within-subject true-experiment can produce a completely within-subject factorial design. The modification consists of the addition of trials. One independent variable is a repeated measure (trials), and the second is the condition or treatment. Subjects are exposed to all trials and conditions. In this case, only the treatment condition can be counterbalanced. Repeated trials preclude use of counterbalancing because trials occur only in one sequence, ordered from first to last.

One example of a completely within-subject factorial is the study conducted by Allen (1987) for the purposes of increasing hospital-based nurses' awareness of research. Because there were two independent variables, each with two values, the design was a 2 × 2 factorial design. The purpose of the study was to examine errors in reading residual fluids in polyvinyl intravenous bags. The two factors were amount of fluid in the bag (either 425 ml or 825 ml) and angle of regard (fluid level was either at eye level or 25 cm above). Because a completely within-subject approach was employed, all subjects participated in four sessions during which they were required to read residual fluids. The four sessions were created by unique combinations of the independent variable values as outlined:

> A—425 ml, at eye level
> B—425 ml, 25 cm above eye level
> C—825 ml, at eye level
> D—825 ml, 25 cm above eye level

These four combinations of the two independent variable values would require 24 sequences for complete counterbalancing or 4 sequences for incomplete counterbalancing (Table 4.3). Subjects must be randomly assigned to one of the four sequences.

A 2 × 2 within-subject factorial analysis of variance (ANOVA) was used to test the three hypotheses that can be formulated with this design (main effect of bag, main effect of angle of regard, and interaction of bag and angle of regard). There was significantly greater error in reading the 425 ml bag compared with reading the 825 ml bag (main effect of bag). There was also a significant interaction. The error was smallest for the 825 ml bag when read at a height of 25 cm and greatest for the 425 ml bag also when read at 25 cm.

Mixed Factorial Designs

These true experiments are considered to be *mixed* because they have at least one within-subject variable and at least one between-subjects variable. Hence, they are both between and within-subject designs.

The mixed factorial within-subject design most often executed is the pre- and posttest true experimental design. It incorporates repeated measures (the pre- and posttests) and a between-groups comparison, representing the independent variable (or treatment) under investigation.

$$O_1 \quad X \quad O_2$$
$$RA$$
$$O_1 \qquad O_2$$

Biddle and Biddle (1985) compared three head coverings to determine which best prevented heat loss in elderly patients during surgery. Patients were randomly assigned to the head cover group (the between-subjects independent variable), and temperature was recorded before and after surgery (0 minutes and 60 minutes after). This was the within-subject variable. When the design used by Biddle and Biddle is employed, data analysis becomes surprisingly complex, as discussed in the next section.

The within-subject component of the mixed-model factorial design can be made elaborate by the addition of trials. Duggleby and Lander (1992) compared patients who were randomly assigned to receive patient-controlled analgesia (PCA) or nurse administered postoperative analgesics. This was the between-subjects variable. Pain was measured at 14 trials spaced over 4 days after surgery. The within-subject variable, trials, consisted of repeated measures.

There are occasions when a mixed-model design is used rather than a full factorial design, such as when it is not possible to expose subjects to all levels of one independent variable. This is especially true when one variable is *measured* rather than *experimental*. Measured independent variables represent subject attributes. A hypothetical example is the assessment of effects of gender and treatment on children's needle puncture pain. Gender would be a measured between-subjects independent variable. Treatment (for example, topical anesthetic versus music distraction) would be an experimental variable. The researcher provides boys and girls with both treatments in counterbalanced order. To be classified as a true experiment, at least one independent variable must be manipulated.

Matched Groups With Randomized Assignment to Treatment

The most elementary version of this design consists of two matched groups, with subjects matched on one or more important variables and then randomly assigned to a group. Each group receives a different treatment condition. This design resembles a between-subjects true experiment, except that the lack of independence among groups must be considered during data analysis. A well-chosen matching variable reduces error.

QUASI-EXPERIMENTAL AND DESCRIPTIVE WITHIN-SUBJECT DESIGNS

Designs discussed in other chapters in this volume include repeated measures designs. They are, therefore, within-subject designs. A familiar example is the nonequivalent pre- and posttest control group design, which is a quasi experiment. This design is often coupled with the matching of subjects in an attempt to increase comparability of groups. Time-series designs are also within-subject because they call for repeated measures.

The one-group pre- and posttest design is a within-subject design, but it is considered to be seriously flawed (for details, see the discussion by Cook & Campbell, 1979). Comparative descriptive designs are also within-subject if groups of subjects are matched.

Data Analysis Issues

Many familiar statistical tests require observations to be independent of one another. Because within-subject designs violate the assumption of independence, specific statistical tests must be used to handle dependence among scores. The paired t test and repeated measures ANOVA are examples.

A detailed discussion about data analysis is beyond the scope of this book; however, several points are worth making. Mixed-model ANOVA (also called split-plot ANOVA) is used for designs with at least one between-subjects variable and one within-subject variable. Separate error variance associated with between-subjects and within-subject factors are computed in the analysis. The appropriate error variance must be used for the determination of F values for main and interaction effects. The more complex the factorial design, the more difficult it is to explain significant interaction effects. Therefore, although there is no ideal limit to the number of variables and values, there is a practical limit.

The approach for analysis of data in pretest-posttest designs is much debated. The pretest score can be used as a covariate. Indeed, this procedure is often recommended (Tabachnick & Fidell, 1989). Individual differences that existed among subjects prior to the intervention can thus be statistically removed. This reduces error variance and achieves a more powerful comparison of the intervention groups (Shavelson, 1988). Thus, analysis of covariance (ANCOVA) or multivariate analysis of covariance (MANCOVA) are suitable.

Some researchers use change scores—pre- to posttest difference scores—for these designs. The acceptability of this strategy has been debated for many years. Use of difference scores may or may not be appropriate, depending on the data set (for details, see Streiner & Norman, 1995).

An alternative approach is a mixed-model ANOVA in which pre- and posttests are the within-subject factor and groups the between-subjects factor. Results of the analysis may not be satisfactory because the important question about posttest differences among groups is ob-

Table 4.5   A Guideline for Choosing Statistical Tests

| Condition | *Statistical Test* | |
	Parametric	*Nonparametric*
IV = 1 IV values = 2 COV = 0	Paired *t* test (i.e., *t* test for dependent measures)	Wilcoxon matched pair test Sign test
IV = 1 IV values = ≥ 3 COV = 0	Repeated measures ANOVA	Friedman test
IV = 1 IV values = ≥ 3 COV = ≥ 1	Repeated measures ANCOVA	
IV = ≥ 2 IV values = ≥ 2 COV = 0	Factorial ANOVA	Friedman test
IV = ≥ 2 IV values = ≥ 2 COV = ≥ 1	Factorial ANCOVA	

NOTE: The table refers to the case of one dependent variable. IV = number of independent variables; IV values = number of independent variable values; COV = number of covariates.

tained only by a circuitous route (through the interaction term and post hoc tests).

A guideline for choosing a statistical test is presented in Table 4.5. In some situations, other tests may also be appropriate. Further details about these and other suitable statistical procedures can be found in Kirk (1982), Marascuilo and McSweeney (1977), and Tabachnick and Fidell (1989).

Strengths and Weaknesses

Using a within-subject design has several advantages. As a general rule, within-subject designs are more economical than between-subjects designs. They require fewer subjects; the total number of subjects needed for a basic within-subject experimental design or a completely within-subject factorial design corresponds to the number required for any one condition. Deiriggi (1990) required 22 infants for her study. If the same study used a between-subjects design, a total of 44 would have been required. Because these designs require fewer subjects, they may be ideal when the population of available subjects is limited. Another aspect of the economy of the within-subject design is that the time, effort, and equipment required to set up some studies need not be repeated or wasted.

A second advantage is that error variance is reduced in within-subject designs. This makes the design most sensitive in the assessment of the independent variable. Generally, the within-subject design provides a more powerful test of the null hypothesis than does the between-subjects design.

On the other hand, there are several obstacles to using the within-subject approach. The factor most likely to dissuade researchers from undertaking a within-subject approach is feasibility. For many studies, it will not be possible to expose subjects to all treatments, either because of permanent carryover effects or because of the possibility of introducing subject bias.

When Lander and Fowler-Kerry (1993) planned a double-blind, placebo-controlled study of transcutaneous electrical nerve stimulation (TENS) for children's procedural pain, they considered the pros and cons of between-subjects and within-subject approaches. They concluded that it would not be possible to maintain a subject-blind about the treatment condition if subjects were exposed to all treatments. Once exposed to TENS, subjects would know they were receiving placebo-TENS. Another factor they considered was that it would be necessary to enroll only children who were certain to have repeated invasive procedures. This would reduce the available population and ultimately slow subject enrollment. They therefore chose a between-subjects design.

Ethical Issues

The same ethical issues that apply to other research designs are pertinent to within-subject designs. For many within-subject designs, it is especially important for the researcher to inform subjects carefully of the required time commitment.

Exemplar Case

Pediatric practitioners faced several dilemmas following the introduction of a new topical anesthetic (EMLA® cream). The drug had the potential to be used for many invasive procedures (especially involving needle pokes) adding greatly to the operating cost of the pediatric units. It was apparent that not all children would require the drug on all occasions but not evident which children should receive the drug. Another question was whether or not a less expensive alternative existed. This last question was addressed as the first of a series of studies (Lander et al., 1996).

Two topical agents were to be compared: 5% Lidocaine, which could be prepared economically in the pharmacy, and EMLA, the new drug. The dependent variable was pain (measured on a 10 cm visual analogue scale). The invasive, pain-inducing procedure was intravenous cannulation.

Several considerations determined the selection of the design. The relatively small number of staff available to participate and the need to constrain study costs favored a within-subject approach. Concern about individual subject differences in past experience with needles and individual differences affecting ease of cannulation also supported a within-subject approach. The potential for carryover effects was balanced against the benefits of a within-subject approach. Because each person had many potential intravenous sites, it was possible to use corresponding sites for the topical drugs, thus minimizing risk of carryover effects. Therefore, a within-subject experimental design was chosen.

Both drugs were applied on all subjects ($N = 7$). One drug was applied to the posterior surface of one hand and the other drug applied to the same site of the other hand. The order of the drugs was counterbalanced, with half of the subjects having EMLA and half having Lidocaine on the right hand. The data collector, intravenous technician, and subjects were all blind about which of the drugs were applied to right or left hand. Moreover, an added precaution was taken by performing intravenous cannulation in a counterbalanced order. The first subject, for example, had the procedure done first on the right hand followed by the left; the second subject had the order reversed.

Using Table 4.5 as a guide, the research conditions were as follows: There was one independent variable, designated as DRUG, that had two values (EMLA and Lidocaine); there were no covariates. Therefore, the paired t test, Wilcoxon matched pair test, or the sign test could be used. Reported cannulation pain was analyzed with a paired t test because the visual analogue scale can be considered to provide interval level data. The paired t test was significant ($p < .05$), and the mean reported pain was greater for Lidocaine than for EMLA. The small sample size was adequate to detect the difference in benefit of the two drugs because the effect was large. The conclusion of the researchers was that EMLA, although more expensive than Lidocaine, was far more effective. They then began planning for the next phase of the research, to identify the children who would most benefit from EMLA.

ADDITIONAL EXAMPLES OF WITHIN-SUBJECT TRUE EXPERIMENTS

Basic Within-Subject

Simms, S. G., Rhodes, V. A., & Madsen, R. W. (1993). Comparison of prochlor-perazine and lorazepam antiemetic regimens in the control of postchemo-therapy symptoms. *Nursing Research, 42,* 232-239.

Mixed Factorial Design

Gift, A. G., Moore, T., & Soeken, K. (1992). Relaxation to reduce dyspnea and anxiety in COPD patients. *Nursing Research, 41,* 242-246.

Lookinland, S., & Appel, P. L. (1991). Hemodynamic and oxygen transport changes following endotracheal suctioning in trauma patients. *Nursing Research, 40,* 133-138.

MacVicar, M. G., Winngham, M. L., & Nickel, J. L. (1989). Effects of aerobic interval training on cancer patients' functional capacity. *Nursing Research, 38,* 348-351.

Marchette, L., Main, R., Redick, E., Bagg, A., & Leatherland, J. (1991). Pain reduction interventions during neonatal circumcision. *Nursing Research, 40,* 241-244.

Miller, P., Wikoff, R., Garrett, M. J., McMahon, M., & Smith, T. (1990). Regimen compliance two years after myocardial infarction. *Nursing Research, 39,* 333-336.

White, H., Thurston, N., Blackmore, K., Green, S., & Hannah, K. (1987). Body temperature in elderly surgical patients. *Research in Nursing & Health, 10,* 317-321.

Completely Within-Subject Factorial Design

Baker, N., Cerone, S., Gaze, N., & Knapp, T. (1984). The effect of type of thermometer and length of time inserted on oral temperature measurements of afebrile subjects. *Nursing Research, 33,* 109-111.

McCain, G. C. (1992). Facilitating inactive awake states in preterm infants: A study of three interventions. *Nursing Research, 41*, 157-160.

Metzger, B. L., & Therrien, B. (1990). Effect of position on cardiovascular response during the valsalva maneuver. *Nursing Research, 39*, 198-202.

Quasi Experiments and Descriptive Research

Heidrich, S., & Cranley, M. S. (1989). Effect of fetal movement, ultrasound scans, and amniocentesis on maternal-fetal attachment. *Nursing Research, 38*, 81-84.

REFERENCES

Allen, M. (1987). *Reading residual IV fluids.* Unpublished manuscript, University of Alberta, Edmonton, Canada.

Biddle, C., & Biddle, W. (1985). A plastic head cover to reduce surgical heat loss. *Geriatric Nursing, 6*, 39-41.

Christensen, L. B. (1991). *Experimental methodology.* Boston: Allyn & Bacon.

Cook, T., & Campbell, D. (1979). *Quasi-experimentation: Design and analysis issues for field settings.* Boston: Houghton Mifflin.

Deiriggi, P. (1990). Effects of waterbed flotation on indicators of energy expenditure in preterm infants. *Nursing Research, 39*, 140-146.

Duggleby, W., & Lander, J. (1992). Patient controlled analgesia for older adults. *Clinical Journal of Nursing Research, 1*, 107-113.

Kirk, R. (1982). *Experimental design procedures for the social sciences.* Pacific Grove, CA: Brooks/Cole.

Lander, J., & Fowler-Kerry, S. (1993). TENS for children's procedural pain. *Pain, 52*, 209-216.

Lander, J., Nazarali, S., Hodgins, M., Friesen, E., McTavish, J., Ouellette, J., & Abel, R. (1996). Evaluation of a new topical anesthetic agent: A pilot study. *Nursing Research, 45*, 50-53.

Marascuilo, L., & McSweeney, M. (1977). *Nonparametric and distribution-free methods for the social sciences.* Monterey, CA: Brooks/Cole.

Shavelson, R. (1988). *Statistical reasoning for the behavioral sciences.* Boston: Allyn & Bacon.

Streiner, D., & Norman, G. (1995). *Health measurement scales: A practical guide to their development and use.* Oxford, UK: Oxford University Press.

Tabachnick, B., & Fidell, L. (1989). *Using multivariate statistics.* Cambridge, UK: Harper & Row.

5

Evaluative Designs

MARILYNN J. WOOD

Evaluative research designs are intended to provide data on the success of action programs. They are of particular interest to policymakers who are responsible for allocating resources in health care. In nursing, we are frequently called on to design program evaluations for many reasons, ranging from developing grant proposals for training or clinical projects to testing the effectiveness of nursing intervention programs in the clinical setting. The value of evaluation has become increasingly apparent to politicians and granting agencies for budget appropriations and funding of programs. In addition, within health care agencies, evaluative research is becoming an important management tool, used to determine whether individual programs are producing benefits that justify their costs.

Evaluative designs do not fit into any one level of research but instead usually have characteristics of more than one level. These research designs are based on the objectives of the program, and therefore, several designs may be combined into one. Evaluation uses the methods and tools of research but applies them in an action setting that may not always fit with the assumptions and principles of traditional research. To conduct evaluation research, we need to be aware of the differences between using research principles for evaluative purposes and using them for projects that are strictly research endeavors.

Evaluative designs are appropriate whenever the research question asks about the effectiveness of a program. For example, the researcher might be interested in whether or not a cardiac rehabilitation program really has an effect on the health and future productivity of the participants and whether or not the cost of the program can be justified in terms of the results. This is a typical evaluative research question. The question could be partially answered using an experimental design with randomly assigned groups. However, an experimental design would be very expensive and would not make use of existing resources (such as a cardiac rehabilitation program already operating in the community). Requiring a control group and random assignment to groups might be unethical if a rehabilitation program is already established. In addition, it is difficult to assess long-range effects (including cost-benefit ratios) through the standard experimental design because of the influence of time on the outcome. Finally, the experimental design is always implemented in an artificial setting and so may not provide an adequate test of the real-life situation. An evaluative design can incorporate some of the control techniques of an experimental design while using both survey and qualitative methods to provide additional data. Its main purpose, however, is to *measure the effects* of the program.

Difficulties may arise in planning evaluative research, stemming largely from the fact that the programs being evaluated are so variable. In health care, the range of programs that need to be evaluated is vast, ranging from small, self-learning modules for teaching students to calculate dosages to complex programs designed to change the image of nursing in the eyes of the general public. Various factors related to the program itself will affect the evaluative approach that can be taken. These have to do with, first, the scope of the program itself in terms of the geographic area affected and the size of the population served by the program. Second, the quality of the program goals will be a significant factor. Can these be explained easily, in precise terms, or are they vague and global in nature? Certainly, goals that are clearly stated in measurable terms will simplify the approach that can be taken, whereas more diffuse goals will require a different approach. Finally, the innovativeness of the approach taken in the program will be a determining factor in the approach that can be taken for evaluation.

In addition to these program factors, however, the politics of evaluation must be kept in mind (Borg & Gall, 1983). In any program, there will be various individuals and groups who have a vested interest in the program and who may try to influence the evaluation accordingly. The reality of the situation is that an evaluation can sometimes do more harm than good, particularly if people feel threatened by the evaluation and their job performance is adversely affected. By including these stakeholders in planning the evaluation, the researcher can include their concerns and issues in the plan and many potential problems can be diffused.

Assumptions of the Design

The following assumptions are implicit in the use of evaluative designs:

1. There are measurable objectives for the program that can be used as a basis for evaluation.
2. There are methods or tools available with which to measure the variables.
3. The objectives can be assigned priorities and weighted in a practical sense according to their value to the project.
4. Adequate control participants can be provided so that a model for statistical testing can be used to establish whether or not the program made a difference.

Basic Design

The question being asked in an evaluative study is, What difference did the program make? The first step in setting up the design is to specify the objectives of the program in measurable terms (Cain & Hollister, 1972). This may have been done when the program was initiated, but it is unlikely that it was if the program was set up as a clinical or social program. Patton (1980) suggests having the program directors develop a set of evaluation questions based on what they would like to know about the results of the program. These questions or objectives must then be listed in order of priority. The process may involve moving from an extensive list of potential questions to a much shorter list of relevant questions to a "focused list of essential and necessary questions" (Patton, 1980, p. 96). Next, a priority list is developed that demonstrates the importance of each objective in relation to the overall mission of the program. For example, for a program designed to provide posthospitalization follow-up care for hypertensives, the primary objective should relate to the actual blood pressure of the participants and how well it is maintained within the normal range for each individual. The attitudes of the participants and their families toward the program, although important to measure, would be given lower priority because they are not directly related to the central mission of the program. Methods of measuring the achievement of the objectives must be demonstrated. If any of the major objectives are intangible in nature, the researcher may recommend qualitative methods for the measurement of these objectives. Once the objectives have been formulated and priorities decided, an appropriate control group must be established. In this respect, the design will usually resemble a quasi-experimental design.

The ideal evaluative design has the major ingredients of an experimental design, but there is one important difference: Because the study is evaluating a specific program, the program participants usually constitute the "experimental" participants rather than a sample of individuals chosen specifically for a research project. This is an important distinction because the selection of these participants is usually determined by the program protocol, not by the researcher. Therefore, they are not randomly assigned, and there is no guarantee of equivalence between experimental and control participants. Cain and Hollister (1972) suggest the following possible alternative methods for obtaining control group data:

Nonequivalent Controls. Controls may be a sample of individuals not participating in the program but are matched with program participants on some significant demographic variables. Although such a matched group can serve as a viable control group, it is likely to be somewhat nonrepresentative; that is, it may differ significantly from the program participant group in some critical ways. It is sometimes possible to construct a control group from persons who have the same disease process as program participants but who have chosen an alternate method of treatment. In this situation, control participants would likely be very similar to the program participants, leading to a significant increase in the internal validity of the study. In other cases, however, the control participants might be persons who were eligible for but chose not to participate in any program of treatment and thus may resemble the participants only in one basic characteristic, such as diagnosis.

An alternative to the matched control group is a large-scale control group from the target population. In this case, the sheer size of the control group increases the validity of the study by ensuring that relevant variables are normally distributed. Large-scale control groups can be randomly selected from the population, thus yielding a sample representative of the population. However, because the program participants are chosen selectively rather than randomly, the unavoidable occurrence of unmeasured variables among experimental participants makes it difficult to compare them to the control group. This problem might prove serious enough to render this type of control group invalid. If so, a matched group will provide a better comparison than a large-scale group.

The Before-and-After Design. In this design, each study participant is expected to be his or her own control. Specifically, a baseline measurement taken on each individual before implementation of the program is used to determine how these persons would perform if there were no program. This method, of course, gives no guarantee of internal validity. Numerous factors other than the program itself could be responsible for any changes observed in the participants. In many situations, one would expect the participant to undergo change irrespective of treatment programs. These anticipated changes, which can reflect either improvement (as in a rehabilitation program) or deterioration (as in a hospice program), can make it impossible to identify the impact of the program itself when participants are used as their own controls.

In addition, other changes in the lives of the participants can occur that have nothing to do with the program but that affect any before-and-after comparison. This design, therefore, should be reserved for use with groups for which the "without treatment" course of events for the participants is well-documented and predictable, thus increasing the possibility of internal validity for the study.

Alternative Experimental Designs. Boruch and Wortman (1979) discuss ways to couple randomized experiments with evaluative studies that try to approximate experiments through the use of statistical analysis. Specifically the evaluative design can incorporate statistical techniques that approximate randomization—and yield comparison groups that are similar to the program population.

It is quite possible, in an evaluation study, that the measurement techniques might involve both quantitative and qualitative data. Qualitative data, such as participant observation, in-depth interviewing, and detailed description, can be of great help to the evaluative researcher in providing a richness of background that puts the data into the context of the participants and the program itself. It can also be of great value in analyzing and interpreting the quantitative data. For example, when analyzing data about dropouts from a particular program, instead of merely interpreting the numbers in light of the demographic characteristics of dropouts versus continuers, it can be very enlightening to have descriptive data on the feelings and perceptions of the participants, including their reasons for either staying with the program or dropping out. In fact, an evaluative design that does not include some of these data would be subject to suspicion. Because the design mimics, but does not equal, the experimental design, it can be tempting to analyze and interpret the results *as though it were a true experiment.* The inclusion of qualitative data prevents this from happening, because the quantitative analysis must then be discussed in light of the qualitative data.

Variations on the Basic Design

An interesting variation on the traditional evaluative design is seen in the case of the *needs assessment.* This type of evaluative research is very important because it puts program design in touch with the realities of the health care system and the consumer. A well-designed needs assessment will also indicate any need to change existing programs.

A needs assessment will normally be designed as a survey, using a questionnaire that collects data from respondents on both the existing and the desired situation (see Chapter 11 on descriptive designs). By defining a need as "a discrepancy between an existing set of conditions and a desired set of conditions," Borg and Gall (1983, p. 753) recommend that a needs assessment be viewed as a discrepancy analysis of current and desired conditions. This sounds quite simple and straight-forward, but some issues with regard to needs assessments should be addressed.

One of these relates to the values underlying needs. These may not be addressed by the assessment tool. For example, Dela Cruz, Jacobs, and Wood (1986) surveyed home health agencies in Southern California to determine the learning needs of home health nurses. The survey items elicited information about the existing educational background of home health nurses and about perceived need for additional knowl-edge in a variety of areas. The resultant data provided the basis for a continuing education program for these nurses. The questionnaire did not, however, address the underlying values of the participants. Partici-pants might differ in how they believe educational deficits among home health nurses should be addressed. Some might believe that a continu-ing education program is not appropriate for nurses who are not adequately prepared to practice home health nursing and that these nurses should be required to obtain bachelor's degrees instead.

Another issue regarding needs assessments stems from the fact that the results are pooled and reported as group trends. Important individ-ual differences can be overlooked, and this could cause problems when a program is implemented.

Examples of Evaluative Studies

Martinson et al. (1986) evaluated a home care alternative to hospital care for children dying of cancer. The program provided care to 64 children referred by oncologists and pediatricians in the north central United States. The children were 17 years of age or younger and dying of cancer. Hospitalization was not planned at time of referral. The design did not include a control group; rather, the progress of each child was evaluated on the basis of the program objectives. The major objec-tive was to allow the child to die at home.

Data were collected from medical records, home care records, ques-tionnaires covering demographic data, grief support lists, care ratings, and progress recordings made by the project nurse coordinators. A 1-month postdeath interview with parents reviewed the process of home care and parent assessment of care, as well as financial aspects of the care. Another interview was conducted 1 year after the child's death.

The home care program successfully provided care to 58 families, 46 of whom experienced the death of a child at home. At 1-month and 1-year intervals after the child's death, the 46 families expressed satisfaction with the experience. This evaluative design is typical in that neither the internal nor the external validity of the design is documented, yet the project objectives are supported.

In a different type of evaluative study, Thurston and Dundas (1985) looked at the effectiveness of an early postpartum discharge program in a large Canadian city. Two major hospitals and the city home care program participated in the study. The major purpose of the program was to provide a safe alternative to hospital care for postpartum patients. Patient safety and satisfaction were high-priority objectives for the project. The program participants were volunteers (both mothers and physicians) who met elaborate admission criteria ensuring that there were no complications related to the delivery. The program was begun as a pilot study with 109 patients and was continued over 7 months for an additional 267 patients. No control group was established, because postpartum complications that might be prevented by longer hospitalization are well-documented. Measurements were established for critical areas of patient safety, including PKU testing of infants, necessity of hospital readmission, and complications for either mother or infant. Patient satisfaction was measured through the use of a questionnaire, for which a return rate of 69% was achieved.

The results demonstrated that the two central objectives of the program were met, in that (a) there were no serious complications for mothers and infants that were attributable to early discharge and (b) the participants expressed satisfaction with the program. Limitations of the design were acknowledged, including the self-selecting, voluntary nature of the participants. As frequently happens with evaluation studies, the positive results led to the incorporation of the program into the routine service of the community prior to the anticipated end of the evaluation study.

Suitable Nursing Problems

Evaluative designs are the best choice for many nursing situations. An evaluative design might even be required, particularly for programs funded by external granting agencies. In these cases, the evaluation must be planned as part of the program. In addition to these mandated evaluations, however, the design can be used by nurses to study phenomena that would otherwise be impossible to study without extensive funding. The evaluative design, unlike the experimental design, can use existing programs and test the effectiveness of various interventions without having to set up special treatment programs. The design could be used, for example, to test the effectiveness with which a weight loss program prepares individuals to maintain their weight loss, the preparedness for bereavement of families of hospice patients, the readiness of graduates of rehabilitation programs to resume product lives, or the professional socialization of students in nursing programs. The criterion for selecting an evaluative design is that the research question be part of the program objectives. If it is, then the evaluative design is appropriate. If not, another design should be selected.

A useful distinction can be made between *formative* and *summative* evaluation. Formative evaluation provides feedback during the progress of the program and is used to improve or modify its operation. Summative evaluation is done after the program is over and attempts to assess how effective the program was in meeting its objectives. Although some programs make use of both types, evaluative research is primarily concerned with summative evaluation (Cain & Hollister, 1972).

The first step in designing an evaluation study is to state the program goals clearly. This can prove to be the most difficult step in the process. For evaluation purposes, the goals must be stated in measurable terms. Thus, the process is enhanced if the researcher assists the project staff to formulate clear, specific, and measurable goals in the development phase of the project. Otherwise, the program goals may be extremely fuzzy, and the staff might not reach a consensus as to what the program is trying to do. The researcher can either work collaboratively with the staff to define the program's goals or formulate goals unilaterally and present them to the staff. In either case, a consensus must be reached. If the views of the staff are extremely diverse, a preliminary exploratory study can be undertaken to describe what the various components of the program are doing; content analysis can then be used to formulate specific objectives for the program.

Once the goals are defined, the investigator must decide which of them to use for evaluation. A priority model can be used to determine which objectives are critical to the program and which are secondary. Although secondary objectives may be easier to measure, the evaluative researcher must first attempt to study the vital goals of the project and not be distracted by interesting but minor concerns. Once the vital goals are identified, some measurable indicators of success must be developed. These outcome criteria will be critically important to the success of the evaluation.

The major concern with evaluative designs is internal validity. We have already discussed how the assignment of study participants to treatment and control groups can compromise internal validity. Just as important, however, are problems with external validity. These concerns arise because the design does not require random sampling of participants, thus creating a potential for selection bias. Sample selection in evaluative research is much more likely to be purposive than random; therefore, the researcher is faced with accounting for possible bias introduced in the selection process. One possible source of bias is self-selection (Bernstein, 1976). Many health care programs are available to the public on a self-selection basis. In this case, the target population must be defined as those who choose to participate in the program. For example, the success of a health screening program designed to identify persons at risk for heart disease and refer them for preventive care cannot be generalized to the entire population of potential heart disease patients. Even if the persons at risk were randomly assigned to different treatment programs, the relative effectiveness of each treatment could be generalized only to those persons who sought health screening. It is tempting to plan programs for the whole population based on the results of evaluation studies, particularly when the demonstrated effects are tremendously successful. However, one cannot assume that persons who voluntarily seek health care from a particular program are indeed representative of the population at large. Only random sampling from the larger population will produce truly generalizable results, but replication of the study with different groups will increase our confidence in the results.

When selecting a program to evaluate, the researcher will frequently choose the one thought to be producing the best results. Similarly, to demonstrate that a program is ineffective, a poorly operated program might be chosen. In this way, the likelihood of obtaining usable results is enhanced. However, this process introduces selection bias. When an exceptionally good program is chosen, the results resemble those of an experimental design in that the researcher has maximized internal validity by eliminating many potential sources of error that might occur in programs less well operated. However, the ability to generalize the positive outcome to other such programs may be limited. This limitation must be recognized when presenting the results. Table 5.1, from Patton (1980), provides an excellent reference for the various types of sampling used in evaluation studies and the key issues accompanying each type.

DATA ANALYSIS

Data analysis has received considerable attention in evaluation studies that use nonexperimental and quasi-experimental designs. Criticism of these designs usually revolves around internal validity (Alwin & Sullivan, 1976). Because randomization is not feasible in most cases, the possibility always exists that the experimental and control groups were not equivalent prior to the start of the program and that these differences have seriously affected the dependent variable.

In designs that incorporate at least one "experimental" group and one control group, an analysis of variance (ANOVA) would normally be used to look for significant differences among the groups. However, because the absence of equivalence among groups in evaluative designs compromises internal validity, ANOVA will not give an accurate picture of those differences. Alwin and Sullivan (1976) recommend that a special form of regression analysis be used to identify pretreatment differences on variables known to be relevant causes of the major outcome measure for the program. When significant pretreatment differences on any of these variables are found, a covariance analysis can hold constant the effects of one or more significant covariates so that the effect of the program on the outcome criterion can be estimated.

When qualitative data have been collected as part of the design, content analysis will be required as part of the analytic process. When performing content analysis on data from control and experimental participant, the researcher should take care that the analysis is done without knowledge of which participants were in the control and which were in the experimental group. The groups can then be compared on

Table 5.1 Sampling Issues in Evaluative Designs

Type	*Purpose*
Random sampling	Avoids systematic bias in the sample; large sample size important for making generalizations
Simple random sample	Achieve a representative sample that permits generalizations to the whole population
Stratified random cluster samples	Increase confidence in making generalizations to particular subgroups or areas
Purposeful sampling	Increase utility of information obtained in small samples; sampling criteria based on the reputation of programs among key decision makers and/or on previous data collected from programs
Sampling extreme or deviant cases	Provide decision makers with information about unusual cases that may be particularly troublesome or enlightening (e.g., outstanding successes/notable failures, programs with long waiting lists vs. programs with recruitment problems, unusually high morale and low morale problems, etc.)
Sampling typical cases	Avoid studying a program for which the results would be dismissed outright because *that* program is known to be special, deviant, unusual, extreme, etc.
Maximum variation sampling—picking three or four cases that represent a range on some dimension (e.g., size, location, budget)	Increase confidence in common patterns that cut across different programs; document unique program variations that have emerged in adapting to different conditions
Sampling critical cases	Permits *logical* generalization and maximum application of information to other cases because if it's true in this one case, it's likely to be true of all other cases
Sampling politically important or sensitive cases	Attracts attention to the study (or avoids attracting undesired attention by purposefully eliminating from the sample politically sensitive cases)
Convenience sampling—take the easy cases	Saves time, money, and effort

SOURCE: Patton (1980). *Qualitative Evaluation Methods.* Beverly Hills, CA: Sage.

the categorizations that were found in the data, in addition to any statistical analysis that has been done.

RELIABILITY AND VALIDITY

Because measurement error jeopardizes both internal and external validity and these two concepts are already compromised in an evaluative design, it becomes critical that the instruments be well-designed and highly reliable so that validity can be maximized. It follows, therefore, that the key objectives of the program must be stated in measurable terms and that the outcome criteria must be easily quantifiable. This is not always easily achieved in evaluative research, because some of the objectives may be vague and difficult to quantify. In this case, employing multiple means of assessment will strengthen the design. The collection of qualitative data can strengthen (or weaken) confidence in the validity of the instruments by providing the perspective of the participants without the restriction of any particular point of view.

ETHICAL ISSUES

The issues surrounding the rights of human subjects in evaluative designs are similar to those involved with experimental designs. The ethical treatment of control groups is of concern, especially when a control group may be randomly selected from among program participants. In this case, informed consent must be obtained from the control participants, and they must be given the opportunity to benefit from the program itself once the data are collected.

Informed consent, in particular free informed consent, is the key issue for all participants in evaluative studies. Usually, the experimental participants have voluntarily sought out the program and have not been recruited by the researcher. They have volunteered for an action program, not for a research project. In funded demonstration projects, however, all program applicants are commonly required to take part in the evaluation study. This can be construed as a form of coercion. Because public money funds these programs, it is generally deemed acceptable for individuals to be asked to participate in the evaluation as their contribution to the public good. Participation may thus be viewed as a form of payment for the benefit they will receive from the program. Nevertheless, participants must clearly understand that they will be research participants as well as program participants, and their rights to confidentiality and anonymity must be protected. In this area, evaluation research differs appreciably from other types of research because the primary emphasis is on the program rather than the research.

RESEARCH PROPOSAL

In many instances, the evaluative design will be part of the program proposal, particularly when the proposal is submitted to a public agency for funding. There may be times, however, when evaluation is planned after a program is well established. Sometimes an evaluation study may be planned to look at only a small portion of the overall program. In these cases, the proposal will be written specifically as a research proposal.

CRITIQUE

When critiquing an evaluation study, internal and external validity must be closely examined. How well the control group was established, whether random assignment was possible, and if not, how much control was achieved over the action of the independent variable are areas of concern. The internal validity of the study will rest on these factors.

External validity may be more difficult to assess. Because the program participants are volunteers, it is seldom possible to resolve the external validity issue. The unknown unique characteristics of a volunteer population are always a limiting factor in evaluative studies. Although this problem exists in experimental designs as well, it is not of equal concern, because the major purpose of an experiment is to test theory, not to provide generalizable results. An evaluative study, on the other hand, should provide usable information about the overall effect of the program. Frequently, the results will affect public policy. External validity, therefore, is much more important in this design than it is in experimental designs. Because evaluation studies rarely involve random selection, external validity must be achieved through replication. Bernstein (1976) believes that multiple replications from different populations greatly increase confidence in the results of evaluation studies. From individual studies, however, results must be interpreted with great caution.

REFERENCES

Alwin, D. F., & Sullivan, M. J. (1976). Issues of design and analysis in evaluation research. In I. N. Bernstein (Ed.), *Validity issues in evaluative research.* Beverly Hills, CA: Sage.

Bernstein, I. N. (Ed.). (1976). *Validity issues in evaluative research.* Beverly Hills, CA: Sage.

Borg, W. R., & Gall, M. D. (1983). *Educational research.* New York: Longman.

Boruch, R. F., & Wortman, P. M. (1979). Implications of educational evaluation for evaluation policy. In D. C. Berliner (Ed.), *Review of research in education* (Vol. 7, pp. 309-361). Washington, DC: American Educational Research Association.

Cain, G. G., & Hollister, R. G. (1972). The methodology of evaluating social action programs. In P. H. Rossi & W. Williams (Eds.), *Evaluating social programs.* New York: Seminar.

Dela Cruz, F., Jacobs, A., & Wood, M. J. (1986). The educational needs of home health nurses. *Journal of Home Health Nursing, 4*(3), 11-17.

Martinson, I. M., Moldow, D. G., Armstrong, G. D., Henry, W. F., Nesbit, M. E., & Kersey, J. H. (1986). Home care for children dying of cancer. *Research in Nursing and Health, 9*(1), 11-16.

Patton, M. C. (1980). *Qualitative evaluation methods.* Beverly Hills, CA: Sage.

Thurston, N. E., & Dundas, J. B. (1985). Evaluation of an early postpartum discharge program. *Canadian Journal of Public Health, 76*(6), 384-387.

PART III

SURVEY DESIGNS

All survey designs specify the relationship of two or more variables without any experimental manipulation of the independent variable. These designs do not control the independent variable and therefore do not have sufficient *internal validity* to support a cause-and-effect relationship. The strength of these designs lies in their *external validity*. They provide the means of examining variables within random samples of target populations and of drawing conclusions about the target populations from the sample data. Because no manipulation of variables occurs in these designs, they provide information about naturally occurring phenomena in a way that is not possible in experimental designs. Survey designs always incorporate statistical analysis of the relationships between and among variables to draw conclusions from the data.

In the case of the comparative survey, the dependent variable is measured and compared across groups, whereas the independent variable is simply observed as it occurs naturally in the population. The comparative design is theory based, as is the experimental design, and research findings derived through this design can be used to strengthen theory. Because, however, the design does not allow the independent variable to be manipulated, it cannot be used to test theory directly.

139

Even when the most sophisticated statistical analysis is applied to data and used to test a predictive hypothesis, the lack of investigator control over the independent variable limits internal validity. The question to be answered using the comparative design is different from that of the experimental design: What are the differences between groups when the groups represent different positions of the independent variable, and why does this difference result? A theoretical framework is used to predict cause and effect, although both the independent and dependent variables are observed as they occur naturally in the environment without investigator interference. These studies are frequently considered preliminary to the experimental design, as a beginning test of theory prior to actual experimentation.

The comparative design is the design of choice when it is either unethical or impossible to manipulate the independent variable. Studies comparing ethnic groups, age cohorts, and people with particular pathologies are all necessarily comparative rather than experimental. In a comparative design, however, such variables must be proposed as independent causative variables with predictive directional hypotheses of the anticipated results. Again, the significant difference between the comparative and experimental design is that in the comparative design the independent variable is *not* manipulated by the researcher.

In the correlational survey, two or more variables are measured as they exist in the population and their relationship is analyzed. Even when one of the variables is known to occur first in time, its effect on the dependent variable may not be predicted with any certainty. The initial question asked is, What is the relationship between or among these variables? The answer is a statistical description of the relationships. The design is supported by a conceptual framework. Although correlational surveys vary greatly in the strength of the framework, they must include potential explanations for the possible relationships between the variables. These explanations are derived from previous exploratory or descriptive studies or from theoretical propositions.

The comparative survey design exerts less control over the independent variable than does the quasi-experimental design but more control than does the correlational survey. The correlational design is frequently used when there is limited knowledge of which variables in the design are independent and which are dependent, whereas in the comparative design the independent variable is used as the basis for formulating the groups. For both types of survey designs, the critical issue is external validity, and for maximum effectiveness, both require large, representative samples of the population. Accuracy of measurement is also critical, with measurement assumed to be primarily at the numeric level. Both designs are inherently descriptive and not directly theory testing, although both have been used by researchers to test and to generate theory.

Structural equation modeling is a useful way to test theory using known or available data sets. The value of this method of examining data is in its computer manipulation. The theory is developed by the researcher or borrowed from another theorist, and a model of the relationship of the variables to one another, as described by the theory, is constructed. The direction of the relationship of each variable to specified other variables is predicted and added to the model. Data are not examined using a computer program such as LISREL until the entire model is constructed. Pamela Ratner, Joan Bottorff, and Joy Johnson examine the validity of the theory in whole and in part in Chapter 8.

We have been intrigued for a very long time with the idea that epidemiologic methods and procedures are natural and appropriate for nursing research. For this reason, we have given special attention to the design by giving it a chapter of its own by Janet Meininger.

Almost every researcher, at one time or another, has felt frustrated by the lack of instrumentation available for specific study purposes and has, as a result, designed a new instrument. Most of these data collection devices have little more than face validity and are tested for reliability within the context of the study itself, if at all, giving little credence to the findings and, often, ruining a perfectly good study (Osguthorpe, Roper, & Saunders, 1983; Risser, Strong, & Bither, 1980). For this reason, the chapter on methodological research has been provided by Merle Mishel to demonstrate how to develop research instruments that are both reliable and valid for the study. It is not a hit-or-miss affair or a "one-shot trial and error"; methodological research is serious business.

REFERENCES

Osguthorpe, N., Roper, J., & Saunders, J. (1983). The effect of teaching on medication knowledge. *Western Journal of Nursing Research, 5*(3), 205-216.
Risser, N. L., Strong, A., & Bither, S. (1980). Postoperative ventilatory function: A self-critique. *Western Journal of Nursing Research, 2*(2), 484-500.

6

Comparative Designs

MARILYNN J. WOOD
PAMELA J. BRINK

The range of designs that examine the relationships between variables as they exist, without attempting to change or manipulate them, provides the backbone of social science research. These designs are a vital part of the establishment of causal relationships and are used to define and describe the relationships between concepts and variables. Comparative designs can provide strong support for causal relationships without manipulation of the independent variable. This chapter focuses on a special comparative design in which the groups are chosen because they represent different positions of an independent variable that we are interested in testing. We recognize that there are a variety of "comparative" designs that do not meet the specifications set forth in this chapter, but we feel strongly that the design described here can be used as a model, and that other comparative designs can be evaluated according to how well they meet these criteria.

The *comparative survey design* is used instead of an experimental design when the theory base for the study meets the criteria for an experimental design (i.e., hypotheses could be tested), but for some reason the investigator cannot manipulate the independent variable and therefore cannot do an experiment. To use this design, it must be possible to find already-existing groups that differ on the independent variable. The action of the dependent variable can be predicted from the theoretical framework. Supposing we are interested in the effect of the social support received from a spouse on the response of cognitively impaired adults to a structured living program. The independent variable (spousal support) cannot be manipulated, it can merely be observed as present or absent or measured in some other sense as strong or weak, positive or negative. It is not possible, therefore, to choose one of the experimental designs, even though there is a strong theoretical framework that can be used to support the study. A comparative design could be used if we could identify two or more groups of cognitively impaired adults in the population who differ on the degree of spousal support they have but who are similar in other characteristics. We can then measure the relevant dependent variables that are indicators of the participants' responses to the structured living program. This design allows theory testing without manipulation of the independent variable, but as is the case with quasi-experiments, the investigator must address the possible threats to internal validity that are likely to arise when there is no random assignment to groups (see Chapter 4).

Two basic situations arise in which the independent variable cannot be deliberately manipulated: (a) when an ethically unacceptable outcome would result from the manipulation, such as creating a toxic condition in the study participants, or (b) when the variable is a trait or characteristic of the participant that cannot be changed, such as age, ethnicity, or place of birth. In these instances, a comparative survey design allows the researcher to look at the effects of an independent variable on a dependent variable without direct intervention or manipulation of the independent variable.

The comparative design is primarily used in field studies. Observations are made in naturalistic environments rather than in controlled laboratory settings to observe cause-and-effect relationships without manipulation or other interference. The design, however, can also be used as a field test prior to the development of an experiment.

BASIC OR CLASSICAL DESIGN

This is a two-group (treatment and contrast) design, similar to the basic experimental design, except that the two groups already exist.

The treatment group has the independent variable and the contrast group does not. A posttest measures only the dependent variable(s), which should yield interval- or ratio-level data. The study will usually be prospective, because the sample is selected based on the independent variable. Two features of this design are critical. First, because random assignment is not possible, the groups must be comparable on the major extraneous variables, ideally differing only in the independent variable. In addition, because the design allows the researcher to predict the effect of the independent variable on the dependent variable, it is essential to have a theoretical framework that explains the cause-and-effect relationship between these variables. The classic example of this design can be found in the studies on smoking and lung cancer. As early as 1950, correlational designs established an association between these two variables. Since that time, many comparative studies have been done using smokers and nonsmokers. In some studies, smokers have been divided into groups based on sex, age, and smoking patterns, such as duration of smoking and number of cigarettes smoked per day (the independent variables). The dependent variable was onset of lung cancer. More recent research has considered the work environment of the smoker as a possible independent variable to determine whether there are certain other persistent daily factors that contribute to the onset and type of lung cancer (U.S. Department of Health and Human Services [DHHS], 1982).

Variations on the Basic Design

Many variations on the basic comparative design can be found. Comparative designs can use multiple groups differentiated on the independent variable. For instance, several types of nurse management systems can be compared on one or more patient outcome measures. Comparative designs can use time-series measurements of the dependent variable. If the study uses available data, such as a chart review, time-series measurements (multiple measures of the dependent variable over time) can occur both before and after the occurrence of the independent variable. Comparative studies can be retrospective if the sample is chosen on the basis of the dependent variable rather than the independent variable. Some studies of smoking and lung cancer are currently being conducted as retrospective studies, with the three types of lung cancer, as ascertained by microscopic examination, being traced back (retrospectively) to amount and type of smoking, age of smoking onset, sex, and work environment (U.S. DHHS, 1982).

Basic Assumptions of Comparative Designs

The following are the assumptions implicit in comparative designs:

1. One can build support for cause and effect without the manipulation of the independent variable.
2. There is enough knowledge about the variable(s) to develop predictive hypotheses based on theory and prior research.
3. One can establish comparable groups using sampling methodology.
4. External validity can be achieved by using a sample that is representative of the population.
5. Measurement of the dependent variable will be accurate.
6. Sampling and data analysis methods will control for extraneous variables so that the difference(s) between or among groups on the dependent variable can be identified.

CONTROL OVER DATA

The data in comparative designs are controlled through sample selection methods, by the conditions under which the independent and dependent variables are measured, and by the statistical techniques used to analyze the data. There is no manipulation of the independent variable because it has already occurred; therefore, the action of the independent variable is observed rather than controlled. Instead, the independent variable is controlled through sample selection. The investigator selects the sample so that it is possible to discriminate between and among groups on the basis of the presence, absence, or amount of the independent variable. All relevant extraneous variables are measured so that their effect on the dependent variable can be estimated.

SAMPLES

A large simple random sample of the population is the ideal and should provide a representative sample from which comparison groups can be formulated unless one or more of the subgroups is expected to be proportionately small. In these cases, stratified random samples are the ideal and are used whenever population parameters are known. The sample is stratified on the independent variable by examining the available population (frequently through census records). The strata are developed and the percentage of the population within each stratum is noted. The sample can have the same proportions as the population, but at times it may be advisable to have equal numbers from each stratum.

Sample Size

The required sample size should be calculated using power analysis, to reduce the possibility of Type II error. It would be futile to carry out a comparative design without ensuring that the sample size is large enough to detect the anticipated effect on the dependent variable. Many published nursing studies have insufficient power to detect real effects because of small sample sizes (Polit & Sherman, 1989). Often, because of the availability of small clinical populations in a given location and the difficulty of organizing multisite studies, nursing studies are based on small sample sizes. As Polit and Sherman note, unless the dependent variables in these studies are those for which a large effect size can be expected, the studies are likely to be underpowered.

For a comparative survey design, the sample size should be planned to achieve a power of .8 for the expected effect size (Cohen, 1988) and would probably be based on either the t-test tables or the analysis of variance (ANOVA) tables, depending on the number of groups being compared. Using Cohen's t-test tables for a one-tail test and a significance level of .05, the sample size required to detect a medium effect size is 50 subjects. This number reduces to 20 for a large effect size and increases to 310 for a small effect size (Cohen, 1988, p. 54). Using fewer subjects than the number required to produce power of .8 increases the likelihood of a Type II error and of failing to reject a null hypothesis that is actually true, which means increasing the likelihood of finding nonsignificant results when a larger sample could produce significant results. The futility of this approach is obvious and brings home the need to seriously address sample size when planning any study, but particularly one in which hypotheses will be tested.

Sample Variations

When the total available population is small, or when the population parameters are unknown, quota samples may be drawn based on the independent variable. These quota samples may sometimes be proportionate to the total population, or sometimes groups of equal size are used. Another sample variation is seen in the use of convenience samples that can be found to exist representing the various positions of the independent variable. For example, in a study of stress in ICU versus non-ICU nurses, the staff of the intensive care units was compared to the staff of general medical-surgical units to see if there was a significant difference in their levels of stress (Keane, Ducette, & Adler, 1985). Comparative designs may also be used to compare total populations to similar total populations. This is common in anthropological research, in which individual populations are studied independently using the single-case descriptive design. The available data obtained through ethnography are then used for secondary analysis in a comparative design. On the assumption that the comparative analysis of single cases builds anthropological theory about human groups, the Human Relations Area Files (HRAF) were developed at Harvard for the sole purpose of providing a database to use in comparing anthropological studies of culture groups. Because human groups cannot be manipulated easily (or, perhaps, ethically), the HRAF provide a needed data set for comparative analysis. Major universities throughout the United States have either complete or partial HRAF in the original paper format or on microfiche.

Another variation on sample selection involves drawing the random sample from two different populations, such as the runners and nonrunners used in the Walsh (1985) study reported below. Although the samples represented their respective populations (runners and students), they did not constitute a representative sample of the desired target population, and the results must therefore be viewed with caution.

The issues that need to be addressed in sample selection procedures are that the sample is representative of the population and that the comparison groups are equivalent on all relevant variables except the independent variable.

METHODS OF DATA COLLECTION

Any method of data collection is acceptable: observation, interview, questionnaire, projective tests, physiological tests, available data. The type of measurement will vary according to the questions asked, the hypotheses being tested, and the situation within which the study is to be conducted. The reliability and validity of the instruments are critical in this design because validity of the results will depend on accurate discrimination among groups. The best or preferred type of measurement is quantitative, using interval and ratio scales to use parametric statistics. Nominal and ordinal scales are used frequently and are quite acceptable so long as they are numerical rather than qualitative.

Possible sources of error in data collection procedures include the possibility of acquiescent response set in interviews, response bias in both interviews and questionnaires, and the Hawthorne effect among participants in comparative studies. Inaccurate transcription of data onto data collection forms or misinterpretation of meaning in written documentation are also possible sources of error in this design, as in all research.

RELIABILITY AND VALIDITY OF MEASUREMENT

In comparative studies, as with experimental designs, the critical issue is determining whether or not the groups differ with regard to the dependent variable. The accuracy of the measurement technique, therefore, becomes paramount. All measurement tools must have at least content validity—that is, they must be based on the known literature on the topic. However, the quality of the study really depends on the quality of measurement, and therefore the use of well-tested instruments is recommended. Because this level of research is built on theory and the findings of previous studies, it is not advisable to proceed without well-developed instruments. The subsequent results would not reflect the desired results in terms of hypothesis testing. The researcher must be able to rely on the measurement tool to measure the dependent variable accurately. Therefore, norm-referenced or criterion-referenced validity of measurement tools is extremely important. Reliability of the instruments must be estimated for the study population. Remember that reliability estimates are not a stable property of an instrument but are specific to the use of that instrument with a particular population under specific measurement conditions (Cronbach, 1970; Lynn, 1985; Nunnally, 1978).

DATA ANALYSIS

The basic question asked by this design is, What are the differences between/among groups on the dependent variable? Assuming probability sampling techniques and interval/ratio levels of measurement, the test of choice in a two group design is the t test. The t test compares the means of two groups and examines the probability of getting this magnitude of difference by chance alone. It is particularly useful in designs requiring the comparison of two groups.

If there are multiple groups based on a categorical independent variable, the quantitative measures of the dependent variable, a one-way ANOVA is appropriate. ANOVA tells us whether the group means differ from one another. It assumes that the independent variable is at the nominal level. A "one-way" ANOVA indicates that there is only one independent variable. (ANOVA can also be used with multiple independent variables.) The dependent variable is assumed to be measured on an interval or ratio scale.

Quite commonly in comparative surveys, however, the comparative groups will be based on a quantitative independent variable, such as level of income or preoperative stress level, and a quantitative dependent variable that may or may not be measured at the interval level. In these cases, the appropriate test will be regression analysis (see Chapter 7 for further discussion of this technique).

Covariance analysis is a useful procedure in comparative as well as experimental designs for statistically removing differences among the comparison groups when they are not equivalent on significant extraneous variables. Through the use of this technique, a statistical control can sometimes be provided for extraneous variables when direct control through experimental design is impossible. The error variance is reduced by controlling for variation in the dependent measure that comes from separate measurable variables that influence all the groupings being compared (Munro, Visintainer, & Page, 1986, p. 218). Analysis of covariance (ANCOVA) is a special case of the linear model. Regression analysis is usually used in survey designs, and ANOVA is used in experimental designs. Wildt and Ahtola (1978) explain ANCOVA as a combination of these two techniques. Therefore, an understanding of these two techniques is expected when discussing covariance. The usual problem in comparative surveys comes when the investigator is interested in the effect of an independent variable, either quantitative or categorical, on a quantitative dependent variable, but one or more "nuisance" variables (covariates) are influencing the dependent variable in a linear fashion. Covariance analysis first removes the effects of the covariates and then examines the relationship between the independent and dependent variable. As with ANOVA, it is assumed that the independent variable is nominal, the dependent variable is continuous, and the covariates are measured at the interval or ratio level. It is also assumed that a covariate has a linear relationship with the dependent variable. If this assumption is violated, the results will be of little value.

Take, for example, a study examining the differences between two techniques of pain management used in two different clinical areas. In a comparative design, the two techniques and their effect on the level of pain perceived by the recipients would be observed as they occur, because no manipulation of treatments would be controlled by the researcher. In this case, individual differences in the participants might influence their responses to the treatment. These differences are then identified as age and prior experience with surgery. By measuring age and prior experience, and treating them as covariates, the researcher is able to adjust for the differences in the participants' level of perceived pain that might be related to these two nuisance variables, thus providing a more accurate assessment of the effect of the two treatments. This approach would remove any bias that might occur because the two groups were not matched on these variables.

CRITIQUE

The first step in critiquing a comparative study is to evaluate whether it sets out to study "differences between and among groups." The next critical step is to determine whether the sample selection technique meets the basic assumptions of the design. A third consideration is the accuracy of the measurement techniques: To what extent are the issues of reliability and validity addressed? Fourth, one must judge whether the data analysis is appropriate to the question asked. Are the limitations of the design recognized? Finally, one must consider whether the findings are interpreted in light of the question asked and in terms of the limitations.

Another important issue in the critique of comparative designs is that of sources of error that might have come from data collection, sample selection, or choice of statistical test, as well as from transcription and coding of data. Each of these sources of error will affect the outcome of the study. The answer to the question, What are the differences between (or among) the groups (or measurements)? should have been accurately predicted by the theoretical framework. If the answer to the question does not support the predictive hypotheses, one should look first for weaknesses in the theory, then for decision errors in sampling, methods, and analysis of data. If the results do support the predictive hypotheses, the author's interpretation of the findings in light of the theoretical framework should be examined. This design cannot be expected to have strong internal validity, and therefore the interpretation of the findings should reflect this limitation.

ETHICAL ISSUES

A major concern with comparative designs is the protection of the anonymity of the groups used for comparisons. Identifying data must be obscured in the final report. When using total populations, each member of the total population must be given the right to refuse to participate even though replacement is not possible in this instance. Another issue that can arise in comparative designs comes from the possibility of serious weaknesses in the design that might negate any findings. In this case, it may be unethical to ask people to participate when there is no possibility of the study's producing valid results.

Finally, if the study examines a sensitive topic, participants may need assistance in coping with the findings. If this is the case, participants should be informed of resources for follow-up support.

EXAMPLES FROM THE LITERATURE

Laffrey (1986) examined perceived weight, perceived health status, health conception, and health behavior choices in normal-weight and overweight adults. Three research questions were addressed:

1. Do perceived weight, perceived health status, health conception, and health behavior choice differ between normal-weight and overweight adults?
2. What are the relationships between perceived health status, health conception, and health behavior choice in normal-weight adults?
3. What are the relationships between perceived health status, health conception, and health behavior choice in overweight adults?

A random sample of 59 households in a midwestern suburban community produced 33 normal-weight and 26 overweight adults (25 men and 34 women). All participants were white and had been born in the United States; ages ranged from 19 to 66 (mean age was 39 for normal weights, 43 for overweights). All overweights were at least 10% to 20% over the normal weight for their height (two were over 20% above normal weight). Education ranged from 5 to 18 years of school (mean 13.5 for normoweights and 13.7 for overweights). The two groups were similar on marital status and reported religious preference. Family income was lower in the normal weight group ($29,000 versus $35,000 for the overweight group).

Perceived weight was measured by asking the participants to rate themselves as underweight, normal, or overweight. This response was validated by also asking them to compare themselves with others of their gender and age on a 3-point scale: weight less than others, weight same as others, or weight more than others. Perceived health status (PHS) was measured using a Cantril ladder, ranging from 1 (*worst health I can imagine*) to 10 (*best health I can imagine*).

Health conception measure (HCM) was a 16-item tool developed for this study. Content validity and a test-retest reliability coefficient of .76

after 1 week were reported. The health behavior choice scale (HBCS) was a 15-item tool to measure the reasons an individual chooses to engage in five health behaviors. Content validity and test-retest reliability coefficient of .93 were reported for this tool.

Body weight was measured using a GE portable digital scale. Participants were asked their height without shoes and were measured if unsure. Weight-height ratios were compared with the norms of the Michigan Department of Public Health to establish normoweight versus overweight groups.

A t-test analysis of the differences between group means demonstrated no significant differences between the two groups on perceived health status, health conception, or health behavior choice. In addition, health conception and health behavior choice were significantly correlated in both groups. The relationship between perceived health status and health conception was positive and significant only in the normoweight group. No other significant relationships were found.

There are two major problems with this study: the weakness of the conceptual framework and the sample size. The author did not distinguish between "overweight" and "obesity" as health hazards, yet the literature states that between 50% and 100% over "normal" weight to height ratios is required before there is any significant difference in health hazard. Therefore, individuals between 10% and 20% overweight are not "at risk" in the epidemiological sense. The prediction that individuals not at risk would perceive themselves to be at risk was somewhat weak. Second, the size of the "overweight" group (26 individuals, with only 2 over 20% overweight) was simply too small to make any predictions about overweight or "obese" participants. Finally, the literature is very clear that American women generally tend to perceive themselves as overweight even when they are of normal weight, so perceived weight for women will be skewed in that direction, regardless of actual weight. The author is to be commended for attempting a random sample, but some populations are so difficult to find that random samples of small populations (59 households) will not yield a sample size sufficient for valid inference. The two groups in the sample were, however, equivalent in origin if not in size. The findings support the weakness in the conceptual framework and in the sample size.

In a study exemplifying an alternative comparative design, Walsh (1985) examined the differences between runners and nonrunners in terms of specific health beliefs. A sample of 150 runners, drawn at random from the membership of a running club, was compared to 150 students randomly chosen from university enrollment. This study demonstrates an alternative to the basic comparative design in the use of a nonequivalent comparison group. In many instances when the design is not an experimental one, it is very difficult to find an equivalent comparison group. Unless another sport is used instead of running, such as tennis or aerobics, it may be impossible to find a comparison group. Because the use of another sport might have confounded the results, these authors elected to draw a random sample of an available population (college students) for comparison. When a comparison group is created in this manner, a complete description of both groups is essential to make assessment of the validity of the design possible.

A total of 140 usable questionnaires were returned (46.7%). In the sample, runners tended to be older, with proportionately more males, more marrieds, and higher household incomes than nonrunners. Of the runners, 53% ran every day and 40% ran more than 50 miles a week.

Responses to the Rokeach Health Value Scale (adapted by Wallston) and the Walsh Health Behaviors Questionnaire were analyzed for the 140 participants. In addition, runners were asked to complete a third questionnaire describing their involvement in running. The two-sample *t* test for independent groups was used to analyze the data. Findings revealed that runners placed significantly more value on personal health than did nonrunners. In addition, health behaviors differed significantly between the two groups, with runners performing more health-related behaviors than nonrunners in the areas of nutrition, exercise, medical awareness, and self-care.

This study demonstrates an alternative to the basic comparative design in the use of a nonequivalent comparison group. In this case, the author was unable to find a comparison group from within the original group and therefore had to seek a comparison group from an entirely different source. This situation is not unusual in comparative studies. A comparison group could have been found from within another sporting group, but the use of another sport may have confounded the results. To minimize bias, the author drew random samples from two totally different populations: college students and a running club. The size of the two samples was held constant. To allow for assessment of the validity of the design, complete descriptions of both groups were provided.

Flaskerud (1984) compared perceptions of problematic behavior among six minority groups and mental health professionals. The theoretical framework for this study was based on culture. The three components of culture were identified as technology, social structures, and ideology or belief system. The author used this framework to predict the differing responses of the minority groups and the mental health professionals about behavior that could be considered to represent mental illness.

A structured interview format was used with all respondents. Twelve nurse investigators in different parts of the country sampled and interviewed each of the minority and professional groups.

The sample of 227 (68 mental health professionals and 159 minority group members) was selected by convenience. All were 18 years of age or over. The mental health professionals included psychiatrists, psychologists, psychiatric social workers, and psychiatric nurses. There were six minority groups represented: Appalachian, black, Native American, Chinese, Filipino, and Mexican American.

The structured interview schedule had two parts: biographical data and vignettes concerning a person experiencing problems. For each vignette, the participant was asked the following: (a) What do you think of this person's behavior? (b) Do you think anything should be done about it? (c) If so, what? Validity and reliability of the instrument were reported. Responses were dichotomized into mental illness/no mental illness and into psychiatric treatment/no psychiatric treatment. A combined score was derived for each participant on the 10 vignettes, and correlations between sample characteristics and response were examined. A stepwise multiple regression was done to determine the strongest predictor of response.

The results indicated significant differences between the two main groups of mental health professionals and minorities. In addition, minority group status proved to be the strongest predictor of both a mental illness and a psychiatric treatment response, explaining .69 and .72 of the variation, respectively.

This provides an excellent example of a comparative survey testing variables that cannot be examined through experimentation. The author provides a theoretical explanation of the relationship between the variables, although it is not a strong framework and does not result in the usual predictive hypotheses. The study hypotheses are global in nature and merely predict "a difference" between the two main groups. Literature is reviewed relating to each cultural group, but predictions are not made on the basis of cultural group within the general category of minorities. Nevertheless, this study provides an example of comparison based on cultural group, and it is well-designed.

SUITABLE NURSING PROBLEMS

Any study of nurses or patients in natural settings is amenable to the comparative design when the independent variable cannot be manipulated or when it is too early in the research protocol for an experiment. Studies of nursing interventions in natural settings on homogeneous patient populations or on specific inpatient units are an excellent use of this method. Other functional uses for this design include studies of nurse management outcomes in natural settings, patient chart reviews, and comparisons of patient population characteristics (ethnicity, education, geography) with particular health care outcomes.

Comparative designs are hypothesis-testing approaches developed to build support for theory. Because the researcher does not manipulate the independent variable, the major weakness of the design is that it does not control internal validity. Its major strengths are that it provides external validity and allows generalizations to be made, thus testing theory in the field setting where people live and work.

SUMMARY OF THIS DESIGN

In writing a research proposal for this design, the most important issues are related to the basic assumptions underlying the design: (a) The independent variable is not manipulable at this time, if ever; (b) probability sampling techniques are based on the independent variable, (c) level of measurement of the dependent variable, and (d) the reliability and validity of the instrument(s). (See Chapter 10, on methodological research.)

To summarize, the essential features of this design are as follows:

1. Theoretical framework and predictive hypotheses
2. Representative (probability) sample
3. Accurate measurement of variables
4. Data analysis appropriate to the level of measurement and sample that answers the question, What are the differences between and among the groups?

Any compromise of these basic assumptions constitutes a limitation of the study.

REFERENCES

Cohen, J. (1988). *Statistical power for the behavioral sciences.* Hillsdale, NJ: Lawrence Erlbaum.

Cronbach, L. J. (1970). *Essentials of psychological testing* (3rd ed.). New York: Harper & Row.

Flaskerud, J. H. (1984). A comparison of perceptions of problematic behavior by six minority groups and mental health professionals. *Nursing Research, 33*(4), 190-197.

Keane, A., Ducette, J., & Adler, D. C. (1985). Stress in ICU and non-ICU nurses. *Nursing Research, 34*(4), 231-236.

Laffrey, S. C. (1986). Normal and overweight adults: Perceived weight and health behavior characteristics. *Nursing Research, 34*(3), 173-177.

Lynn, M. (1985). Reliability estimates: Use and disuse. *Nursing Research, 34*(4), 254-256.

Munro, B. H., Visintainer, M. A., & Page, E. B. (1986). *Statistical methods for health care research.* Philadelphia: J. B. Lippincott.

Nunnally, J. C. (1978). *Psychometric theory* (2nd ed.). New York: McGraw-Hill.

Polit, D. F., & Sherman, R. E. (1989). Statistical power in nursing research. *Nursing Research, 39*(6), 365-369.

U.S. Department of Health and Human Services. (1982). *The health consequences of smoking: A report of the surgeon general.* Rockville, MD: Public Health Service.

Walsh, V. R. (1985). Health beliefs and practices of runners versus nonrunners. *Nursing Research, 34*(6), 353-356.

Wildt, A. R., & Ahtola, O. T. (1978). *Analysis of covariance.* Beverly Hills, CA: Sage.

ADDITIONAL EXAMPLES OF STUDIES USING COMPARATIVE DESIGNS

Ferketich, S. L., & Mercer, R. T. (1995). Predictors of role competence for experienced and inexperienced fathers. *Nursing Research, 44*(2), 89-95.

Jones, E. G. (1995). Deaf and hearing parents' perceptions of family functioning. *Nursing Research, 44*(2), 102-105.

LaMontagne, L. L. (1987). Children's preoperative coping: Replication and extension. *Nursing Research, 36*(3), 163-167.

Mynatt, S. (1985). Empathy in faculty and students in different types of nursing preparation programs. *Western Journal of Nursing Research, 7*(3), 333-348.

Ouellette, M. D., MacVicar, M. G., & Harlan, J. (1986). Relationship between percent body fat and menstrual patterns in athletes and non-athletes. *Nursing Research, 35*(6), 330-333.

Reed, P. G. (1986). Developmental resources and depression in the elderly. *Nursing Research, 35*(6), 368-378.

Taylor, M. S., & Covaleski, M. A. (1985). Predicting nurses' turnover and internal transfer behavior. *Nursing Research, 34*(4), 237-241.

7

Correlational Designs

MARILYNN J. WOOD
PAMELA J. BRINK

The state of knowledge in many areas within nursing is at the point where the investigator needs to look for relationships between variables. These variables may have been identified in a number of ways. An exploratory study using a qualitative design may have produced a number of variables from a description of a particular patient population. Friesen (1988), for example, in a qualitative study of spouses of patients on home dialysis, identified four categories of spouses. Within these four categories, the variables that appeared to make the difference for the spouse were issues such as level of involvement, marital adjustment, career commitment, and age of children. Alternatively, variables may have come to light during a review of the literature on a particular topic. For example, in a review of disaster studies, Murphy (1987) reports a number of variables that have been suggested to be related to health status in disaster victims. Descriptive studies have also brought to light a number of variables that seem to be related to a given topic. For example, McCloskey and McCain (1988) identified a number of variables related to nurse performance in a study of newly hired nurses at a large midwestern hospital. Identification of variables and determination of their relevance in the study of particular concepts or populations leads to the need to establish more definitive relationships and patterns of relationships to begin to explain what is happening in the situation.

A correlational design is used when investigators have reason to suspect a relationship between variables and can support their suspicions through literature or previous research. These variables are known to exist in the population and a conceptual framework can be devised to provide justification for studying them. This design differs from the comparative survey because the framework does not usually have the substance of a theoretical explanation. It merely proposes, based on previous study of the concepts represented by the variables under study, possible connections between these concepts. The purpose of a correlational study is to describe the relationship between the variables rather than to test theory, but the results may provide support for a particular theoretical perspective, and there is a wide range of situations for which correlational studies are appropriate. These studies vary greatly in the strength of their theoretical bases. On the one hand, although a conceptual framework may be developed to explain possible associations between variables, sometimes the investigator is not sure which variables are independent and which are dependent and may also be unsure of the direction of the relationship. Even if a variable occurs first in time, the investigator may not know whether it directly influences the other variables, whether it is affected by the other variables, or whether any relationship exists at all. This design, therefore, might be used to explore cases in which certain variables have associations with one another, but the nature of the associations is unknown. In essence, such studies can be "fishing expeditions," although the researcher can always provide at least a tentative conceptual framework to support the examination of these particular variables in the population under study.

On the other hand, an investigator may have a fairly well-developed theoretical framework but may want to refine the precise relationships between a number of variables. For instance, Mishel and Braden (1987) attempted to delineate the impact of social support on uncertainty in women with gynecologic cancer, using a correlational design to determine the relationship among the variables. A model was proposed to predict psychosocial adjustment in the study participants. This study supported the model and the influence of social support and uncertainty on psychosocial adjustment. This design covers a wide range of theoretical perspectives, from tentative conceptual frameworks to well-developed theories. The commonality among these is that to progress further, they all require precise description of the relationships between variables.

Correlational designs make use of quantitative data collection methods and multivariate statistical techniques and may result in the development of causal models. Techniques such as factor analysis, causal modeling, canonical correlation analysis, path analysis, and residual analysis are designed to answer questions about the strength and direction of the relationships between groups of independent and dependent variables and to generate support for conceptual explanations of variable relationships (Asher, 1983; Berry, 1984; Ferketich & Verran, 1984; Levine, 1977; Thompson, 1984). Because of easy access to computer programs that aid data analysis, these techniques are readily available to researchers. The results are expected to support the development of theory to explain how concepts relate to one another. Correlational designs are at least one step beyond descriptive designs in that the investigator does not examine variables at random but, rather, looks at specific variables selected because of the conceptual framework.

There is no control over the independent variables in these designs. All variables are measured as they exist, with no manipulation. In this respect, the correlational design resembles the comparative survey. In the correlational survey, however, the investigator may scrutinize the relationships between several variables without knowing which variables are dependent until data analysis is complete and the results are known.

Complex questions—such as, What are the relationships between body mass index; location of surgery; number and type of previous surgeries; types of anesthesia; gender; intensity and duration of pain; and type, route, and amount of medication among general surgery adult patients?—are appropriately tested using a correlational design. Although gender and body mass index both occur first in time, there is no way to predict whether these variables relate in any way to pain perception or medication usage. Although there may be some literature to support the relationship between pain perception and effect of pain medication, there is no theoretical explanation for such a relationship.

In addition, the other variables must be assessed to determine whether they enter into the equation. This is a typical question leading to a multiple-variable correlational design.

As pointed out in Chapter 6, early research into the causes of lung cancer used correlational designs to look at broad questions such as, What are the relationships between onset of lung cancer, family history of lung cancer, environmental pollution, diet, smoking, and other personal health habits of U.S. citizens? The dependent variable was known to be lung cancer, so the search was for the independent, intervening, and extraneous variables. The correlational design was chosen to explore the relationships between these variables.

In some correlational research, the independent variable is thought to be known but evidence supporting exactly how it influences other variables is not available. For example, obesity is thought to create a number of different health problems, yet exactly what obesity causes is not really known. In some cases, obesity may actually be a result rather than a cause. Actuarial tables on which standards for weight by height have been established for the American population have been derived from individuals who carry life insurance. Yet height/weight standards alone without body mass indicators, muscle-to-fat ratios, ethnicity, amount or degree of obesity, age of onset of obesity, length of time the participant was obese, placement of adiposity, and age of participant may not be predictive of specific health problems. A correlational design would therefore be useful for finding other variables, in association with the independent variable, that might account for the variance found in participants with obesity.

BASIC ASSUMPTIONS UNDERLYING CORRELATIONAL DESIGNS

The following assumptions are implicit in the use of correlational designs:

1. The study variables have not been shown to covary in previous studies of similar populations.
2. A conceptual framework can be proposed to support the possibility of relationships between the variables.

3. There is no tested theory on which to predict the possible relationships between the variables.

4. The variables exist in the population and are amenable to study.

5. The sample is representative of the population.

6. There is no manipulation of variables; they are studied as they exist naturally.

BASIC OR CLASSICAL DESIGN

The classic correlational design includes all of the following:

■ A large random sample of the population is assembled.

■ A conceptual framework is proposed to explain potential relationships.

■ Research questions rather than hypotheses are posed regarding possible relationships between variables.

■ Cross-sectional data are collected on each variable from each participant.

■ Data are measured using tools designed to measure quantitative or numerical data.

■ Correlational analysis is used to examine the relationships between the variables.

It may be necessary to develop tools to measure some of the variables if no tools are available. In this case, a methodological study is combined with, or done prior to, the correlational survey to provide accurate measurement of the variables.

The best sample for a correlational study is a large random sample of the population. The same is a critical element in all designs, but in a correlational design, it is of utmost importance that the sample be representative. The whole idea of a correlational study is to determine whether changes in one variable correspond to changes in another variable. The relationships that emerge have no meaning if they cannot be generalized from the sample to a population. The representativeness of the sample, therefore, determines the value of a correlational design, and a large random sample is the best means of ensuring representativeness.

Another issue in the basic correlational design is the conceptual framework. It has already been noted that the investigator does not usually have a theoretical foundation to explain the relationships between the variables under study. However, it is important to develop a possible explanation for covariation between the variables to support the need for the study. It helps to place the study in perspective among other nursing studies and to justify asking people to participate. It is possible, for example, to consider seeking a correlation between the intellectual performance of elementary school children and the prenatal nutrition of their mothers. But unless a fairly strong case can be built for a direct relationship between these two variables that would still exist in school-age children despite all the intervening events since the prenatal state, it would not be worthwhile to ask mothers and children to invest time and energy providing data for the study. The relationship postulated in this example could be biological, or it could be psychosocial in nature. If no conceptual framework is provided, there is no indication of where this study might fit in the universe of nursing research, and thus the value of the study is questionable. Unless a conceptual framework can be developed, an exploratory descriptive study could handle this topic much more effectively by exploring *all* family variables in a group of elementary school children.

Because the conceptual framework for the correlational survey is usually one posed by the investigator and not one that has been tested in other studies, it makes better sense to summarize the framework in the form of questions rather than hypotheses for study. This supports the tentative nature of the framework and does not give it the appearance of unwarranted strength. The research questions can easily be converted to null hypotheses for statistical testing, without giving them the stature of predictive hypotheses. Predictive hypotheses, then, can be left for designs that actually test theory. Occasionally, a correlational design will be used to test theory when the investigator wishes to look at the interactions between multiple variables as part of theory development. In these cases, the design will be supported by a theoretical framework, and the study integrated into a series of studies planned for testing a particular theoretical perspective.

The data for this design must be primarily quantitative because of the necessity of statistically testing for significant relationships. In the basic design, the data are collected cross-sectionally. At one data collection period, the investigator measures all variables on all participants and then tests them statistically, looking for significant relationships. No attempt is made to manipulate any of the variables, but all are measured as they exist. One of the strengths of this design is its ability to look at the interactions between several variables at the same time and to see which of them vary together.

Common Variations in the Classical Design

In studies in which the researcher is unable to use a random sample, systematic sampling techniques or convenience samples may be used. Remember, this design will be judged on the representativeness of the sample. When nonprobability sampling is used, the researcher must provide detailed information about the sample to allow others to assess its representativeness. External validity in this case would come under question.

Time-series designs can be developed to look at changes in the variables over time. These can be done retrospectively or prospectively and are sometimes used to predict future events. Using this technique, variables such as changes in health care beliefs can be studied over generations. Ostrom (1978) has provided an in-depth discussion of regression analysis as it applies to time-series designs. This classic work is an excellent guide for designing a correlational study using a time-series approach, because the quality of the inferences drawn from the results will depend heavily on the researcher's having met the assumptions of the time-series analysis.

EXAMPLES FROM THE LITERATURE

Woods (1985) studied the relationship of socialization and stress to perimenstrual symptoms, disability, and menstrual attitudes. The researcher looked at perimenstrual symptoms (PS) as symptoms rather than disease, from the standpoint of illness behavior and understanding how people adapt to recurring, *cyclic* symptoms. The purpose of the study was to assess the extent to which a woman's environment and socialization influence her experiences of PS, related disability, and menstrual attitudes.

The study population resided in five neighborhoods in a southeastern U.S. city and consisted of women who were 18 to 35 years old, who were not pregnant, and who had not had hysterectomies. Of 241 potential subjects, 179 agreed to participate. The instruments used to measure the variables were as follows:

1. Moos Menstrual Distress Questionnaire (MDQ)
2. 42-item Schedule of Recent Events (SRE)
3. 16-item Index of Sex Role Orientation (ISRO)
4. Debilitation scale from the Menstrual Attitudes Questionnaire (MAQ)

Path analysis used a multiple regression procedure to test the relationships between stressful life events (STR), socialization (SOC), menstrual attitudes (DE), and disability (DI) for three groups of symptoms: negative affect (NA), pain (PN), and water retention (WR). Pain was first regressed on STR and SOC, then NA on STR and SOC, and WR on STR and SOC. Finally, DI on STR, SOC, PN, NA, and WR and DE on STR, SOC, PN, NA, WR, and DI were regressed. All predictor variables were entered into the equations simultaneously.

Simple correlations for all variables were reported. Stressful life events were positively related to negative affect, and nontraditional socialization was negatively related to debilitation scores. Women who scored high on one symptom scale tended to score high on others. Perimenstrual pain and NA were positively related to DI and DE scores; WR was unrelated to either.

A path model was developed among the concepts that indicated that socialization plays a minor role in explaining severity of perimenstrual symptoms, but traditional socialization was shown to be related to seeing menstruation as debilitating. The influence of a stressful social milieu was important for negative affect symptoms but had only a minor influence on water retention and pain symptoms. Of all symptom clusters, negative affect was most influential with respect to disability.

This report provides an excellent example of a correlational survey that results in the proposal of a causal model. The major assumptions of a correlational design are met. There is a well-developed conceptual framework, which is proposed as a theoretical model because of the relationships found in the study. The sample was randomly selected and should provide accurate representation of the population. Several variables were measured on each participant, and these are examined first to establish their correlations with each other, and then a path analysis model is used to examine the pattern of their relationships to each other as independent and dependent variables and to determine whether or not this pattern supports the conceptual framework. The author explains that a longitudinal study is currently under way to determine whether these causal models will be confirmed. The conceptual framework for this study was chosen from a large number of possibilities representing the immense variability in the research in the area of perimenstrual symptoms and the multitude of theoretical explanations from different fields of study.

In a different study, Majewski (1986) examined the relationship between the maternal role for woman and other roles they may occupy concurrently. This study was based on a conceptual framework derived from role and family development theories, in particular, the idea that role conflict may create a problem for women who occupy several roles—such as spouse and mother roles in addition to occupational roles. This concept was explored in relation to the developmental stage of expansion in which children are born and raised.

The sample consisted of 86 first-time mothers between 20 and 39 years old, currently married, living with spouse, and with a live first-born infant between 5 and 18 months of age. The sample was nonrandom, consisting of recruits from a variety of agencies and institutions.

Data from a semistructured interview were used to measure transition to the maternal role on a 7-item scale adapted from Blank and Mercer (TMRS). Role conflict was measured using a scale developed by Holahan and Gilbert (RCS). Marital satisfaction was measured with a scale adapted from Roach (MSS). The Employment Role Attitude Scale (ERAS) was developed by Parry and Warr for use with mothers of young children.

The results revealed no significant differences between employed and unemployed mothers on role conflict. This did not differ when work was divided into "career" versus "job." There was, however, a significant relationship for all mothers between perceived role conflict and ease of transition into the maternal role. This correlation was significant for all subscales of the RCS (spouse versus parent, spouse versus self, parent versus self). In addition, there was a significant correlation between perceived marital satisfaction and ease of transition into the maternal role for all mothers. No relationship was found between employment role attitude and ease of transition into the maternal role.

This report provides a good example of a correlational survey that does not use a random sample and in which the independent and dependent variables are not clearly distinguishable. In the analysis of data, transition into the maternal role is presumed to be the dependent variable, yet there is no theoretical foundation for this assumption; this variable could as easily be the independent variable affecting marital satisfaction, role conflict, and employment satisfaction. Role conflict is used by Majewski as both an independent and a dependent variable (independent in relation to transition to the maternal role and dependent in relation to employment and career versus job orientation). Thus, the "fishing expedition" orientation of the correlational survey is nicely illustrated by this study.

SUITABLE NURSING PROBLEMS

An enormous number of studies can be done using this design. Any study that looks at the interaction between the patient and the institutional environment can be done with a correlational design. For example, studies about the institutional care of Alzheimer patients that look at elements such as level and intensity of noise, colors, and number of people in the environment in relation to selected patient behaviors have yielded new nursing care plans for this group entirely different from the care and environment of other geriatric problems. Specific nursing diagnoses would benefit from correlational studies of the antecedent conditions. Studies examining variables such as social support, locus of control, spiritual well-being, ethnic background, and coping mechanisms of both patients and nurses are appropriate for the correlational design. In nursing education, studies of student characteristics and progress through educational programs are suitable correlational studies. Studies of staffing patterns, nursing care delivery systems, and job satisfaction, burnout, and turnover are good examples of administrative studies using correlational designs. We have just begun to touch on the wealth of questions that need to be addressed using this design. Much of our body of knowledge in nursing is at the level where this is the design of choice.

Studies using correlational designs are classified as descriptive studies because they do not manipulate any variables and do not primarily
test theory but study and describe variables as they exist naturally.
These types of studies frequently are based on findings from single-
variable studies. The results contribute to the development of theory.

SAMPLES

Because the major goal in a correlational study is to describe relationships between variables in a population, external validity, or generalizability, is of paramount importance. There is little value in describing statistical relationships that do not generalize to any population.
Hence, it is crucial that the sample be one that represents a given
population. The best sample is one that is randomly selected from the
target population to which the findings will be generalized.

The size of the sample needed for correlational survey designs is
closely related to the method of data analysis that will be used. The
sample must be large enough to make it possible to observe the full
range of variance on all the variables under study and must fit the
particular needs of the statistical techniques to be used with the data.

Sample size in correlational studies can be calculated using power
analysis, as discussed in the previous chapter. More often, however,
simpler methods are used to project an adequate sample size, such as
counting the number of independent variables and ensuring an adequate number of subjects per variable.

Tabachnick and Fidell (1989) have recommended that for multivariate analysis it is ideal to have 20 subjects for each independent variable.
At a minimum, a 5:1 ratio of subjects to independent variables (IVs)
must be ensured (Tabachnick & Fidell, 1989, pp. 128-129). In deciding
what figure between 5 and 20 to choose as a basis for subject-to-IV ratio,
consider the expected size of the effect on the dependent variable and
use a 5:1 ratio for a large effect size and a 20:1 for a small effect size; plan
for the smallest number of cases that has a good chance of finding a
significant relationship when there is one. Remember that it is also
possible to have too large a sample; almost any multiple correlation will
show significant departure from zero if the sample is large enough
(Tabachnick & Fidell, 1989, p. 129).

The use of certain statistical techniques such as factor analysis, step-wise regression, or LISREL will require larger samples. Unless you are knowledgeable about the requirements, consultation should be sought on the necessary sample size before beginning a study of this kind.

METHODS OF DATA COLLECTION

Measurement must be numeric, preferably at the interval or ratio level, although ordinal and nominal data are frequently used. The methods of data collection and the procedures used need to be maintained or standardized. The researcher should use tools that have been tested for reliability and validity on similar populations and should take steps to control anything that may affect reliability of data during data collection. The value of a correlational survey is directly related to the accurate measurement of the variables.

DATA ANALYSIS

This is the design for which multivariate statistical techniques were intended. We will discuss a few of the most commonly used techniques. All of these require interval data. When ordinal scales are used to measure variables, they must be at least metric in nature if any of these methods of analysis are to be used. If categorical or dichotomous (nominal) variables are used, the type of statistical analysis that can be used is significantly changed.

Correlational Analysis

The correlation coefficient measures the degree of linear association between two variables. This means that increases in one variable will create like increases (or decreases) in the other variable. The correlation coefficient always lies between the values of +1 and −1. When the two variables are unrelated, or have little effect on each other, the correlation coefficient will be close to zero. A positive correlation, meaning that increases in one variable are associated with increases in the other variable, will lie somewhere between zero and +1. The closer to +1 that the coefficient approaches, the more clearly it can be associated with increases in the other variable. Negative correlation occurs when an increase in one variable is associated with a decrease in another. The correlation coefficient, in this case, would lie somewhere between zero and –1. The correlation coefficient measures only the degree of association between two variables and does not indicate a cause-and-effect relationship. Although the two variables may appear to affect each other, it is always possible that both could be related to a third variable that has not been considered.

Multiple Correlation

Correlation, as described in the previous paragraphs, is used to test the degree of linear association between two variables: one independent (X) and one dependent (Y). Multiple correlation extends this concept to include relationships between more than one independent variable (X^1, X^2, and so on) and one dependent variable (Y). In multiple correlation, the coefficient can range from zero to +1. There are no negative correlations because the method of least squares is used to calculate the correlation coefficient. Multiple correlation is used to measure the relationship between a dependent variable and a weighted combination of independent variables (Munro, Visintainer, & Page, 1986, p. 82).

Regression Analysis

Linear regression analysis is used to test the validity of functional relationships. A functional relationship exists when one variable is thought to be affected by changes in another. Regression uses the correlation between variables to make predictions about one variable based on what is known about another. For example, the statement "The stress level of hospitalized patients is greater when they are unsure of their diagnoses" reflects an inference that stress level is a function of uncertainty in hospitalized patients. Regression analysis assumes that the relationship between stress and uncertainty is linear—that is, an increase in uncertainty creates a proportional increase in stress so that if the scores were depicted on a graph they would show a straight line with an upward slope. Correlational analysis tells us the amount of variance the two variables share. In regression analysis, however, we can determine whether the actual scores we obtain from our sample on the two variables, uncertainty and stress, are sufficiently close to forming a straight line to support the idea of a functional relationship between them. Linear regression requires that one variable be specifically designated as the dependent variable and that the variables be measured on interval scales. Ordinal variables can be used if they are continuous (not categorical).

Multiple Regression

Linear regression, as discussed above, deals with one independent and one dependent variable. If the study is based on a conceptual framework proposing that several factors might simultaneously affect a dependent variable, multiple linear regression analysis provides a means of measuring the effects of several factors concurrently. According to Schroeder, Sjoquist, and Stephan (1986), "The concept is the same as that of simple linear regression except that two or more independent variables are used simultaneously to explain variations in the dependent variable" (p. 30). The results will indicate the effect of any given independent variable on the dependent variable while holding the effects of the other independent variables constant. It is a method of recognizing that multiple factors may influence an observed process and measuring the relative effect of each factor.

Factor Analysis

Factor analysis actually includes statistical techniques, the goal of which is to determine if a large number of variables can be represented by a smaller number of underlying concepts or factors. In a correlational study, the investigator may have measured a number of variables thought to be predisposing to obesity on each member of the sample. It is not known whether there are underlying dimensions to the data that would reduce the number of variables into some common factors, but factor analysis will determine whether there are such underlying dimensions to the data. If they exist, these factors, rather than the individual variables, are assumed to be the actual causes of obesity. Factor analysis provides a way of examining the data to ascertain the minimum number of hypothetical factors that can account for the covariation among the variables (Kim & Mueller, 1978). This use of factor analysis is exploratory and may result in the development of a theoretical explanation for the covariance among the variables.

Factor analysis can also be used to test a more fully developed conceptual framework. The investigator can hypothesize that there are three underlying dimensions to the data, and that specific variables belong to each of these three dimensions. In this case, factor analysis is used to test theory rather than to develop it, and the results will show the degree to which the predicted underlying factors actually account for the observed covariation among the variables.

RELIABILITY AND VALIDITY

In correlational designs, the concepts of reliability and validity take on critical importance. Because the outcome of the study is determined by the statistical analysis of the data, the measurement of each variable must produce an accurate representation of the true value of the trait being measured. Instrument development, as described by Mishel in Chapter 10, is an important prerequisite of all studies at this level. In addition to using instruments with documented validity and reliability, reliability estimates should be established for all instruments with the population under study. This can be done in a pilot study, or these estimates can be calculated using the study data.

HUMAN SUBJECTS

If the major method of data collection is through the use of questionnaires, personal issues may be raised, leading to self-discovery that may be unpleasant for the study participants. This possibility must always be considered when studying variables representing personal attributes. The investigator should be prepared to assist respondents with feelings about self-revelation. In a study that can be viewed as a fishing expedition, there should be a sufficiently sound conceptual framework to warrant asking participants to contribute their time and energy to providing data for the research. Along these same lines, the design should be sound; it is an infringement on the rights of participants to waste their time contributing to a study that is based on a flawed design.

Studies that have correlational designs frequently use questionnaires and are therefore thought to be exempt from review by institutional review boards. This is a practice that should be considered carefully by colleges and universities because of the exploratory nature of some correlational studies. Research participants have a right to expect that their time and effort is not being wasted by inferior designs that are unlikely to produce any usable results.

RESEARCH PROPOSAL

An adequate conceptual framework is necessary for a correlational survey. Attention must be paid to the establishment of reliability and validity for the instruments. An adequate description of the population and the sampling procedures to be used will provide evidence of a representative sample, ensuring external validity. An adequate description of each tool to be used should be included, along with a rationale for its use, and a relationship should be established between each tool and the study's conceptual framework. The data analysis techniques must be appropriate for establishing relationships between the variables and should be chosen carefully in light of the kind of data (level of measurement) and sample available (sample selection techniques) for the study.

CRITIQUE

A critique of a correlational survey should focus on two areas: sample and measurement. A large random sample of the population forms the basis for this design, and any deviation from this ideal will serve to limit the study. In the area of measurement, those conducting a critique will look for precise quantitative measurement and for the use of instruments that have demonstrated reliability and validity for the population under study.

ESSENTIAL FEATURES OF THIS DESIGN

These designs are used to examine relationships between variables. There is a wide variation in the levels of knowledge that we have for correlational designs and, therefore, in theoretical perspectives, ranging from a very tentative conceptual framework to well-developed theories. The essential features are as follows:

1. Large random sample of the population
2. Conceptual framework
3. Quantitative data collected using valid and reliable measures
4. Statistical analysis focused on correlation between variables

In its essential form, this is one of the simplest designs, collecting data on two or more variables on the same group of participants and then computing a correlation coefficient—for example, collecting data on age and blood pressure on a random sample of shoppers at a shopping mall. The merit of this design is determined by the depth of the rationale and theoretical constructs that guide the study.

Although these designs are used to explore possible cause-and-effect relationships between variables, the results must be viewed with caution. There are always alternative explanations for the relationships observed in correlational designs.

REFERENCES

Asher, H. B. (1983). *Causal modeling* (2nd ed.). Beverly Hills, CA: Sage.

Berry, W. D. (1984). *Nonrecursive causal models.* Beverly Hills, CA: Sage.

Ferketich, S. L., & Verran, J. A. (1984). Residual analysis for causal model assumptions. *Western Journal of Nursing Research, 6*(1), 41-60.

Friesen, D. (1988). *Experience of spouses of dialysis patients.* Unpublished master's thesis, University of Alberta.

Kim, J.-O., & Mueller, C. W. (1978). *Introduction to factor analysis: What it is and how to do it.* Beverly Hills, CA: Sage.

Levine, M. S. (1977). *Canonical analysis and factor comparison.* Beverly Hills, CA: Sage.

Majewski, J. L. (1986). Conflicts, satisfactions, and attitudes during transition to the maternal role. *Nursing Research, 35*(1), 10-14.

McCloskey, J. C., & McCain, B. (1988). Variables related to nurse performance. *Image, 20*(4), 203-207.

Mishel, M. H., & Braden, C. J. (1987). Uncertainty: A mediator between support and adjustment. *Western Journal of Nursing Research, 9*(1), 43-57.

Munro, B. H., Visintainer, M. A., & Page, E. B. (1986). *Statistical methods for health care research.* Philadelphia: J. B. Lippincott.

Murphy, S. A. (1987). Self-efficacy and social support. *Western Journal of Nursing Research, 9*(1), 58-73.

Ostrom, C. W., Jr. (1978). *Time series analysis: Regression techniques.* Beverly Hills, CA: Sage.

Schroeder, L. D., Sjoquist, D. L., & Stephan, P. E. (1986). *Understanding regression analysis.* Beverly Hills, CA: Sage.

Tabachnick, B. G., & Fidell, L. S. (1989). *Using multivariate statistics* (2nd ed.). New York: HarperCollins.

Thompson, B. (1984). *Canonical correlation analysis.* Beverly Hills, CA: Sage.

Woods, N. F. (1985). Relationship of socialization and stress to perimenstrual symptoms, disability, and menstrual attitudes. *Nursing Research, 34*(3), 145-149.

8

Structural Equation Modeling

PAMELA A. RATNER
JOAN L. BOTTORFF
JOY L. JOHNSON

Structural equation modeling, or LInear Structural RELations (LIS-REL) modeling is not a research design per se but is best described as a statistical technique used in the analysis of theoretical models. Most simply, structural equation modeling (SEM) probes the covariances (or correlations) among variables to determine whether the hypothesized relationships between concepts within a theoretical system or model are plausible. It is perhaps the best example of how "theory and research are inextricably intertwined" (Brink & Wood, 1989, p. 11) in that it provides a means of testing theories that specify relationships be-

AUTHORS' NOTE: The authors acknowledge the thoughtful comments offered by their reviewers, Dr. Leslie Hayduk and Dr. Ivo Abraham, and the support they have received from the Canadian National Health Research and Development Program and the Medical Research Council of Canada through doctoral and postdoctoral fellowships.

tween theoretical constructs (Jöreskog, 1993). SEM can be used with data from survey, quasi-experimental, and experimental research designs. SEM (a) allows for the consideration of relationships between multiple variables, (b) incorporates measurement error in the variables, (c) permits multiple indicators of theoretical constructs, and (d) facilitates the study of reliability and validity (Bollen & Long, 1993a).

To highlight some examples in nursing research, SEM has been used, with varying degrees of finesse, to test causal models of postmyocardial infarction patients' coping effectiveness (Bennett, 1993), nurses' job satisfaction (Blegen & Mueller, 1987; Dodds, Lawrence, & Wearing, 1991), health behavior (Cox & Roghmann, 1984), mother-adult daughter relationships and mental health (Davis & Jones, 1992), adolescent girls' perceived health status (De Maio-Esteves, 1990), maternal self-efficacy (Gross, Conrad, Fogg, & Wothke, 1994), work performance among persons with multiple sclerosis (Gulick, 1992), leisure time physical activity (Hawkes & Holm, 1993), health promotion (Bottorff, Johnson, Ratner, & Hayduk, 1996; Johnson, Ratner, Bottorff, & Hayduk, 1993; Ratner, Bottorff, Johnson, & Hayduk, 1994, 1996), workers' use of hearing protection (Lusk, Ronis, Kerr, & Atwood, 1994), the health consequences of loneliness (Mahon, Yarcheski, & Yarcheski, 1993), birth and family functioning (Mercer & Ferketich, 1990), nurses' documentation behavior (Renfroe, O'Sullivan, & McGee, 1990), older adults' social participation (Wright, 1990), and positive health practices (Yarcheski & Mahon, 1989). It has also been used in confirmatory factor analyses of the Family Environment Scale (Loveland-Cherry, Youngblut, & Leidy, 1989) and the Perceived Self-Care Agency Questionnaire (Weaver, 1987).

SOME UNDERLYING ASSUMPTIONS

Sophisticated statistical techniques such as SEM, to some extent, are double-edged swords. On one hand, they provide us with a powerful mechanism for testing and modifying theories; on the other, their application can be complex, be prone to numerous pitfalls, and lead to intricate and perplexing interpretations. Consequently, there may be a tendency to naively accept the results of such analyses. Too often our models are taken as expressing something more real or meaningful than our experiences themselves. Gould (1981) points out that because of the pervasiveness of the Platonic assumption that "what we can see and measure in the world is merely the superficial and imperfect representation of an underlying reality" (p. 239) we have come to reify models and to view statistical techniques as a means of evincing that underlying reality. Consequently, there is a potential danger of viewing our statistical findings as somehow "more real" than the data from which they arise. To counterbalance this tendency, we offer a brief summary of what we believe to be pertinent epistemological assumptions underlying SEM. In discussing these assumptions, we hope to underscore the position that statistical techniques such as SEM are merely techniques from which we hope to gain an understanding of how things operate in the real world.

One assumption relates to the place of causation within SEM. SEM is grounded on the notions that causation exists and that we can model causative connections between concepts. Clearly, however, the inference of a causal relationship must be derived from something other than the mere occurrence of a statistically significant covariance within a variance/covariance matrix. In that structural equation models (SEMs) are putatively "causal," we are, in essence, indicating the potential rather than the actual flow of causation; we are positing that causation is conceivable or possible (Davis, 1985). Evidence in the form of time order, logical relationships, predictability, and experimental data may further support the warrantability of such causal claims.

A second epistemological assumption relevant to our understanding of the contributions of SEM concerns the question of whether theories can be confirmed. What can be gained by empirical tests of our theories? We take the position that all theories are tentative, conjectural, or hypothetical and subject to modification or refutation. Our theories cannot be proven to be true; rather, techniques such as SEM allow us to reject or modify those theories that conflict with our observations. Through the withstanding of repeated tests of a model, we may become more confident in our conjectures. This does not, however, rule out the possibility that competing theories may more adequately explain the causal relationships between the phenomena under consideration. There is always the possibility that an unspecified, competing theory may more adequately explain our observations.

Our belief that causal models represent our current "best guess" regarding that which occurs in reality is reflected in the process we recommend for developing and testing SEMs. We concur with Bollen and Long (1993a) who characterize the process of SEM as involving five steps: model specification, identification, estimation, testing fit, and respecification. By including respecification as part of the modeling process, we acknowledge that our initial models may not accurately capture the relationships reflected in the data. The five steps are inter-related, of course, and some are more statistically dense than others. We intend to touch on each of these steps, although most of the emphasis in this chapter is placed on the specification of models.

THE PROCESS OF STRUCTURAL EQUATION MODELING

Prior to describing the five steps, however, it is appropriate to consider the specification of theories deemed suitable for SEM.

Specifying Theories

Sufficient explication of our theories includes a full accounting of the relevant concepts, including specification of their dimensions and their interrelationships and classification of their causal role as either causal (*exogenous*, independent) or caused (*endogenous*, dependent). Further-more, for each concept postulated to be caused by one or more of the other concepts, a clear specification is required of which of those other concepts are, and are not, involved. In some cases, the researcher may be able to specify the direction (sign) or magnitude (relative size) of the postulated effects.

Most scientific theories relevant to nursing and of interest to nursing researchers consist of abstract concepts that cannot be measured di-rectly. Rather, such concepts are measured indirectly through responses obtained through questionnaires, interviews, observations, and so forth. These quantified measures, or indicators, are assumed to be representative of the concepts (Jöreskog, 1993). How, then, do we know if our theories correspond with the real world? Because we cannot observe or measure our abstract concepts directly, we cannot test the veracity of our theories directly. As Jöreskog (1993) points out, all we can do is examine the theoretical validity of our hypothesized relation-ships between concepts within a given context.

Before we can undertake an empirical test, we must define a set of observable or measurable indicators for each dimension of each concept. And we must make very clear how each indicator, often referred to as the *manifest variable,* corresponds with its respective concept or dimension of a concept, the *latent variable.* This correspondence, which Blalock (1968, 1979, 1982) suggests be expressed in an auxiliary theory, should narrow the gap between our abstract conceptions and concrete events, our measurements.

One advantage of SEM is made most evident in the necessity that the researcher fully specify her or his model prior to any statistical maneuvering. Admittedly, the researcher can unadvisedly "cheat" by examining correlation matrices prior to the specification of a model, but ultimately, the model must make good theoretical sense. We cannot emphasize strongly enough that knowledge of substantive, empirical matters, not statistical analyses, underlies the appropriate specification of causal models.

A second advantage of SEM is its ability to incorporate measurement error. Most other statistical techniques, by nature, assume perfect measurement; that is, the measures or indicators become the concepts. In SEM, researchers must not only lay out their theories describing the causal connections between concepts, but they must also describe how they have operationalized or measured those concepts and link the two by specifying the relations between the indicators and the concepts (Herting, 1985). That is, they must describe how their error-ridden indicators relate to their respective latent, abstract concepts. This auxiliary theory is as significant as the specification of the interrelationships between abstract, theoretical concepts. In research, the two are inextricably linked.

Specifying Models

The first step in SEM is the specification or formulation of a model, based on extant research findings and theory. The specified model represents an explicit statement of a researcher's assumptions about the nature of the causal relationships between exogenous and endogenous variables, about the behavior of error or unexplained components within the model, and about the presence of measurement error (Marsden, 1981).

In essence, there are two parts to SEMs: the structural equation part and the measurement part. The structural equation part contains the theoretical relationships between the unobservable or latent concepts. The measurement part contains the connections between the latent concepts and the measured, observed, or manifest indicators. All relationships specified in an SEM, whether correlations or directed effects, are quantifiable, and their magnitude can be estimated or specified. Collectively, the relationships, or effects to be estimated, are referred to as *coefficients*.

Translating Verbal Theories
Into Mathematical Models

Basically, the first step of the SEM process takes a verbal theory and translates it into a mathematical model. The translation procedure used in the LISREL statistical package relies on terms and Greek letters that may seem tedious; however, a grasp of the LISREL language (defined below) is necessary for one to read statistical output, research reports, and related literature. The two parts to an SEM are represented by three matrix algebra equations: (a) the structural equation part:

$$\eta = B\eta + \Gamma\xi + \zeta$$

(b) the measurement part for the endogenous variables:

$$y = \Lambda_y\eta + \varepsilon$$

and (c) the measurement part for the exogenous variables:

$$x = \Lambda_x\xi + \delta.$$

Note, the three equations take the form of regression equations. These equations specify the sources of variance, or causes, of the endogenous latent concepts (η's), the endogenous manifest variables (y's), and the exogenous manifest variables (x's), respectively.

The terms in the three equations are defined as follows:

η (eta)	is a vector or list of endogenous latent concepts;
ξ (ksi)	is a vector or list of exogenous latent concepts;

B (Beta)	is a matrix of effect coefficients linking the endogenous latent concepts (η's) to one another;
β (beta)	a lower-case β (beta) represents a particular coefficient from the B matrix;
Γ (Gamma)	is a matrix of effect coefficients linking the exogenous latent concepts (ξ's) to the endogenous latent concepts (η's);
γ (gamma)	a lower-case γ (gamma) represents a particular coefficient from the Γ matrix;
ζ (zeta)	is a vector or list of errors representing as yet unknown sources of each of the endogenous latent concepts (η's);
y	is a vector or list of manifest indicators of the endogenous latent concepts;
x	is a vector or list of manifest indicators of the exogenous latent concepts;
Λ_y (Lambda$_y$)	is a matrix of directed effect coefficients arising from the regression of y on η, or factor loadings;
λ_y (lambda$_y$)	a lower-case λ_y (lambda$_y$) represents a particular coefficient from the Λ_y matrix;
Λ_x (Lambda$_x$)	is a matrix of directed effect coefficients arising from the regression of x on ξ, or factor loadings;
λ_x (lambda$_x$)	a lower-case λ_x (lambda$_x$) represents a particular coefficient from the Λ_x matrix;
ε (epsilon)	is a vector or list of measurement errors in the manifest indicators of the endogenous latent concepts (y's);
δ (delta)	is a vector or list of measurement errors in the manifest indicators of the exogenous latent concepts (x's).

To facilitate your understanding of the presentation here, it is perhaps useful to think of the Γ, B, and Λ matrices as containing the *relationships* between causes and consequences or results. The ξ, η, δ, ε, ζ, y and x vectors contain the names or identities of either the *causes* or their *consequences* (Herting, 1985).

Two types of error terms are included in SEMs. The first, the ζ's, are connected to the endogenous latent concepts. We cannot expect to account for all the variance in each of the endogenous latent concepts. For various reasons, we often fail to include all of those variables that are associated with or that determine the concepts of interest. The aggregation of those omitted variables is represented in SEMs by a set of ζ error terms, one for each endogenous latent concept (Jöreskog, 1993). Those error terms represent the unexplained variance or the variance of each of the endogenous latent concepts not accounted for by the variables included in the model. The second type of error term, the ε and δ error terms, occurs in the measurement part of the SEM. These error terms are defined as random measurement errors, or specific factors, associated with the indicators; they represent sources of variance in the indicators other than the desired theoretical or latent concepts.

Two additional matrices occur within the structural equation part of an SEM: the Φ (Phi) matrix consisting of the covariances among the exogenous latent variables (ϕ's) and the Ψ (Psi) matrix consisting of the variances and covariances among the error terms, the ζ's, attached to the endogenous latent variables. Two additional matrices also occur in the measurement part of the SEM; the variances and covariances among the error terms, the δ's and ε's, appear in the Θ_δ (theta$_{delta}$) and Θ_ε (theta$_{epsilon}$) matrices. The following section describes the conventional nomenclature and depiction of SEMs.

Path Diagrams

It has become common practice for the "causal flow," or effects, within a model to be represented in path diagrams (flow graphs, pictograms). If properly drawn and labeled, path diagrams fully illustrate all parameters in a model. Although frequently omitted in published figures, convention has established that the indicators, or manifest variables, the x's and y's, are represented in boxes, and concepts, or latent variables, the ξ's and η's, are represented in circles. Error terms, ζ's, δ's, and ε's, are depicted as short arrows with unnamed sources. The relationships between variables are indicated by longer arrows. A one-way arrow between two variables indicates a direct effect of one variable on the other. Exogenous latent variables are generally allowed to covary among themselves. Such covariances are depicted by curved double-headed arrows. Finally, each coefficient is given two subscripts:

the first represents the number of the variable to which the arrow is pointing; the second represents the number of the variable from which the arrow originated. For example, if a latent exogenous variable ξ_1 causes the latent endogenous variable η_2, the resultant coefficient would be designated $\gamma_{2,1}$.

Figure 8.1 depicts a theory developed to assist us in describing SEM and is not necessarily grounded in extant research findings. This theory suggests that individuals' likelihood of engaging in regular exercise programs is determined, in part, by their evaluations of their health status and by perceptions of their self-efficacy. Furthermore, the theory postulates that age indirectly influences the likelihood of engaging in exercise by influencing individuals' thoughts regarding their health status and self-efficacy and by processes that are, as yet, undetermined. Gender also influences exercise behavior by indeterminate processes and by influencing individuals' perceptions of their health. Gender, however, is not believed to influence perceptions of self-efficacy. Note that the theory also suggests that the causal relationship between exercise behavior and health status is reciprocal, in that exercise affects one's perceptions of one's health status. The effect of exercise on perceived health status also allows for a connection between perceived self-efficacy and perceived health status. Although there is no direct link between these two concepts, perceived self-efficacy indirectly affects perceived health status by influencing exercise.

In this model (Figure 8.1), there are two exogenous latent concepts, *gender* (ξ_1) and *age* (ξ_2). Each is measured by a single, manifest variable or indicator, *reported gender* (x_1) and *reported age* (x_2), respectively, which are linked to their respective concepts by λ's. Each indicator has an associated error term, a δ, represented by the short arrows, whose variances and covariances will eventually appear in the Θ_δ matrix. The two exogenous latent concepts (gender and age) are allowed to covary, as represented by the curved two-headed arrow ($\phi_{1,2}$). Note that no error terms are attached to these two concepts. This is because these concepts are introduced only as causes of other concepts and are not, themselves, represented as consequences of other concepts within this model. This model includes, but does not attempt to explain, the fluctuations in, or background covariances among, the exogenous latent concepts. Collectively, the variances and covariances of the exogenous latent concepts form the Φ matrix.

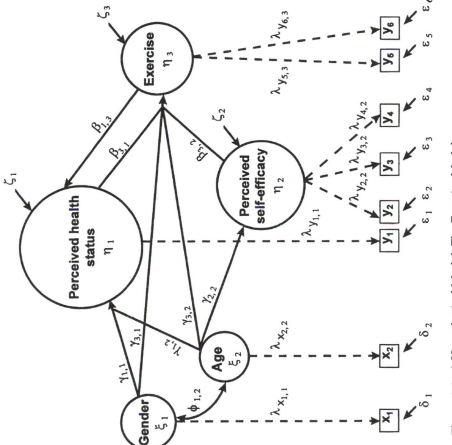

Figure 8.1. A Hypothetical Model: The Exercise Model

187

There are three endogenous latent concepts in the model, *perceived health status* (η_1), *perceived self-efficacy* (η_2), and *exercise* (η_3). Each endogenous latent concept has an associated error term (ζ_1, ζ_2, and ζ_3), represented by a short arrow, which serves to acknowledge that we do not expect to explain all the variance in any of these concepts. Admittedly, other likely determinants of the endogenous variables are not included in the model. The variances of the error terms (ζ's), collectively, appear in the Ψ matrix.

Again, the latent concepts are connected to their respective indicators by λ's. *Perceived health status* (η_1) is measured by participants' reports of their current health status (y_1). *Perceived self-efficacy* (η_2) has three indicators: reported confidence in achieving exercise goals (y_2), reported confidence in developing an exercise routine (y_3), and reported confidence in ability to carry out one's favored exercise (y_4). *Exercise* (η_3) has two indicators: the number of kilocalories per kilogram expended daily, on average, in voluntary exercise (y_5) and the number of times a week, on average, participants engage in calisthenics or physical exercise (y_6). Each of the endogenous variable indicators has an associated error term, an ε, whose variance appears in the Θ_ε matrix. Covariances among error variables are permitted in SEM, but none appears in this particular model.

The basic structure of the theory consists of the effects among the exogenous and endogenous latent variables. These are represented by the single-headed arrows between the latent concepts. The effects of the exogenous variables on the endogenous variables are γ's. The effect of gender on perceived health status is labeled $\gamma_{1,1}$ because this is the effect going to η_1 from ξ_1. Gender was also postulated to have an effect on exercise through a process other than through the two specified cognitive processes. This effect is represented as $\gamma_{3,1}$. Recall that the theory further postulated that gender has no effect on perceived self-efficacy; hence, there is no arrow from ξ_1 to η_2. The absence of this effect can be thought of as an effect whose magnitude is fixed at zero; $\gamma_{2,1} = 0.0$. The hypothesized influences of age on the three endogenous latent variables are represented as single-headed, straight arrows labeled $\gamma_{1,2}$, $\gamma_{2,2}$, and $\gamma_{3,2}$, respectively.

The effects among the endogenous latent concepts constitute the B matrix, and hence, the specific effects appear as lower-case β's with subscripts indicating the identity of the consequence and the cause. Both *perceived health status* and *perceived self-efficacy* were postulated to influence *exercise*. These effects are labeled $\beta_{3,1}$ and $\beta_{3,2}$, respectively. Exercise was postulated to have an effect on perceived health status, labeled $\beta_{1,3}$. Note that the theory made no mention of a direct causal connection between *perceived health status* and *perceived self-efficacy*. Some spurious covariance is expected between these concepts because they arise from a common source, *age*. The absence of any direct causal connection between these concepts corresponds to the "missing" arrow between these concepts and is identical to specifying $\beta_{2,1}$ and $\beta_{1,2}$ as fixed at zero.

As is the case in this model, hypothesized direct effects can sometimes connect into chains of effects, the so-called indirect effects that connect variables. For example, as depicted in Figure 8.1, gender has an indirect effect on perceived health status, in addition to its direct effect ($\gamma_{1,1}$), by having an effect on exercise ($\gamma_{3,1}$), which, in turn, has an effect on perceived health status ($\beta_{1,3}$). All indirect effects specify the mechanism carrying the effect (the intervening variable), which is exercise in the example, and are calculated as the product of the basic direct effects, once these have been calculated. The indirect effect of gender on perceived health status would equal $\gamma_{3,1} \times \beta_{1,3}$. The sum of the direct and indirect effects is the total effect. The total effect of gender on perceived health status equals $\gamma_{1,1} + (\gamma_{3,1} \times \beta_{1,3})$.

Using matrix notation, the three equations associated with this specific model are represented in Table 8.1. (For those readers unfamiliar with matrix algebra, Hayduk, 1987, Bollen, 1989, and Searle, 1982 provide excellent introductory level treatments of the subject.) Breaking down the equations in Table 8.1, we see, for instance, that the latent concept, exercise (η_3) is specified by the equation

$$\eta_3 = \beta_{3,1}\eta_1 + \beta_{3,2}\eta_2 + \gamma_{3,1}\xi_1 + \gamma_{3,2}\xi_2 + \zeta_3.$$

Similarly, the endogenous indicator, reported current health status (y_1) is specified by the equation

$$y_1 = \lambda_{y1,1}\eta_1 + \varepsilon_1,$$

and the exogenous indicator, reported gender (x_1) is specified by the equation:

$$x_1 = \lambda_{x1,1}\xi_1 + \delta_1.$$

TABLE 3.1   Matrix Representations of the Exercise Model

$$\eta = B + \Gamma\xi + \zeta$$

$$\begin{vmatrix} \eta_1 \\ \eta_2 \\ \eta_3 \end{vmatrix} = \begin{vmatrix} 0 & 0 & \beta_{13} \\ 0 & 0 & 0 \\ \beta_{31} & \beta_{32} & 0 \end{vmatrix} \begin{vmatrix} \eta_1 \\ \eta_2 \\ \eta_3 \end{vmatrix} + \begin{vmatrix} \gamma_{11} & \gamma_{12} \\ 0 & \gamma_{22} \\ \gamma_{31} & \gamma_{32} \end{vmatrix} \begin{vmatrix} \xi_1 \\ \xi_2 \end{vmatrix} + \begin{vmatrix} \zeta_1 \\ \zeta_2 \\ \zeta_3 \end{vmatrix}$$

$$y = \Lambda_y\eta + \varepsilon$$

$$\begin{vmatrix} Y_1 \\ Y_2 \\ Y_3 \\ Y_4 \\ Y_5 \\ Y_6 \end{vmatrix} = \begin{vmatrix} \lambda_{y11} & 0 & 0 \\ 0 & \lambda_{y22} & 0 \\ 0 & \lambda_{y32} & 0 \\ 0 & \lambda_{y42} & 0 \\ 0 & 0 & \lambda_{y53} \\ 0 & 0 & \lambda_{y63} \end{vmatrix} \begin{vmatrix} \eta_1 \\ \eta_2 \\ \eta_3 \end{vmatrix} + \begin{vmatrix} \varepsilon_1 \\ \varepsilon_2 \\ \varepsilon_3 \\ \varepsilon_4 \\ \varepsilon_5 \\ \varepsilon_6 \end{vmatrix}$$

$$x = \Lambda_x\xi + \delta$$

$$\begin{vmatrix} x_1 \\ x_2 \end{vmatrix} = \begin{vmatrix} \lambda_{x11} & 0 \\ 0 & \lambda_{x22} \end{vmatrix} \begin{vmatrix} \xi_1 \\ \xi_2 \end{vmatrix} + \begin{vmatrix} \delta_1 \\ \delta_2 \end{vmatrix}$$

Identification

Despite our best efforts at combining a promising, substantive theory and a data set possessing the calculated variances and covariances among the manifest indicators, we may fail to find a unique solution for the estimates of the coefficients within a model. This problem, known as the "identification problem," results when there are too many coefficients to be estimated (i.e., the "unknowns") in a model relative to the number of variances and covariances in the data set (i.e., the "knowns"). This type of model is referred to as an underidentified model. Little confidence can be placed in the estimates that result from an underidentified model because they can take on a range of values, and the selection of an acceptable estimate from that set of possible values is purely arbitrary; the analysis is statistically indeterminate (Carmines, 1986; Cuttance, 1985; Hayduk, 1987). Alternatively, when a model is "just" identified, the researcher has specified a model in such a way that there are exactly the right number and combination of unknown parameters or coefficients to be estimated in the model and a unique solution is a likely result (Hayduk, 1987). Most simply explained, the researcher desires an "overidentified" model in which the number of coefficients to be estimated is smaller than the number of knowns. That is, the number of coefficients to be estimated (t) must be less than the number of observed variances and covariances among the data set, or $t < 1/2(p + q)(p + q + 1)$, where p is the number of endogenous indicators (y's) and q is the number of exogenous indicators (x's) (Carmines, 1986).

Ensuring that the number of coefficients to be estimated is less than the number of knowns is a fairly simple condition to meet. However, identification is also related to other conditions within a model, including the specified relationships between the concepts and the nature of the data. Unfortunately, few guidelines or procedures exist for the comprehensive assessment of model identification (Bollen, 1989; Bollen & Jöreskog, 1985; Carmines, 1986; Hayduk, 1987). Because of the difficulties inherent in assessing identification problems prior to model estimation, Hayduk suggests that we be vigilant for signs of identification problems, be alert to the kinds of models in which we can expect problems, and use strategies to prevent the problem from occurring. There may be clues in the LISREL output that lead a researcher to suspect identification problems, including (a) the presence of large standard errors (because "acceptable" estimated values of a coefficient can vary considerably, the standard error will be large); (b) the estimates obtained are unreasonable or impossible (although this may also be a sign of other problems, such as mistakes in programming); and (c) the correlations between some coefficient estimates exceed ± 0.9 (Hayduk, 1987).

Some modeling strategies lend themselves to identification problems (Hayduk, 1987). For example, when researchers insert effects simply because they are possible (or, in the extreme, they let every concept affect every other concept), they run the risk of specifying models with too many coefficients to be estimated. All hypothesized effects (including the absence of effects) should be based on substantive theory. Taking this approach, the number of coefficients to be estimated is potentially minimized and each of the resulting significant and insignificant effects will have direct implications for supporting or refuting theoretical claims. Similarly, the practice of estimating all coefficients that link the latent concepts to their indicators (λ's) introduces additional unknowns into the model and can lead to identification problems. The solution to this problem is simply to fix (assign a specific value to) at least one λ for each concept. Such an approach is described in greater detail in our discussion of measurement. Finally, Hayduk points out that the inclusion of reciprocal or causal loops in a model can lead to identification problems. In the case of reciprocal effects, the problem may be minimized by including concepts that are thought to cause one concept and not the other within the reciprocal relationship—although finding additional concepts that meet this requirement may not always be possible.

Identification problems, however, can be prevented by taking advantage of theoretical constraints (Hayduk, 1987). For example, theory can be used to identify where the absence of effects might be expected. In these instances, fixed zero coefficients can be included. In some instances, researchers can take advantage of postulated equality constraints to reduce the number of unknowns. In testing gender differences in relation to health promoting behaviors, Ratner et al. (1994) included equality constraints for those effects theorized to be the same (both in direction and magnitude) for men and women. This effectively reduced the number of coefficients to be estimated in their model. Fixing measurement error variances, based on reliability estimates or the known strengths and weaknesses of measurements (e.g., Bottorff et al., 1996; Johnson et al., 1993; Ratner et al., 1994, 1996), and fixing the magnitude of effects based on previous research are other ways to reduce the number of unknowns in models.

Ultimately, our main objective is to develop strongly overidentified models—that is, models that have many concepts linked with a few structural coefficients.

> Researchers inclined to let everything influence everything else are not only headed for identification problems, but they have abandoned the parsimony canon of science. The fewer the structural coefficients required to achieve an acceptable data fit, the more parsimonious is our explanation of the observed data. (Hayduk, 1987, p. 154)

Estimation

Model development and estimation have been approached in at least two ways. Some methodologists advocate a two-step procedure (Anderson & Gerbing, 1988; Jöreskog, 1993), and some nursing scholars support this approach (Aaronson, Frey, & Boyd, 1988; Hickey, 1993). In a two-step procedure, the first step involves the estimation of the "measurement model," comprising an exploratory or confirmatory analytic process in which the indicators of the latent concepts are evaluated with respect to how well they load on their latent factors. Combining the measurement model obtained in Step 1 and the theoretically postulated structural effects between latent concepts, the full model is then estimated in Step 2. Alternatively, model development and estimation can be completed using a one-step procedure (Fornell & Yi, 1992a; Hayduk, 1987, 1996, chap. 2) as demonstrated in our research (Bottorff et al., 1996; Johnson et al., 1993; Ratner et al., 1994). The major premise underlying this approach is that measurement issues cannot be neatly separated from theory—all measures are theory-laden (e.g., Ratner et al., 1996). In addition, if you accept that concepts are granted meaning both through the links to their indicators and by their links to other concepts, then to proceed with separate tests of the measurement and structural models puts one in the position of defending "partially-determined meanings" (Hayduk, 1996, chap. 2)

A full explication of the debate concerning the relative merits of the one-step and two-step approaches (Anderson & Gerbing, 1988, 1992; Fornell & Yi, 1992a, 1992b; Hayduk, 1996, chap. 2) is beyond the scope of this chapter. We will proceed by describing model estimation and development using the one-step procedure. We do this for several reasons. First, the one-step procedure accommodates a wider variety of modeling styles, and it ensures that the meanings of concepts are clearly specified within the context of a structural model solidly connected to its manifest variables. Furthermore, a two-step procedure can lead to biased estimates of the λ's if the analysis fails to acknowledge that some of the concepts influencing the indicators are correlated with one another. That is, if an exploratory factor analysis is conducted for each concept separately, any indicator that may be influenced by more than one of the concepts is not well estimated. In addition, the connections between latent concepts and their indicators depend on the nature of the structural effects between the concepts. If one evaluates the measurement of all latent concepts simultaneously, by allowing the concepts to covary, one can obtain different values for the λ's, or factor loadings, compared with when one specifies specific directional effects among the latent concepts. Finally, the chi-square (χ^2) tests employed to determine the fit of the first model, the measurement structure, and the second model, the structural model, are not independent. If the second model is specified on the basis of information obtained during the first step, the χ^2 test is compromised (Hayduk, 1987, 1996, chap. 2).

In using the one-step procedure, the measurement and structural equation parts of a model are subject to an omnibus analysis. The resultant estimated coefficients are calculated based on the covariances among the indicators (which are known) and the constraints within the model. Historically, maximum likelihood procedures have been used most often as the estimation method in SEM. However, many other estimators exist and are likely to be used with greater frequency in the future (Tanaka, 1993).

Several SEM computer programs are currently available, including EQS (Bentler, 1992), LISREL (Jöreskog & Sörbom, 1989), LISCOMP (Muthén, 1987), and LINCS (Schoenberg, 1987). The most commonly used statistical package to estimate SEMs seems to be LISREL, and its notation has become the common terminology for SEM. Clearly, this chapter cannot provide the full computational details of the program. Readers are advised to refer to more comprehensive works (Hayduk, 1987; Jöreskog & Sörbom, 1989). In essence, the LISREL program obtains estimates of a model's coefficients by comparing the observed covariances among the indicators (as reflected in the data set) with the covariances implied by the model. Maximum likelihood estimates, therefore, are directly linked to a combination of model and data constraints. The structural equation part of a model constrains estimates by virtue of the number of concepts that are included in the model and the location of free coefficients (or effects), which link the concepts to one another and to the indicators. In addition, the estimates are constrained by the data, because it is through a comparison of the model-implied covariances and the observed covariances (data) that the best set of estimates is selected. Therefore, error in either the theoretical specification of a model or in the data collection process can lead to invalid results.

The estimates obtained for the free coefficients within a model result in an implied covariance structure for the indicators or manifest variables that is as nearly identical to the observed data covariance matrix as possible. The program does this by creating an initial estimate for each model coefficient (with absent effects set at zero). Once the first set of estimates or initial values is created, the program then iteratively checks the fit of the implied covariance matrix to the observed matrix and adjusts the estimated values in ways that might reduce or eliminate any ill fit. The iterative process concludes when the smallest differences between the implied and actual covariances are found (Cuttance, 1985). This may not necessarily lead to a well-fit model, but any other solution would lead to larger differences and have a worse fit (Hertig, 1985). In addition to the estimates of the coefficients within a model, standard errors, *t* values, and other statistics are provided. The adequacy of the estimated model can be determined from the LISREL output. This is described in more detail in the following section.

Testing Fit

Although a full discussion of the various techniques for assessing the consistency of a model with its data is beyond the scope of this chapter, it is important to note that the goal of such techniques is to determine if the statistical relationships implied by the postulated model are compatible with the variance and covariance matrix one has observed as data. If one finds that the implications of one's specified model (the implied covariance structure) depart from the covariance matrix of the observed variables, doubt is cast on the model specification and therefore on the obtained estimates. Such departures are determined by various goodness-of-fit tests of the model or "fit" indices, including the χ^2 test and the adjusted goodness-of-fit index, and by examining other information provided in the LISREL output, such as the residuals (the discrepancies between the observed covariances and the implied covariances).

In using the χ^2 test to evaluate estimated models, it is important to note that smaller χ^2 values are an indication of better fitting models and that an insignificant χ^2 is desirable. The latter indicates that the implied covariance matrix is nearly identical to (does not differ significantly from) the observed data set and that the remaining differences are likely to be due to sampling fluctuations. It is also important to recognize the sample size dependency associated with the χ^2 test. If a sample is too small, even an inadequate model is likely to fit the data. On the other hand, if the sample is too large, even the best theoretical explanation can be rejected because of minor random fluctuations (Carmines, 1986). Hayduk (1987) recommends that, depending on the type of model estimated, the χ^2 test is a useful indicator of fit for samples of 50 to 500 cases.

Although researchers most commonly report χ^2 tests and adjusted goodness-of-fit indices, almost 20 goodness-of-fit indices are currently available (Gerbing & Anderson, 1993). Bollen and Long (1993b) provide an excellent discussion of the issues related to testing fit.

In addition to considering the overall fit of a model, investigators are advised to consider the "components" of the model, including the R-square values of the equations (the proportion of variance accounted for in each endogenous latent concept), the magnitude of the coefficient estimates, and the sign of the coefficients (Bollen & Long, 1993a). It is possible to obtain a model with acceptable overall fit but to find that little of the variance is explained and that all coefficients are weak (e.g., Johnson et al., 1993). In addition, we are reminded by Hayduk (1987) that obtaining successful estimation is not the end of the modeling process, but it provides the necessary foundation for a detailed investigation of the estimates and their implications. "The *results are the substantive implications of the estimates* obtained through the combined force of the best available theory and data" (Hayduk, 1987, p. 155).

Respecification

Frequently, following the initial estimation of a specified model, one finds that the model fits poorly. That is, there is evidence pointing to significant departures between the covariances implied by the model and the observed covariances among the manifest variables. At this point, decisions about what to do next rest on the initial purpose of one's study. Jöreskog (1993) identifies three possible situations. If a study is strictly confirmatory in nature—that is, a single model is tested against some empirical data—and a poor fit is obtained, the model should be rejected. If several alternative, competing models are proposed, the best model should be identified, based on the analysis of a particular data set. The third situation, the most common approach in nursing research (to date) is one in which the researcher has specified a tentative, initial model with the aim of generating a model that can best fit the data. In this case, when the initial model does not fit the empirical data, the model should undergo modification and retesting.

The LISREL package provides statistical output to assist in the location of modifications that can improve the fit of a model. One should consider the standardized residuals, the modification indices, and the expected parameter change statistics, which are provided for every pair of observed variables. In a perfectly fitting model, one would find no differences between the observed and implied covariance matrices; the residuals would all equal zero. In less than perfectly fitting models, standardized residuals are calculated by determining the number of standard deviations the residuals are away from zero (Hayduk, 1987). Large positive standardized residuals indicate underestimation of the covariance between the indicators, whereas large negative standardized residuals indicate overestimation. Many solutions to such problems may exist; however, typically, both underestimation or overestimation of a covariance may require the addition of one or more effects.

Modification indices provided in the statistical output of LISREL indicate how much the χ^2 value can be expected to decrease if a particular constrained effect (fixed to equal 0) is freed and the model is reestimated. The "expected parameter change" values are associated with the modification indices and indicate how much a particular coefficient estimate is expected to change in size if the effect is indeed freed (Jöreskog, 1993).

Of course, the examination of standardized residuals and modification and expected change indices is, at best, an ad hoc procedure that can provide hints for model respecification but that cannot guarantee the best fitting model or the "true" model (Long, 1981). Furthermore, when one incrementally improves the fit of a model by adding or eliminating effects, based on statistical output (and substantive claims), one runs the risk that the enhanced fit may have been obtained by chance (Jöreskog, 1993). The final model, and any competing models, should be "cross-validated" on an independent data set. We recommend that if the initial data set is sufficiently large, one should randomly split the data set in half. One half can be used for the exploratory phase of model development. The second half can be used for an uncompromised test, or cross-validation, of the final model (Anderson & Gerbing, 1988; Long, 1981). The best guide to respecification of a model, however, must be strong substantive theory. Does a proposed modification make good theoretical sense? If not, it would be futile to defend the model, even if it provided a superior fit to the data.

When respecifying a model, we may be tempted to seek a single model that obtains the best fit possible. However, because much of nursing knowledge is in the early stages of development, a better approach might be to consider several, alternative models rather than examining one particular model. In this manner, researchers can explore and compare several plausible structures (Bollen & Long, 1993a). It would be naive to assume that a particular structural equation model represents the "definitive explanation of a phenomenon under investigation. Models represent 'best guesses' that are subject to further verification or refutation" (Tanaka, 1993, p. 34). As Hayduk (1990) says,

> If one adopts the philosophy that structural equation models are supposed to be prods to sluggish imaginations, sparks that ignite insight, keys that unlock advancement, or hammers that forge progress from burning issues, we will have to do better than merely searching through the list of potentially-freeable coefficients, no matter how diligently and with how much technical sophistication we conduct the search. (p. 196)

OTHER CONSIDERATIONS

SEM is a complex procedure that incorporates numerous methodological and theoretical considerations. Indeed, all those topics included in an introductory research text are relevant to a discussion of SEM. In the following section, we highlight some key issues and some innovative strategies in SEM.

Power

Researchers must consider whether the number of cases constituting a data set are sufficiently large to reliably evaluate a model. Unfortunately, no simple power equations or guidelines are available for the structural equation modeler. Statisticians have yet to determine the asymptotic statistical theory of SEM and the conditions under which samples are sufficiently large (Tanaka, 1987, 1993). However, as in other statistical techniques, there is an interplay between excessive statistical power and sufficient power to test a model. In SEM, too much power can result in the rejection of a model for minor or trivial deviations from the data, whereas insufficient power can make the poorest fitting model look good. A guiding principle in the determination of sample size is to use as large a sample as feasible (Borg & Gall, 1989; Fowler, 1984;

Sudman, 1983). Several factors, including the anticipated margin of error, the degree of external validity, the number of subgroups or strata within the population the researcher desires to study, and cost-efficiency should be considered. Post facto, the best approach, as discussed previously, is to report several indices and indications of the fit of a model because most currently available fit indices depend on sample size (Bollen & Long, 1993a; Tanaka, 1993).

Measurement

We have recommended that the measurement and structural equation parts of a model be specified and estimated simultaneously. In this way, we acknowledge the "theory-laden" nature of measurement and force researchers who choose to follow this approach to make explicit their conceptualizations rather than merely relying on factor analytic techniques to determine the dimensionality and nature of their concepts. When one specifies the measurement structure of a model, both the scales for the latent concepts and the error variance associated with measuring those concepts should be specified by the researcher (Hayduk, 1987) (e.g., Bottorff et al., 1996; Johnson et al., 1993; Ratner et al., 1994). That is, the connection between each latent concept and one of its indicators, a λ, should be fixed at 1.0. Values of 1.0 in these equations simply specify that the latent concepts are scaled in the same manner as are the respective scaling indicators. In the case of multiple indicators, the indicator believed to be the best, that is the least error prone, should have its λ fixed at 1.0, whereas the remaining λ's are free to be estimated. The error variances for the scaling indicators, the Θ_δ's and Θ_ϵ's, should be fixed at a value equivalent to a research-specified proportion of the variance in the respective indicators. The remaining variance is provided by the corresponding underlying latent concept. One strength of this approach is that there can be an adjustment for measurement error even with single indicators. But it is even more important that this forces researchers to be clear about the meaning they attach to the latent concepts; these can be altered by the decisions made related to the error variances of the indicators (Hayduk, 1987; Ratner et al., 1996). This results in meanings for the concepts that are not arbitrarily accomplished, as often is the case when λ's are freely estimated and subject to change with structural modifications. That is, it forces a stable, researcher-determined designation of meaning onto each concept (Hayduk, 1996, chap. 1).

What kind of indicators are appropriate? Admittedly, our measures are never perfect. Even the most mundane concept, such as age, can be fraught with random measurement error. Some may honestly not know their actual date of birth. Some define age in terms of their age at their nearest birthday, while others define age in terms of their last birthday. Others may exhibit preferences for specific digits, most often those ending in zero or five, and may round their age or avoid certain numbers (Stockwell, 1976). Once the data are collected, other sources of error emerge during the coding and data entry processes. In our research, to accommodate specific sources of error, we assigned 5% of the variance in age as error (Johnson et al., 1993).

We know that the error proneness of our measurements becomes increasingly marked as the concepts we are attempting to measure become increasingly abstract and subjective. The standard approach to this problem is to use multiple measures or indicators. The thinking underlying this approach assumes that if several indicators measure the same concept, the influence of the concept is common to all the indicators, whereas the errors associated with each indicator or measure are random. All we must do, it is argued, is capture the common thread running through the set of indicators (Hunter & Gerbing, 1982). Usually, this is accomplished by summing the responses to several items, demonstrated by factor analysis to be indicative of a concept, and using the total score or average score as "the measure." We, however, take issue with such an approach. First, if there is considerable error in each of the items and few items constitute the aggregate score, a great deal of error may persist. Second, an aggregate score, by its very nature, assumes that a concept is unidimensional. However, the assumption is not subject to further testing if the aggregate score is used (Hayduk, 1996). Furthermore, if the concept is indeed multidimensional and erroneously treated as unidimensional, the indicator, the aggregate score, is likely to display complex and obscure associations with other concepts in one's model. Finally, a specific item within the aggregate score may not only be an indicator of the concept it is intended to measure but may additionally be an indicator of another concept in the model. Aggregate scores complicate this sort of modeling.

We recommend that each constituent of a scale be modeled. For example, in our hypothetical model (see Figure 8.1), rather than measure *perceived self-efficacy* with a single aggregate score obtained by summing items, we modeled three items as multiple indicators of *perceived self-efficacy*. However, in so doing, one is likely to encounter several problems, particularly as the number of indicators increases. Models with multiple indicators are subject to what Hayduk (1987, 1996) calls "a proportionality requirement" and what Hunter and Gerbing (1982) call "an external consistency or parallelism criterion". What this means, in terms of our exercise model, is that the three indicators for perceived self-efficacy must possess a strict pattern of covariance with, for example, both *reported age* and the indicators for exercise. Age and exercise are an antecedent and a consequence of perceived self-efficacy, respectively. Hence, each indicator of perceived self-efficacy must have proportional covariances with the indicators for exercise and age. This requirement is often difficult to meet, and models with such inherent requirements are likely to fail (e.g., Ratner et al., 1996). Hayduk (1987) recommends that if one chooses to use multiple indicators, a researcher should begin with the single best indicator and incrementally add more indicators. This approach not only simplifies the initial model but is likely to provide the clearest conceptual definitions.

In most statistical analyses, there is an underlying assumption that error terms are uncorrelated. This constraint is not present in SEM in that, if a model is not underidentified, two error terms can be specified as covarying. Despite this feature, we generally expect measurement error terms to be independent of one another. This is where the strength of our claim that an indicator is a measure of a concept lies. If the error terms for two or more indicators covary, we can conclude that the indicators measure something in addition to, or other than, the concepts that we have specified. That is, we must acknowledge the presence of an unspecified factor or concept in the face of covariance among these error terms (Gerbing & Anderson, 1984). In some instances, the a priori specification of covariance among error terms can be meaningful—for example, an acknowledgment of a method factor. However, Jöreskog (1993) correctly admonishes that the use of correlated error terms in the measurement part of SEMs for the *sole* purpose of obtaining a better fit in a model is inappropriate. As Bagozzi (1983) says, "Correlated measurement residuals are fall-back options nearly always detracting from the theoretical elegance and empirical interpretability of a study" (p. 450). Every correlation between error terms has significant theoretical or methodological implications and, if incorporated in a model, should be accompanied by a substantive interpretation (Fornell, 1983).

Exploring Interaction Effects

It is naive for us to assume that the causal effects we model will remain constant for all groups and all conditions. Causal effects between variables may differ depending on the value of a third variable, such as one's gender, age, education, locus of control, or beliefs about health. In cases in which the magnitude of an effect differs between two variables depending on the value possessed by a third variable, *interaction* is said to exist (Hayduk, 1987). For example, in the exercise model (Figure 8.1), a plausible interaction could exist between the variables age and gender. It is reasonable that the effect of age on exercise differs depending on one's gender. This could occur because we suspect that young men, on average, are more regularly active than young women. The aging effect and its consequent reduction in exercise, therefore, may be more profound in men. That is, the magnitude of the effect of age on exercise may be different for men and women.

One approach to modeling an interaction in SEM is similar to the multiple regression procedures for handling interactions. In our example, wherein an interaction is hypothesized between age and gender, we would require an additional concept, ξ_3, to represent the interaction term, the product of ξ_1 (gender) and ξ_2 (age) (i.e., $\xi_3 = \xi_1\xi_2$) (Hayduk, 1987).

A second approach to interaction is to specify separate models for each group of interest. For example, we could develop an exercise model for men and one for women. However, by developing and testing two completely separate models, we could not allow for the claim that there are other effects that we expect to remain equivalent between the two groups. For example, we could expect the effect of age on perceived self-efficacy to be the same for men and women. An alternative and preferred approach to developing and testing separate models is to "stack" the groups in a single LISREL run (Hayduk, 1987; Jöreskog & Sörbom, 1989). Stacking groups together allows us to constrain some of the effect coefficients to be equal between the groups, while leaving other coefficient estimates free to vary between the groups. This approach is very useful when one suspects numerous interactions within a model (e.g., Ratner et al., 1994).

The program for a stacked model is basically composed of two or more separate programs stacked one behind the other. LISREL then treats the multiple models as a single model. When the program is run, all models are simultaneously estimated. One can determine if interaction is present by examining the effects to see if there is a difference in the magnitude or direction of those effects that were allowed to differ across the groups. One can readily anticipate additional advantages in LISREL's ability to stack models. Multiple-group or multiple-sample analysis, conducted in this manner, can be very useful in experimental designs (stacking experimental and control groups), validation studies (stacking two halves of a data set), or longitudinal or panel designs (stacking time-lagged measures) (Lomax, 1983).

Reporting LISREL Findings

Because of the complexity of SEM, it is often difficult to determine what should be included in research reports of such analyses. On the basis of our review of the literature and on our own experience in attempting to present coherent pictures of complex analyses, we make several recommendations.

First, the purpose of the research endeavor must be clearly stated. Readers should have little difficulty in identifying whether a study was undertaken to confirm a model, test alternative or competing models, or generate a model based on a tentative theory. Clearly, the purpose of the study will determine the appropriate criteria for evaluation of the findings. Such explication should clearly demonstrate the theoretical position held by the researcher.

It is essential that the theoretical model be clearly described. This description includes the nature and direction of the hypothesized effects within a model. Clear explication of the latent concepts is imperative, including their dimensionality. One "complex concept" might appear as the several specific dimensions required to span all of the relevant aspects of the complexity (e.g., Ratner et al., 1996). Furthermore, the operationalization of the concepts must be specified. This specification includes the theory underlying the connections between the latent concepts and their indicators, frequently referred to as epistemic correlations, rules of correspondence, or operational definitions (Costner, 1985). In addition, the measurement structure must be described, including the nature of the indicators. Ideally, this would include the wording of the instrument or questionnaire items, previous assessments of their reliability and validity, the coding or recoding of the values, the treatment of missing and outlier cases, descriptive statistics of the indicators, and so forth. Furthermore, researchers are advised to report how they approached measurement error and whether factor loadings were estimated or specified. Path diagrams that include all latent and manifest variables and structural and measurement effects provide a succinct specification of one's model. Researchers are advised to verify that their verbal language corresponds to their mathematical language as implied by the path diagram.

As space permits, a detailed discussion of the study sample is useful. Such discussion should include a description of the sampling procedure and the size of the sample. Furthermore, the nature of the data set should be described, including whether the matrix is a covariance matrix, correlation matrix, or some other matrix and how missing cases were deleted—that is, whether listwise or pairwise deletion was used. Publication of the actual data matrix is ideal.

Turning to the findings, we are convinced that all model modifications should be described. Even a summary description of the modifications will give the reader an indication of the degree to which the researcher may have capitalized on chance. If the process of revising models is incremental in nature and each step is outlined, the theoretical underpinnings of models can be more easily discerned.

Furthermore, it is advisable to provide a path diagram of the final model, along with a description of the coefficient estimates (organized in tabular format) and indications of the model's goodness of fit (χ^2 test, degrees of freedom, probability, and adjusted goodness-of-fit indices). Such description should include both significant and nonsignificant coefficients, the proportion of variance attributed to measurement error, whether error terms (either structural or measurement) were allowed to covary, the proportion of variance explained in each endogenous concept, and areas in which the model-implied covariance structure departed from the observed data. That is, indication of the largest residuals should be provided in a manner in which the reader can determine the magnitude of such departures. Ideally, this would be expressed as correlations.

Clearly, an overwhelming amount of information can be reported. We recommend that researchers isolate and highlight three or four significant or key substantive findings in their discussion. Such an approach aids readers in interpreting the significance of the findings and in isolating the key elements of the modeling process. For example, one may want to discuss whether the sign or magnitude of coefficients is consistent with what is currently known or with what was anticipated. Furthermore, any new insights about the behavior of particular indicators or concepts can be emphasized. Finally, too often, we expect to see well-fit models with relatively large explanatory power published. Yet those models that fail can be equally informative. Accordingly, we encourage researchers to share their failed attempts at explaining their observations or at confirming theories.

CONCLUSION

We have attempted to highlight the key elements of SEM. This overview cannot sufficiently inform readers of the intricacies of SEM. Accordingly, review of more comprehensive texts is advised for those who plan to conduct such research. Furthermore, advances continue to be made in the area of SEM. Readers are alerted to the fact that numerous questions related to model development and testing remain controversial, so no simple cookbook approach to SEM is possible. We anticipate that, in the future, we will encounter greater and wider use of SEM techniques and subsequent refinements of modeling techniques. The strength in SEM lies in its ability to marry theory and observation in a demonstrable fashion. No longer must we merely keep in the back of our minds notions about unreliability, less than ideal measurement, and the simultaneity or causal flow of effects. SEM provides us with a mechanism to fully expose the theory-laden nature of our measurements and the consequences of our less than perfect measures, in addition to exploring the causal mechanisms underlying the covariance structures of our observations.

REFERENCES

Aaronson, L. S., Frey, M. A., & Boyd, C. J. (1988). Structural equation models and nursing research: Part II. *Nursing Research, 37,* 315-318.

Anderson, J. C., & Gerbing, D. W. (1988). Structural equation modeling in practice: A review and recommended two-step approach. *Psychological Bulletin, 103,* 411-423.

Anderson, J. C., & Gerbing, D. W. (1992). Assumptions and comparative strengths of the two-step approach: Comment on Fornell and Yi. *Sociological Methods and Research, 20,* 321-333.

Bagozzi, R. P. (1983). Issues in the application of covariance structure analysis: A further comment. *Journal of Consumer Research, 9,* 449-450.

Bennett, S. J. (1993). Relationships among selected antecedent variables and coping effectiveness in postmyocardial infarction patients. *Research in Nursing and Health, 16,* 131-139.

Bentler, P. M. (1992). *EQS structural equations program manual.* Los Angeles: BMDP Statistical Software.

Blalock, H. M., Jr. (1968). The measurement problem: A gap between the languages of theory and research. In H. M. Blalock, Jr. & A. B. Blalock (Eds.), *Methodology in social research* (pp. 5-27). New York: McGraw-Hill.

Blalock, H. M., Jr. (1979). Measurement and conceptualization problems: The major obstacle to integrating theory and research. *American Sociological Review, 44,* 881-894.

Blalock, H. M., Jr. (1982). *Conceptualization and measurement in the social sciences.* Beverly Hills, CA: Sage.

Blegen, M. A., & Mueller, C. W. (1987). Nurses' job satisfaction: A longitudinal analysis. *Research in Nursing and Health, 10,* 227-237.

Bollen, K. A. (1989). *Structural equations with latent variables.* New York: John Wiley.

Bollen, K. A., & Jöreskog, K. G. (1985). Uniqueness does not imply identification: A note on confirmatory factor analysis. *Sociological Methods and Research, 14,* 155-163.

Bollen, K. A., & Long, J. S. (1993a). Introduction. In K. A. Bollen & J. S. Long (Eds.), *Testing structural equation models* (pp. 1-9). Newbury Park, CA: Sage.

Bollen, K. A., & Long, J. S. (Eds.). (1993b). *Testing structural equation models.* Newbury Park, CA: Sage.

Borg, W. R., & Gall, M. D. (1989). *Educational research: An introduction* (5th ed.). New York: Longman.

Bottorff, J. L., Johnson, J. L., Ratner, P. A., & Hayduk, L. A. (1996). The effects of cognitive-perceptual factors on health promotion behavior maintenance. *Nursing Research, 45,* 30-36.

Brink, P. J., & Wood, M. J. (1989). Introduction. In P. J. Brink & M. J. Wood (Eds.), *Advanced design in nursing research* (pp. 11-24). Newbury Park, CA: Sage.

Carmines, E. G. (1986). The analysis of covariance structure models. In W. D. Berry & M. S. Lewis-Beck (Eds.), *New tools for social scientists: Advances and applications in research methods* (pp. 23-55). Beverly Hills, CA: Sage.

Costner, H. L. (1985). Theory, deduction, and rules of correspondence. In H. M. Blalock, Jr. (Ed.), *Causal models in the social sciences* (2nd ed., pp. 229-250). New York: Aldine de Gruyter.

Cox, C. L., & Roghmann, K. J. (1984). Empirical test of the Interaction Model of Client Health Behavior. *Research in Nursing and Health, 7,* 275-285.

Cuttance, P. (1985). A general structural equation modeling framework for the social and behavioral sciences. In R. B. Smith (Ed.), *A handbook of social science methods: Vol. 3. Quantitative methods: Focused survey research and causal modeling* (pp. 408-463). New York: Praeger.

Davis, B., & Jones, L. C. (1992). Differentiation of self and attachment among adult daughters. *Issues in Mental Health Nursing, 13,* 321-331.

Davis, J. A. (1985). *The logic of causal order* (Sage University Paper series on Quantitative Applications in the Social Sciences, series No. 07-055). Beverly Hills, CA: Sage.

De Maio-Esteves, M. (1990). Mediators of daily stress and perceived health status in adolescent girls. *Nursing Research, 39,* 360-364.

Dodds, A. E., Lawrence, J. A., & Wearing, A. J. (1991). What makes nursing satisfying: A comparison of college students' and registered nurses' views. *Journal of Advanced Nursing, 16,* 741-753.

Fowler, F. J. (1984). *Survey research methods.* Beverly Hills, CA: Sage.

Fornell, C. (1983). Issues in the application of covariance structure analysis: A comment. *Journal of Consumer Research, 9,* 443-448.

Fornell, C., & Yi, Y. (1992a). Assumptions of the two-step approach to latent variable modeling. *Sociological Methods and Research, 20,* 291-320.

Fornell, C., & Yi, Y. (1992b). Assumptions of the two-step approach: Reply to Anderson and Gerbing. *Sociological Methods and Research, 20,* 334-339.

Gerbing, D. W., & Anderson, J. C. (1984). On the meaning of within-factor correlated measurement errors. *Journal of Consumer Research, 11,* 572-580.

Gerbing, D. W., & Anderson, J. C. (1993). Monte Carlo evaluations of goodness-of-fit indices for structural equation models. In K. A. Bollen & J. S. Long (Eds.), *Testing structural equation models* (pp. 40-65). Newbury Park, CA: Sage.

Gould, S. J. (1981). *The mismeasure of man.* New York: Norton.

Gross, D., Conrad, B., Fogg, L., & Wothke, W. (1994). A longitudinal model of maternal self-efficacy, depression, and difficult temperament during toddlerhood. *Research in Nursing & Health, 17,* 207-215.

Gulick, E. E. (1992). Model for predicting work performance among persons with multiple sclerosis. *Nursing Research, 41,* 266-272.

Hawkes, J. M., & Holm, K. (1993). Gender differences in exercise determinants. *Nursing Research, 42,* 166-172.

Hayduk, L. A. (1987). *Structural equation modeling with LISREL: Essentials and advances.* Baltimore, MD: Johns Hopkins University Press.

Hayduk, L. A. (1990). Should model modifications be oriented toward improving data fit or encouraging creative and analytical thinking? *Multivariate Behavioral Research, 25,* 193-196.

Hayduk, L. A. (1996). *LISREL® issues, debates, and strategies.* Baltimore: Johns Hopkins University Press.

Herting, J. R. (1985). Multiple indicator models using LISREL. In H. M. Blalock Jr. (Ed.), *Causal models in the social sciences* (2nd ed., pp. 263-319). Hawthorne, NY: Aldine de Gruyter.

Hickey, M. L. (1993). Structural equation models: Latent variables. In B. H. Munro & E. B. Page (Eds.), *Statistical methods for health care research* (2nd ed., pp. 295-319). Philadelphia: J. B. Lippincott.

Hunter, J. E., & Gerbing, D. W. (1982). Unidimensional measurement, second order factor analysis, and causal models. *Research in Organizational Behavior, 4,* 267-320.

Johnson, J. L., Ratner, P. A., Bottorff, J. L., & Hayduk, L. A. (1993). An exploration of Pender's health promotion model using LISREL. *Nursing Research, 42,* 132-138.

Jöreskog, K. G. (1993). Testing structural equation models. In K. A. Bollen & J. S. Long (Eds.), *Testing structural equation models* (pp. 294-316). Newbury Park, CA: Sage.

Jöreskog, K. G., & Sörbom, D. (1989). *LISREL®7 user's reference guide.* Mooresville, IN: Scientific Software.

Lomax, R. G. (1983). A guide to multiple-sample structural equation modeling. *Behavior Research Methods and Instrumentation, 15,* 580-584.

Long, J. S. (1981). Estimation and hypothesis testing in linear models containing measurement error: A review of Jöreskog's model for the analysis of covariance structures. In P. V. Marsden (Ed.), *Linear models in social research* (pp. 209-256). Beverly Hills, CA: Sage.

Loveland-Cherry, C. J., Youngblut, J. M., & Leidy, N. W. K. (1989). A psychometric analysis of the Family Environment Scale. *Nursing Research, 38,* 262-266.

Lusk, S. L., Ronis, D. L., Kerr, M. J., & Atwood, J. R. (1994). Test of the Health Promotion Model as a causal model of workers' use of hearing protection. *Nursing Research, 43,* 151-157.

Mahon, N. E., Yarcheski, A., & Yarcheski, T. J. (1993). Health consequences of loneliness in adolescents. *Research in Nursing and Health, 16,* 23-31.

Marsden, P. V. (1981). Multiequation models. In P. V. Marsden (Ed.), *Linear models in social research* (pp. 117-122). Beverly Hills, CA: Sage.

Mercer, R. T., & Ferketich, S. L. (1990). Predictors of family functioning eight months following birth. *Nursing Research, 39,* 76-82.

Muthén, B. (1987). *LISCOMP: Analysis of linear structural equations with a comprehensive measurement model.* Mooresville, IN: Scientific Software.

Ratner, P. A., Bottorff, J. L., Johnson, J. L., & Hayduk, L. A. (1994). The interaction effects of gender within the Health Promotion Model. *Research in Nursing and Health, 17,* 341-350.

Ratner, P. A., Bottorff, J. L., Johnson, J. L., & Hayduk, L. A. (1996). Using multiple indicators to test the dimensionality of concepts in the Health Promotion Model. *Research in Nursing and Health, 19,* 237-247.

Renfroe, D. H., O'Sullivan, P. S., & McGee, G. W. (1990). The relationship of attitude, subjective norm, and behavioral intent to the documentation behavior of nurses. *Scholarly Inquiry for Nursing Practice: An International Journal, 4,* 47-60.

Schoenberg, R. (1987). *LINCS: Linear covariance structure analysis users guide.* Kensington, MD: RJS Software.

Searle, S. R. (1982). *Matrix algebra useful for statistics.* New York: John Wiley.

Stockwell, E. G. (1976). *The methods and materials of demography* (condensed ed.). San Diego, CA: Academic Press.

Sudman, S. (1983). Applied sampling. In P. H. Rossi, J. D. Wright, & A. B. Anderson (Eds.), *Handbook of survey research* (pp. 145-194). San Diego, CA: Academic Press.

Tanaka, J. S. (1987). "How big is big enough?" Sample size and goodness of fit in structural equation models with latent variables. *Child Development, 58,* 134-146.

Tanaka, J. S. (1993). Multifaceted conceptions of fit in structural equation models. In K. A. Bollen & J. S. Long (Eds.), *Testing structural equation models* (pp. 10-39). Newbury Park, CA: Sage.

Weaver, M. T. (1987). Perceived self-care agency: A LISREL factor analysis of Bickel and Hanson's questionnaire. *Nursing Research, 36,* 381-387.

Wright, L. K. (1990). Mental health in older spouses: The dynamic interplay of resources, depression, quality of the marital relationships, and social participation. *Issues in Mental Health Nursing, 11,* 49-70.

Yarcheski, A., & Mahon, N. E. (1989). A causal model of positive health practices: The relationship between approach and replication. *Nursing Research, 38,* 88-93.

9

Epidemiologic Designs

JANET C. MEININGER

What is epidemiology? The literal definition of epidemiology is very broad: the study of (*logos*) what comes upon (*epi*) the people (*demos*). It can be defined as the study of the distribution and determinants of health and disease in human population groups.

One of the distinguishing features of epidemiology is that the outcome of interest, the dependent variable, is health or disease status. As the interests of epidemiologists have expanded to include chronic as well as infectious diseases and health as well as disease, models used to explain the incidence of diseases have become more complex. Although the environment has always been an important component in epidemiologic investigations, we now understand that lifestyle factors and the social milieu are related to health status and to the prevention, cause, and course of disease.

Another distinguishing feature of epidemiology is that it is population based. Although individuals are usually the units of analysis, they are studied in the effort to understand the dynamics of health and disease in populations. Characteristically, the epidemiologist measures the frequency of cases in relation to the population in which they occur. The contribution that epidemiologists can make to clinical investigations is increasingly appreciated by both epidemiologists and clinicians. Even in a hospital-based study of patients, the relationship between the sample studied and the target population is of prime interest to the epidemiologist.

Epidemiologists use experimental and observational research designs. Epidemiologic methods have been applied in human experiments involving large populations to test the effectiveness of an intervention on a communitywide basis. The large-scale trial of the polio vaccine is a classic example of this approach (Francis et al., 1955). The Multiple Risk Factor Intervention Trial (MRFIT) is a more recent example of an epidemiologic experiment (Multiple Risk Factor Intervention Trial Group, 1982). The experimental method, in which the investigator has control over the independent variable and study participants are randomly assigned to concurrent groups, is not always an ethical or feasible approach to studying health outcomes in human populations. For this reason, epidemiologists have developed and adopted rigorous observational approaches to control the myriad sources of bias that can invalidate the study of naturally occurring events. In observational studies, participants are exposed to the independent variable because of self-selection, genetic endowment, or occupational exposures or those due to geographic location, such as naturally occurring fluoride in the water supply. Participants otherwise similar who have not been exposed are used for comparison. This emphasis on comparison is another distinguishing feature of epidemiology, but it is by no means unique to it. Because experimentation is not always feasible, epidemiologists rely on careful selection and rigorous comparison of groups that are observed concurrently while controlling extraneous sources of variation. They have also developed guidelines for making causal inferences from epidemiologic studies (Hill, 1965, 1971).

Selected observational designs and methods will be the focus of this chapter. Observational designs are divided into those that are longitudinal and those that are cross-sectional. In a cross-sectional study, all the measurements relate to one point in time, in contrast to the longitudinal approach, in which measurements relate to at least two points in time. In this chapter, two longitudinal designs will be discussed: cohort and case-comparison (case-control) studies. The emphasis will be placed on cohort studies because they are much more prevalent in the nursing research literature than case-comparison studies (Jacobsen & Meininger, 1985).

THE LOGIC OF COHORT AND CASE-COMPARISON STUDIES

Although the investigator does not manipulate the independent variable, the logic or flow of reasoning in a cohort study is the same as the logic of an experiment. Participants are measured or categorized on the basis of the independent variable and are followed forward for observation of the dependent variable. In a cohort study, it is established at the outset that all participants have not already experienced the outcome of interest (dependent variable). Thus, the time sequencing of events can be established; that is, it can be demonstrated that the independent variable preceded the occurrence of the dependent variable.

In a case-comparison study, the logic or flow of reasoning is in the opposite direction. Participants are categorized on the basis of the dependent variable (the outcome of interest). The purpose of the study is to search for factors in the past (independent variables) that may explain the outcome.

RETROSPECTIVE AND PROSPECTIVE APPROACHES

Formerly, it was common to equate cohort studies with the prospective approach and case-comparison studies with the retrospective approach. This is an oversimplification and is incorrect. *Prospective* and *retrospective* are terms that refer to the timing of the occurrence of the study variables in relation to the investigator's place in time.

A case-comparison study is always retrospective. The investigator begins the study after the occurrence of the dependent variable. Cohort studies, on the other hand, can be conducted prospectively or retrospectively, or a combination of both approaches can be used. In a retrospective cohort study (also known as a nonconcurrent follow-up study or a historical cohort study), the dependent variable has already occurred at the time the investigator initiates the study. The sequence of events can be reconstructed through records. Specifically, it can be established that individuals free of the outcome of interest were measured and classified on the basis of the independent variables and can be followed forward in time through the records for documentation of the occurrence of the dependent variable.

COHORT STUDIES

Overview

In a cohort study, participants are selected from a population and then examined to exclude those who have the outcome of interest. In other words, only those at risk of developing the outcome are studied. These individuals are measured and classified in terms of their characteristics (risk factors, exposures, independent variables). The participants are followed over time to observe the occurrence of the outcome. In the classical epidemiologic study, incidence of disease is the outcome of interest. The analysis consists of comparison of groups with different characteristics (values of the independent variables, risk factors, exposures). The incidence of disease among the exposed is compared with the incidence of disease among the nonexposed. A flowchart for a cohort study is presented in Figure 9.1.

The use of epidemiologic terminology to classify study designs in nursing research is not common. Although the dependent variable is often some aspect of health status, it is not usually a disease entity. Examples of studies that have cohort design features published by nurse researchers include Ballard and McNamara (1983), Jones (1981), Moore (1983), Norbeck and Tilden (1983), and Woods (1980).

Selection of Participants

Although we usually think of cohorts as birth cohorts—that is, individuals born in a particular year—there are many other kinds of cohorts. Three sources of cohorts are frequently sampled for epidemiologic investigations (MacMahon & Pugh, 1970):

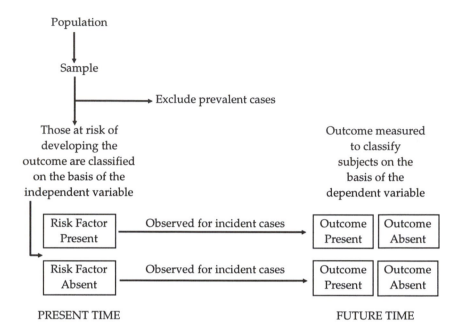

Figure 9.1. Flowchart for a Prospective Cohort Study

1. *Special exposure groups* are those receiving especially high doses of a substance hypothesized to have an impact on health outcomes. Examples include occupational groups exposed to chemicals, military groups exposed to herbicides, and survivors of the atomic bomb exposed to radiation.

2. *Captive participants* are those who are members of well-defined groups and can be readily contacted and/or followed through records. Examples include members of prepaid health plans, members of professional organizations or other occupational groups, insured persons, obstetric populations receiving prenatal care from a particular source, and students.

3. *Geographically defined cohorts* are often used in epidemiologic studies. For example, classic studies of cardiovascular disease were based in Framingham, Massachusetts; Evans County, Georgia; and Tecumseh, Michigan.

Those exposed to the independent variable in a cohort study are compared with participants from the same population who have not been exposed. Sometimes a comparison group is not readily available. This is the case when an entire group or community has been exposed to something such as an occupational hazard or radiation. In this case, another special cohort is selected on the basis of its being similar to the exposed group. Alternatively, rates for the exposed cohort are compared with rates for the general population. However, even with adjustment for age, sex, and race, comparison of a special cohort with the general population can be invalid because of selection bias.

After an appropriate source of study participants has been decided on, methods for selecting individuals from these sources are designed. Kelsey, Thompson, and Evans (1986) describe sampling procedures common to epidemiologic studies. The same principles of sample selection apply in this situation as in any other. A random procedure should be used in selection to ensure that each potential study participant has the same probability of being selected into the sample. This is not the same as randomization in an experimental study, and it does not achieve the same purpose. Random sampling is done to achieve a representative sample in relation to the target population. This is the basis for making statistical inferences about the population from sample data. Application of a statistical test allows the investigator to quantify the likelihood of error due to the chance process of sampling. Randomization, on the other hand, is a procedure used to ensure the internal validity of a study. The purpose of randomization is to use a chance process to decide group assignment and to distribute extraneous sources of variation evenly among the groups.

In an observational study, the investigator may want to include and exclude participants on the basis of certain characteristics to control for extraneous sources of variation. This is done as a means of ensuring internal validity, acknowledging that generalizability of the findings (external validity) will be limited to individuals similar to those studied. If participant restriction is used, it should be applied to the sampling frame. That is, the restriction should take place before the random selection of participants is carried out.

A common procedure is stratified sampling from mutually exclusive subgroups of the population. This is usually done for efficiency at the analysis stage to ensure that there are adequate numbers of participants in all categories of interest.

Table 9.1   Usual Data Presentation for a Cohort Study

Independent Variable	Dependent Variable		Total
	Outcome Occurs During Follow-up Period	Outcome Does Not Occur During Follow-up Period	
Exposed	a	b	a + b
Not exposed	c	d	c + d

Incidence among those exposed
to the independent variable $\quad = \quad \dfrac{a}{a+b} \times 1{,}000$ per unit time

Incidence among those not exposed
to the independent variable $\quad = \quad \dfrac{c}{c+d} \times 1{,}000$ per unit time

Relative risk = ratio of incidence rates $\quad = \quad \dfrac{\dfrac{a}{a+b}}{\dfrac{c}{c+d}}$

Measures of Effect

The basic structure of the analysis in a cohort study is the comparison of subgroups with different characteristics (independent variables, risk factors, exposures). Comparison of the incidence rates of the outcome in the exposed and unexposed groups is the key feature of the analysis. Table 9.1 displays a 2 × 2 table for dichotomized independent and dependent variables, calculation of the incidence rates for exposed and unexposed groups, and the relative risk, which is one of the measures of effect that can be calculated from cohort data.

The numerator of an incidence rate indicates the number of new cases of the outcome developing over a certain period of time (length of the follow-up period). The denominator in the calculation of an incidence rate indicates the number of individuals at risk of developing the outcome during the follow-up period. Obviously, the denominator does not usually remain stable over the length of the follow-up period, particularly if this period is lengthy. Individuals may drop out, die, or move away and will no longer be under observation. In addition, individuals may enter the study at slightly different times. For these reasons, the denominator in the calculation of an incidence rate can be expressed as person-time, which takes into account the number of participants followed and the duration of follow-up for each individual. In a study in which participants are followed over very long periods of time for the development of chronic diseases with long latency periods such as heart disease and cancer, the denominator is expressed as person-years. In studies with shorter follow-up periods such as investigation of pregnancy outcomes, person-weeks may be the appropriate unit. Person-days is suitable for epidemiologic investigations of acute outbreaks of health problems.

As demonstrated in Table 9.1, relative risk is based on the ratio of incidence rates. Other measures of effect that can be calculated from cohort data are those based on rate differences as opposed to rate ratios. Only the simplest forms of analysis of cohort data are presented to illustrate the structure of an epidemiologic follow-up study and its chief measure of effect, the relative risk. The reader is referred to Elandt-Johnson (1975) for further details on rates, and Fleiss (1981); Kelsey et al. (1986); Kleinbaum, Kupper, and Morgenstern (1982); Miettinen (1985); and Rothman (1986) for methods of adjustment for confounding, testing for interaction, analysis of matched data, and subgroup analysis.

Measurement of the Variables

Sources of information about the variables include physical exams; measurements of the environment; self-reports (interviews or responses to standardized tests); clinical, occupational, and school records; and records of births and deaths. As in any other empirical study, the investigator is concerned with the reliability and validity of the measurements. Reliable measures will minimize random errors; valid measures will minimize systematic errors. Methods for assessing reliability and validity depend on the type of instrument used and the level of the resulting measurement. The reader should refer to psychometric texts for background on reliability and validity.

TOWARD AN INTERNALLY VALID STUDY: MINIMIZING BIAS

The design of a study and the methods for carrying it out are aimed at minimizing bias. A study that is sufficiently unbiased is internally valid.

Likewise, the research report should include information necessary for a skilled reader to evaluate potential sources of bias and the degree to which internal validity is questionable. It follows that the critique should be targeted toward evaluating these same sources of potential bias.

First, bias will be defined. Three major sources of bias will then be described. Finally, specific examples will be presented to illustrate particular types of bias and steps that can be taken to avoid or minimize it.

Bias refers to a distortion in the estimate of an effect measure; that is, it is higher or lower than it would be if we could obtain a less biased or unbiased estimate. In a cohort study, the effect measure of major interest is the relative risk. If a study is biased, the relative risk is higher or lower than it should be, and if the distortion is large enough, this can lead to an erroneous inference about the importance of the relationship between a risk factor and a health outcome.

Long lists of potential sources of bias have been published (Feinstein, 1985; Sackett, 1979). Others have taken a more streamlined approach, subsuming the myriad sources of bias under major categories (Kleinbaum et al., 1982; Rothman, 1986). The latter approach will be used here. In the following sections, three major sources of bias will be discussed: selection, measurement, and confounding.

Selection Bias

Selection bias is a distortion in the estimate of effect resulting from the manner in which participants are selected into the study population.

In a cohort study, potential sources of selection bias include (a) flaws in the choice of groups to be compared; (b) inability to locate or nonresponse of participants selected into the sample, resulting in differential effects on the comparison groups; and (c) because the design is longitudinal, subsequent attrition of those who had initially agreed to participate, which changes the composition of comparison groups. Knowledge of these likely sources of selection bias in a cohort study leads to two questions that can be used in the design, execution, reporting, and critique of such a study.

Are the cohorts that are being compared drawn from the same or similar populations? A well-known source of selection bias, "the healthy worker effect," occurs when employed individuals are compared with those not employed (Fox & Collier, 1976; McMichael, 1976). Because individuals are selected in and out of the labor force on the basis of health status, employed people are healthier than the general population of the same age, race, and sex. Therefore, estimates of risk for adverse health outcomes based on comparisons of employed groups with the general population are biased toward the null hypothesis. Waldron, Herold, Dunn, and Staum (1982) demonstrate empirically that this effect operates for women. In a study of the effects of women's roles on their health status as reflected in their reports of illness episodes in a health diary, Woods (1980) took steps to avoid this source of bias. She excluded from the analysis those women who were currently unable to work due to illness or injury, those who had been unable to work for more than 6 months due to the illness or injury, and those who had to change the kind or amount of work due to some illness or injury.

Has there been differential selection or loss to follow-up from the study groups? In a follow-up or cohort study, the initial sample selection procedures are not as likely to introduce bias as is subsequent attrition of participants during the follow-up period. In cross-sectional and case-comparison studies, a major issue is selective survival—that is, over- or underrepresentation of exposure among those who survive long enough to be selected into the sample. On the other hand, the major source of selection bias in a cohort study is subsequent attrition of participants initially selected for study. The overall number of participants lost is not as critical as the differential loss from study subgroups consisting of particular independent-dependent variable combinations, as illustrated in the following numerical example.

Assume that an investigator hypothesized that high exposure to a factor would be associated with increased incidence of a health problem. In her sample of 100 participants, 50 were categorized as high on the exposure variable and 50 as low on this variable.

- *Scenario 1:* no attrition. If every participant remained in the study for the entire follow-up period of 1 year and in each category of the independent variable 10 new cases of the health problem developed, the incidence rate would be 20% per year in each group. The relative risk would be 1.00, as shown in Table 9.2A.
- *Scenario 2:* loss of four participants without differential loss from study subgroups. If one participant was lost from each of the four cells of the

table, as illustrated in Table 9.2B, the incidence rate would be 18.75% in each group. Although this result differs from that obtained in the previous scenario, in which no attrition occurred, an unbiased estimate of effect is obtained. The relative risk is 1.00 because there has been no differential loss of participants from the cells of the 2 × 2 table.

■ *Scenario 3:* loss of four participants with differential loss from study subgroups. If four participants were lost from one of the four cells of the table, as illustrated in Table 9.2C, the incidence rate would be 20% per year in the exposed group and 13% per year in the unexposed group. The relative risk in this case is biased upward. It is 1.54 instead of 1.00, which it would have been had there been no differential attrition from the groups. This is how selection bias operates.

In summary, even the loss of a large percentage of study participants would not introduce bias unless the loss were distributed differentially as illustrated above. This assumes, of course, that there are still enough observations for statistical precision.

Measurement Bias

Measurement bias, sometimes referred to as information bias, occurs when the exposure variable (independent variable) or outcome (dependent variable) is measured in a way that is systematically inaccurate and results in distortion in the estimate of effect.

The major sources of measurement bias are (a) a defective measuring instrument; (b) a procedure for ascertaining the outcome that is not sufficiently sensitive, specific, or both; (c) the likelihood of detecting the outcome dependent on exposure status; (d) selective recall of participants; and (e) lack of blind measurements. See Kelsey et al. (1986, pp. 285-352) for an overview of measurement issues in epidemiology.

Sensitivity and Specificity. In the classic epidemiologic study, both the exposure and the outcome are categorical variables, very often a dichotomy. In this case, concurrent validity can be expressed as sensitivity, specificity, predictive value positive, and predictive value negative. In making a decision about the source of information to use and the methods of data collection, a methodological pilot study is conducted to determine the best method when alternatives are available. A memo-

Table 9.2A   Illustration of Selection Bias in a Cohort Study: Scenario 1, No Attrition

	Dependent Variable		
	---	---	---
Independent Variable	*Health Problem Develops*	*Health Problem Does Not Develop*	*Total*
Exposed	10	40	50
Not exposed	10	40	50

NOTE: Incidence rate exposed group, 10/50 = .20 or 20 per 100 per year; incidence rate not exposed group, 10/50 = .20 or 20 per 100 per year; relative risk, .20/.20 = 1.00.

Table 9.2B   Illustration of Selection Bias in a Cohort Study: Scenario 2, Loss of Four Subjects Without Differential Loss From Study Subgroups

	Dependent Variable		
	---	---	---
Independent Variable	*Health Problem Develops*	*Health Problem Does Not Develop*	*Total*
Exposed	9	39	48
Not exposed	9	39	48

NOTE: Incidence rate exposed group, 9/48 = .1875 or 18.75 per 100 per year; incidence rate not exposed group, 9/48 = .1875 or 18.75 per 100 per year; relative risk, .1875/.1875 = 1.00.

Table 9.2C   Illustration of Selection Bias in a Cohort Study: Scenario 3, Loss of Four Subjects With Differential Loss From Study Subgroups

	Dependent Variable		
	---	---	---
Independent Variable	*Health Problem Develops*	*Health Problem Does Not Develop*	*Total*
Exposed	10	40	50
Not exposed	6	40	46

NOTE: Incidence rate exposed group, 10/50 = .20 or 20 per 100 per year; incidence rate not exposed group, 6/46 = .13 or 13 per 100 per year; relative risk, .20/.13 = 1.54.

Table 9.3   Validity of Self-Reported Circumcision Status

| | Physical Exam | | |
Subject's Statement	Circumcised	Not Circumcised	Total
Circumcised	38	6	44
Not circumcised	50	72	122
Total	88	78	166

NOTE: Sensitivity = 38/88 × 100% = 43.2%; specificity = 72/78 × 100% = 92.3%; predictive value positive = 38/44 × 100% = 86.4%; predictive value negative = 72/122 × 100% = 59.0%.

rable example is provided by Lilienfeld and Graham (1958) in their study of the relationship between cervical cancer and circumcision of the partner. The decision was whether to determine circumcision status on the basis of physical exam or to rely on participant report of circumcision status. Obviously, the method used would make a great deal of difference in the facilities, time, personnel, and participant cooperation necessary for data collection. An empirical comparison of the two methods was undertaken to determine the accuracy of the self-report approach compared with the superior but more costly physical exam; the results are presented in Table 9.3.

The specificity indicates that a high percentage of those who were not circumcised (on the basis of physical exam) said that they were not (92.3%). Sensitivity was much lower; less than half of those who were circumcised reported that they were (43.2%). Predictive values indicate how well the participant's statement reflects actual circumcision status as categorized by physical exam. The predictive value positive indicates that a relatively high percentage of those who said they were circumcised actually were (86.4%). The predictive value of a negative statement was lower; of those who said they were not circumcised, only 59% were not, as indicated by physical exam.

The purpose of this type of analysis is to quantify the magnitude and describe the direction of bias in the measurement of a dichotomous variable. Further information can be obtained from epidemiology texts (e.g., Mausner & Kramer, 1985; Weiss, 1986). See Meininger (1985) for an illustration of its use in methodological research.

Blindness. In an observational design, the investigator does not have control over the independent variables, so the issue of blindness in its manipulation is not relevant. What is extremely important in an observational study is blindness in the measurements. Participants should not be alerted to the specific hypotheses being investigated. In the process of obtaining informed consent from participants, the researcher should be certain that they understand the nature of the data collection procedures that will be used. However, there are usually several groups of variables measured in addition to the independent and dependent variables, such as those that will be used to describe the sample and control variables. It is not advisable to alert participants as to which ones are the key variables.

To maintain interviewer or observer blindness, the outcome should be measured without knowledge of the exposure status of the participant. This can be accomplished by using different data collectors for each set of variables and keeping them blind as to the status of the variable they are not measuring. Another approach that is often recommended is to keep data collectors blind as to the specific hypotheses under investigation.

Selective Recall. The potential for selective or biased recall by participant is not as great in a follow-up or cohort study as it is in a case-comparison study. This is because with the case-comparison approach, participants are asked to recall their history of exposure after the outcome has already occurred. If the outcome has not yet occurred, as is the case in a prospective cohort study, the nature of the outcome cannot distort the reporting of the exposure. In a retrospective cohort study, the outcome has occurred at the time the data collection begins. However, the measurements of the independent variable were recorded previously and thus cannot be biased by the outcome (although they may be invalid or unreliable measurements for other reasons). Comparability of quality of information in the study subgroups should be a major consideration in planning data collection (MacMahon & Pugh, 1970, pp. 257-261). The circumstances of obtaining information from participants (setting, length of interview, amount and content of probing) should be the same for all participants. Although comparability can never be ensured, the investigator can present evidence that there are no glaring differences between the groups. Noncomparability should be suspected if there are vastly different response rates for cases and controls (or exposed and unexposed participates in a cohort study).

Confounding Bias

Confounding bias occurs when the exposure-outcome relationship under investigation is interrelated with an extraneous (or confounding) factor. Unless the confounding factor is controlled in the design of the study or in its analysis, distortion in the estimate of effect will result. A confounding factor operates through its association with both the independent (exposure) and dependent (outcome) variables, producing an indirect statistical association.

In the planning phase of a research project, the investigator should identify factors that have the potential to confound the exposure-outcome relationship under investigation and propose strategies for eliminating or controlling their effects. Knowledge of the subject matter and a thorough review of the literature are essential for the identification of these potentially confounding factors.

An important distinction between confounding bias and other types of bias is that confounding is correctable at the analysis stage, whereas selection and information biases are usually difficult if not impossible to correct at that stage. Confounding bias can be eliminated, controlled, or minimized at (a) the design stage by restricting the study sample to participants with certain characteristics or by matching the comparison groups and (b) at the analysis stage by using a multivariable approach to the statistical analysis to adjust for the confounding factors or by examining the exposure-outcome relationship within specified levels or categories of the confounding factor (stratified analysis).

A study by Woods (1980) illustrates control of potentially confounding variables by restriction of participant characteristics and by statistical analysis of data with multiple regression. The independent variables were role proliferation, sex role norm traditionalism, role reinforcement, and failure. The dependent variable was number of illness episodes as recorded in a health diary over a 3-week period. Age, marital status, and source of health care were controlled by restricting the sample to married women between 20 and 40 years of age who were registrants at a particular family health clinic and lived within a 10-mile radius of it. At the analysis stage, multiple regression was used to examine the effects of the independent variables while controlling for other factors that could be correlated with number of illness episodes recorded: age, education, income, race, and number of children. Note that age was partially controlled at the design stage by restriction of the sample to those 20 to 40 years old. Any residual confounding due to age within this range was handled by adjusting for its effect statistically at the analysis stage.

Robarge, Reynolds, and Groothuis (1982) used sample restriction and matching to control for potentially confounding factors in their study of the relationship between twin births and child abuse. Sets of twins delivered at a specific hospital were included if their average birth weights exceeded 2,000 grams and if their 5-minute apgars were greater than or equal to 6; 38 sets of twins met these criteria. Two or three single-birth infants who met the same criteria were individually matched to each set of twins for race, socioeconomic status, and maternal age. Although several differences between the characteristics of the twins and single births were noted by the authors, these variables were not evaluated for their confounding effects as reported in the article. If these other variables had confounding effects on the relationship under investigation, it would have been appropriate to control for them in the analysis.

Matching. Although matching is generally considered a powerful tool for achieving control in an experimental or observational study, it should be pointed out that a matched design has disadvantages as well as advantages. Matching is a very useful strategy for managing variables that would have a strong confounding effect. It is particularly useful in a small study in which there is little hope of controlling for the factor in the analysis because of lack of overlap between the study groups on the confounding factors.

A major disadvantage of matching is the time and effort it can take to find appropriate matches, particularly when several matching factors are specified and close matches are desired. Of course, the time and effort required to find appropriate matches depends on the size of the participant pool available and on access to information on variables that constitute selection criteria. If matching participants are drawn from hospital records, a large pool of participants and information about them may be readily available, provided access to the records is not a problem. On the other hand, if neighborhood controls are sought and several matching factors are involved, an extensive search may be necessary to find appropriate matches. A disadvantage of individual matching in a case-control study is that it precludes the ability to examine the effects of the matching factor. The implication is that a matching factor should be a well-known confounder, one that has been thoroughly demonstrated in previous studies. One should never match intervening variables—that is, those that are intermediate in the causal pathway between the risk factor and the disease (MacMahon & Pugh, 1970, p. 256). Matching on the intervening variable would eliminate the ability to detect a relationship between the risk factor and the disease.

A final caution about matching: There is a possibility of overmatching (MacMahon & Pugh, 1970, p. 256; Miettinen, 1985, p. 77; Schlesselman, 1982, p. 110). One can think of overmatching as a loss of efficiency. Recall that in a matched analysis, information for testing the hypothesis is gained only from discordant pairs. If there is a strong relationship between outcome status and the matching factor (in a case-control study), this overmatching will inflate the number of concordant pairs that are discarded from the analysis.

In considering the pros and cons of matching, the researcher should keep in mind that individual matching (or matched pairs, triplets, and so on) is not the only alternative. Frequency matching should also be considered. The goal of frequency matching is to achieve balance between the comparison groups in the proportion with or without given characteristics. If there are similar distributions of age, sex, and race in the comparison groups, the confounding effects of these variables are controlled.

TOWARD A STATISTICALLY RELIABLE STUDY: MINIMIZING CHANCE ERROR, MAXIMIZING POWER

The second aim of research design is to minimize random error to ensure a reliable study, one that maximizes precision. Validity, the lack of systematic error, is of overriding concern to the researcher because a highly reliable but invalid study would yield a very precise estimate of the wrong answer. Assuming that a valid study is being designed, how would the researcher decide how large a sample is required to achieve statistical reliability? Sample size formulas and tables for epidemiologic studies are available (Schlesselman, 1974, 1982; Walter, 1977). These formulas relate the size of the sample to the following elements (Rothman, 1986):

1. Level of statistical significance (alpha error)
2. Chance of missing a real effect (beta error)
3. Magnitude of effect
4. Disease rate in the absence of exposure (or exposure prevalence in the absence of disease)
5. Relative size of the compared groups (i.e., ratio of cases to controls)

Holding everything else constant, the power of a study can be increased by increasing the sample size.

A major advantage of a case-control design over a cohort design is the number of participants required. Schlesselman (1982) provides the following illustration of a study designed to determine whether maternal exposure to estrogens around the time of conception results in an increased risk of congenital heart defects among offspring. If 8 heart defects occurred per 1,000 births among unexposed women, a cohort study would require observation of the pregnancy outcomes of 3,889 women exposed to estrogens and 3,889 unexposed women to detect a relative risk of 2.0 or greater. A case-control study would require only 188 cases and 188 controls if approximately 30% of women were exposed to estrogens around the time of conception. If one were interested in a specific heart defect that occurred at a rate of 2 cases per 1,000 births, a cohort study would require follow-up on approximately 15,700 women exposed to estrogens and 15,700 women not exposed to detect a twofold or greater increase in risk. The case-control approach would require only 188 cases and 188 controls. This illustration points out the advantages of a case-control study in terms of sample size, particularly for studying outcomes that occur rarely.

Keep in mind that sample size estimates are not nearly as accurate as they appear. They are based on figures that are "estimates"—more accurately described as "guesses." Furthermore, the simplest formulas do not take into account design and analysis nuances such as confounding, interaction, nonresponse, subgroup analysis, and matching.

HUMAN SUBJECTS ISSUES

Epidemiologic design issues that have the potential to impinge on the rights of human subjects are similar to those encountered in other types of research. An issue that has particular relevance to the design of epidemiologic studies is the use of records to define a population from which to sample or to find particular types of participants.

CAUSAL INFERENCES BASED ON EPIDEMIOLOGIC EVIDENCE

One of the major aims of epidemiologic research is to study the etiology of disease. Implicit in this aim is the need to infer cause-and-effect relationships. Because epidemiologists often investigate problems that cannot be studied experimentally with human subjects and because animal models are not always appropriate, rigorous observational designs are the specialty of the epidemiologist. Rarely is there certainty about the link between a putative cause and an adverse health outcome. Rather, risk factors are studied in relation to the probability of a specified change in health status.

In addition to critiquing the internal and external validity of each individual study, the following criteria are used to review, evaluate, and synthesize findings from more than one study on the same topic (Hill, 1965, 1971).

1. *The strength of the association:* The magnitude of an effect is used in evaluating the strength of an association. The measure of effect in most epidemiologic studies is the relative risk. It is more difficult to find alternative explanations for strong associations. Note that a probability value does not convey information about the strength of an association; a very weak relationship can be highly statistically significant if the sample size is large enough.

2. *Dose-response effect:* An increasing frequency of disease with an increasing level of exposure to the risk factor (dose) points toward a causal association, but there may be alternative explanations for this finding (Weiss, 1981). On the other hand, its absence is not evidence against a causal association. For instance, a causal relationship may take the form of a threshold effect rather than a dose-response effect.

3. *Lack of temporal ambiguity:* The risk factor must precede the development of the outcome. For instance, if an association is observed between depression and chronic illness, one could not consider depression a risk factor unless it preceded the occurrence of the disease. In other words, a purported risk factor must be identifiable as an antecedent to the outcome rather than a consequence.

4. *Consistency:* If findings are replicated, this is good evidence for a causal association, but it is neither necessary nor sufficient evidence. Lack of consistency may be due to differences in methods and samples and to secular changes. On the other hand, consistent results may be found in several studies that are biased in the same direction.

5. *Coherence of the evidence:* This means that the results are not inconsistent with known facts. However, ignorance about a problem may impede the ability to evaluate inconsistencies.

6. *Biological plausibility:* This evidence is helpful, but an association may be judged to be causal before we have enough knowledge to state how the cause leads to the effect. In meeting this criterion, we often need to rely on laboratory studies of disease models to understand the pathways through which the risk factor operates.

7. *Specificity of the association:* This criterion implies that a risk factor is associated with only one disease, and/or a disease is associated with one risk factor. Specificity is not usually an appropriate criterion because most health outcomes have multiple causes and many risk factors have multiple effects.

These criteria should be used as guidelines for organizing evidence of causality rather than as a checklist. A recent example is provided by Matthews and Haynes (1986). This discussion serves only as an introduction to views held by some epidemiologists. The reader is referred to the following references for more extensive background on the topic: Evans (1976, 1978), Lilienfeld and Lilienfeld (1980), MacMahon and Pugh (1970), and Susser (1973).

SUMMARY

Experimental and observational designs are used in epidemiology, although the emphasis is on observational approaches. Even when an experimental design is employed in an epidemiologic study, it is usually carried out in an uncontrolled environment. Because experimentation is not always an ethical or feasible approach to studying health outcomes in human populations, epidemiologists have developed and adopted rigorous observational approaches to control the myriad sources of bias that can invalidate the study of naturally occurring events.

The emphasis in this chapter has been on cohort designs. Studies with cohort design features are much more prevalent in the nursing literature than are case-comparison studies. The major advantage of a cohort study is that study participants are observed for the occurrence of the outcome. Thus, the risk factor can be identified as an antecedent to the outcome rather than as a consequence. The major advantage of a case-comparison study is in the much smaller sample size required. If carefully designed and executed, this can be a very powerful approach.

Three sources of bias that could threaten the internal validity of an epidemiologic study have been discussed: selection, measurement, and confounding. Approaches to avoiding or adjusting for these biases have been delineated. Finally, guidelines for drawing causal inferences from epidemiologic data were presented.

REFERENCES

Ballard, S., & McNamara, R. (1983). Quantifying nursing needs in home health care. *Nursing Research, 32,* 236-241.

Elandt-Johnson, R. C. (1975). Definition of rates: Some remarks on their use and misuse. *American Journal of Epidemiology, 102,* 267-271.

Evans, A. S. (1976). Causation and disease: The Henle-Koch postulates revisited. *Yale Journal of Biology and Medicine, 49,* 175-195.

Evans, A. S. (1978). Causation and disease: A chronological journey. *American Journal of Epidemiology, 108,* 249-258.

Feinstein, A. R. (1985). *Clinical epidemiology: The architecture of clinical research.* Philadelphia: W. B. Saunders.

Fleiss, J. L. (1981). *Statistical methods for rates and proportions.* New York: John Wiley.

Fox, A. J., & Collier, P. F. (1976). Low mortality rates in industrial cohort studies due to selection for work and survival in the industry. *British Journal of Preventive and Social Medicine, 30,* 225-230.

Francis, T. J., Korns, R. F., Voight, R. B., Biosen, M., Hemphill, F. M., Napier, J. A., & Tolchinsky, E. (1955). An evaluation of the 1954 poliomyelitis vaccine trials: Summary report. *American Journal of Public Health, 45,* 1-63.

Hill, A. B. (1965). The environment and disease: Association or causation? *Proceedings of the Royal Society of Medicine, 58,* 295-300.

Hill, A. B. (1971). *Principles of medical statistics* (9th ed.). New York: Oxford University Press.

Jacobsen, B. S., & Meininger, J. C. (1985). Designs and methods of published nursing research: 1956-1983. *Nursing Research, 34,* 306-312.

Jones, C. (1981). Father to infant attachment: Effects of early contact and characteristics of the infant. *Research in Nursing and Health, 4,* 193-200.

Kelsey, J. L., Thompson, W. D., & Evans, A. S. (1986). *Methods in observational epidemiology.* New York: Oxford University Press.

Kleinbaum, D. G., Kupper, L. L., & Morgenstern, H. (1982). *Epidemiologic methods: Principles and quantitative methods.* Belmont, CA: Wadsworth.

Lilienfeld, A. M., & Graham, S. (1958). Validity of determining circumcision status by questionnaire as related to epidemiological studies of cancer of the cervix. *Journal of the National Cancer Institute, 21,* 713-720.

Lilienfeld, A. M., & Lilienfeld, D. E. (1980). *Foundations of epidemiology.* New York: Oxford University Press.

MacMahon, B., & Pugh, T. F. (1970). *Epidemiology: Principles and methods.* Boston: Little, Brown.

Matthews, K. A., & Haynes, S. G. (1986). Type A behavior pattern and coronary disease risk: Update and critical evaluation. *American Journal of Epidemiology, 123,* 923-960.

Mausner, J. S., & Kramer, S. (1985). *Epidemiology: An introductory text* (2nd ed.). Philadelphia: W. B. Saunders.

McMichael, A. J. (1976). Standardized mortality ratios and the "healthy worker effect": Scratching beneath the surface. *Journal of Occupational Medicine, 18,* 165-168.

Meininger, J. C. (1985). Validity of Type A behavior scales for employed women. *Journal of Chronic Diseases, 38,* 375-383.

Miettinen, O. S. (1985). *Theoretical epidemiology: Principles of occurrence research in medicine.* New York: John Wiley.

Moore, D. (1983). Prepared childbirth and marital satisfaction during the antepartum and postpartum period. *Nursing Research, 32,* 73-79.

Multiple Risk Factor Intervention Trial Group. (1982). Multiple Risk Factor Intervention Trial: Risk factor changes and mortality results. *Journal of the American Medical Association, 248,* 1465-1477.

Norbeck, J. S., & Tilden, V. P. (1983). Life stress, social support and emotional disequilibrium in complications of pregnancy: A prospective multivariate study. *Journal of Health and Social Behavior, 24,* 30-46.

Robarge, J. P., Reynolds, Z. B., & Groothuis, J. R. (1982). Increased child abuse in families with twins. *Research in Nursing and Health, 5,* 199-203.

Rothman, K. J. (1986). *Modern epidemiology.* Boston: Little, Brown.

Sackett, D. L. (1979). Bias in analytic research. *Journal of Chronic Diseases, 32,* 51-63.

Schlesselman, J. J. (1974). Sample size requirements in cohort and case-control studies of disease. *American Journal of Epidemiology, 99,* 381-384.

Schlesselman, J. J. (1982). *Case-control studies: Design, conduct and analysis.* New York: Oxford University Press.

Susser, M. (1973). *Causal thinking in the health sciences: Concepts and strategies in epidemiology.* New York: Oxford University Press.

Waldron, I., Herold, J., Dunn, D., & Staum, R. (1982). Reciprocal effects of health and labor force participation among women: Evidence from two longitudinal studies. *Journal of Occupational Medicine, 24,* 126-132.

Walter, S. D. (1977). Determination of significant relative risks and optimal sampling procedures in prospective and retrospective comparative studies of various sizes. *American Journal of Epidemiology, 105,* 387-397.

Weiss, N. S. (1981). Inferring causal relationships: Elaboration of the criterion of "dose-response." *American Journal of Epidemiology, 113,* 487-490.

Weiss, N. S. (1986). *Clinical epidemiology: The study of the outcome of illness.* New York: Oxford University Press.

Woods, N. F. (1980). Women's roles and illness episodes: A prospective study. *Research in Nursing and Health, 3,* 137-145.

ADDITIONAL READINGS

Textbooks and Study Guides

Fletcher, R. H., Fletcher, S. W., & Wagner, E. H. (1987). *Clinical epidemiology: The essentials.* Baltimore: Williams & Wilkins.

Friedman, G. D. (1987). *Primer of epidemiology* (3rd ed.). New York: McGraw-Hill.

Hennekens, C. H., & Buring, J. E. (1987). *Epidemiology in medicine.* Boston: Little, Brown.

Morton, R. F., & Hebel, J. R. (1984). *A study guide to epidemiology and statistics.* Rockville, MD: Aspen.

Sackett, D. L., Haynes, R. B., & Tugwell, P. (1985). *Clinical epidemiology: A basic science for clinical medicine.* Boston: Little, Brown.

Slome, C., Brogan, D., Eyres, S., & Lednar, W. (1982). *Basic epidemiological methods and biostatistics: A workbook.* Monterey, CA: Wadsworth Health Sciences.

Designing Observational Studies

Cole, P. (1979). The evolving case-control study. *Journal of Chronic Diseases, 32,* 15-27.

Copeland, K. T., Checkoway, H., McMichael, A. J., & Holbrook, R. H. (1977). Bias due to misclassification in the estimation of relative risk. *American Journal of Epidemiology, 105,* 488-495.

Feinleib, M. (1987). Biases and weak associations. *Preventive Medicine, 16,* 150-164.

Feinstein, A. R. (1985). Experimental requirements and scientific principles in case-control studies. *Journal of Chronic Diseases, 38,* 127-133.

Freeman, J., & Hutchinson, G. B. (1980). Prevalence, incidence and duration. *American Journal of Epidemiology, 112,* 707-723.

Greenland, S. (1977). Response and follow-up bias in cohort studies. *American Journal of Epidemiology, 106,* 184-187.

Hartge, P., Brinton, L. A., Rosenthal, J. F., Cahill, J. I., Hoover, R. M., & Waksberg, J. (1984). Random digit dialing in selecting a population-based control group. *American Journal of Epidemiology, 120,* 825-833.

Hayden, G. F., Kramer, M. S., & Horwitz, R. I. (1982). The case-control study: A practical review for the clinician. *Journal of the American Medical Association, 247,* 326-331.

Kalish, L. A., & Begg, C. D. (1987). Evaluation of efficient designs for observational epidemiologic studies. *Biometrics, 43,* 145-167.

Kramer, M. S., & Boivin, J. F. (1987). Toward an "unconfounded" classification of epidemiologic research design. *Journal of Chronic Diseases, 40,* 683-688.

McKinley, S. M. (1977). Pair matching: A reappraisal of a popular technique. *Biometrics, 33,* 725-735.

Miettinen, O. S. (1970). Matching and design efficiency in retrospective studies. *American Journal of Epidemiology, 91,* 111-117.

Nair, R. C. (1984). Statistical problems associated with cohort studies of workers in an industry. *Annals of the Academy of Medicine, 13* (suppl.), 317-320.

Schlesselman, J. J. (1974). Sample size requirements in cohort and case-control studies of disease. *American Journal of Epidemiology, 99,* 381-384.

Spitzer, W. O. (1985). Ideas and words: Two dimensions for debates on case controlling. *Journal of Chronic Diseases, 38,* 541-542.

Szklo, M. (1987). Design and conduct of epidemiologic studies. *Preventive Medicine, 16,* 142-149.

Thompson, W. D., Kelsey, J. L., & Walter, S. D. (1982). Cost and efficiency in the choice of matched and unmatched study designs. *American Journal of Epidemiology, 116,* 840-851.

Walter, S. D. (1976). The estimation and interpretation of attributable risk in health research. *Biometrics, 32,* 829-849.

Designing Clinical Trials

Chalmers, T., Smith, H., Blackburn, B., Silverman, B., Schroeder, B., Reitman, D., & Ambroz, A. (1981). A method for assessing the quality of a randomized control trial. *Controlled Clinical Trials, 2,* 31-49.

Ellenberg, S. S. (1984). Randomization designs in comparative clinical trials. *New England Journal of Medicine, 310,* 1404-1408.

Friedman, L. M., Furberg, C. D., & DeMets, D. L. (1985). *Fundamentals of clinical trials* (2nd ed.). Littleton, MA: PSG.

Frieman, J. A., Chalmers, T. C., Smith, H., Jr., & Kuebler, R. (1978). The importance of beta, the Type II error and sample size in the design and interpretation of the randomized control trial: Survey of 71 "negative" trials. *New England Journal of Medicine, 299,* 690-694.

Meinert, C. (1986). *Clinical trials.* New York: Oxford University Press.

Mosteller, F., Gilbert, J. P., & McPeek, B. (1980). Reporting standards and research strategies for controlled trials: Agenda for the editor. *Controlled Clinical Trials, 1,* 37-58.

Pocock, S. J. (1983). *Clinical trials: A practical approach.* Chichester: John Wiley.

Pocock, S. J. (1985). Current issues in the design and interpretation of clinical trials. *British Medical Journal, 296,* 39-42.

10

Methodological Studies: Instrument Development

MERLE H. MISHEL

Instrumentation, the process of developing a measure of a concept, is of major importance in the structure of a scientific investigation. As discussed in prior chapters, all decisions concerning the structure and conduct of a research study are done to enhance control. The more control evidenced in the methodology of a study, the more confidence the researcher can have in the validity of the findings. The more control that exists over sources of extraneous variables, the fewer alternative explanations can be posited for the study findings.

The strength of study findings is not based solely on choice of design, sampling decisions, and other means of controlling extraneous vari-

AUTHOR'S NOTE: I would like to thank Dr. Carrie Jo Braden for her expert assistance in the discussion of scaling methods and Dr. Mary R. Lynn for her outstanding skill in editing this chapter.

ables; it is also due to the amount of control that exists within the indexes of the conceptual variables. When the concept of control is applied to measurement, it refers to the ability of instruments to index the concepts with precision, accuracy, and sensitivity. *Precision* refers to the exactness with which the instrument defines the concept, *accuracy* refers to the correctness or truthfulness with which the instrument reports the concept, and *sensitivity* refers to the ability of the instrument to discriminate levels of the concept. The more precise, accurate, and sensitive the instrument is, the more control exists within the study. If the instrument is not very precise, then interpretation of the findings will be confounded. When instruments lack accuracy, the hypothesized relationships between variables will appear weaker than if the variables were measured by more accurate tools.

In the arena of instrumentation, the concept of control is translated into the term *measurement error,* the aspect of scores that does not reflect how participants differ in the amount of the concept being indexed but that reflects scores due to some other influence. Observed scores on a measure equal true score plus error ($x = T + e$). Inaccuracy and imprecision in a measure refer to the amount of measurement error in that instrument. The net effect of measurement error is to lower the degree of correlation. The errors in a set of measures are not correlated, and they make up the portion of the relationship that the set of tests do not have in common. Thus, they reduce or attenuate the degree of relation (Guilford, 1936). Because of the attenuation effect, it is necessary to construct instruments with as little measurement error as possible to enhance the strength of the findings.

This chapter will discuss instrument development from the perspective of enhancing control—that is, of decreasing measurement error. Each step in the process of instrument development will be presented in terms of how the activity should be approached to enhance the accuracy, precision, and sensitivity of the final instrument, thereby minimizing measurement error. Measurement error is not an issue to be considered only when reliability and validity testing enter the process of instrument development. Rather, enhancing control by minimizing measurement error permeates each step of the instrument development process. How each step in the instrumentation process relates to the issue of measurement error will be discussed. Published nursing instrumentation studies will be used as examples of specific instrumentation topics, but I take no position concerning the overall quality of any study used as an example.

The field of instrument development is too varied and complex to be presented in a single chapter; thus, only major portions of the instrument development process will be discussed here. The reader is referred to other authors for further information throughout the discussion.

Measures in nursing can be used for different purposes, such as discriminating between participants, predicting the results of some tests, or evaluating change over time. Norm-referenced measures are constructed for the purpose of discriminating between participants. A specific characteristic is measured in such a way that differences among people who possess differing quantities of that characteristic will be evidenced on the scale. A major feature of this type of measure is variance—that is, the spread of people across a possible range of scores. The goal is to achieve a distribution of scores that resembles a normal curve (Waltz, Strickland, & Lenz, 1984). A predictive index, often referred to as a *criterion-referenced measure,* is constructed for the purpose of determining whether an individual has or has not achieved a predetermined set of target behaviors. The test categorizes individuals into a set of predefined behaviors and can use an external criterion, available either concurrently or prospectively, to determine whether individuals have been classified correctly. A third possible purpose of a nursing instrument is as an evaluation index, for measuring the magnitude of longitudinal change in an individual or a group on a dimension of interest. Such instruments are often used in determining treatment benefit in clinical trials (Kirshner & Guyatt, 1985).

Because the major steps in scale development differ for these different measurement frameworks, it is important that a chapter such as this limit its scope to one framework. The norm-referenced approach, which is the construction of a discriminative index, includes the majority of personality, attitudinal, affective, and cognitive constructs that are developed in nursing. This chapter will focus on methods of test construction based on the summative or linear model (Nunnally, 1978). In this model, items are summed to produce a test score. According to Nunnally (1978), there is no general competitor to the linear model. Any measure that is a linear combination of individual responses will fit the principles to be discussed even if the measure has dichotomous items or items scorable on more than 2 points.

MEASUREMENT ERROR

Zeller and Carmines (1980) present an observation by Hauser in which he proposes that it is inadequate measurement, more than inadequate concepts or hypotheses, that has tormented researchers and that accounts for mediocre explanations from investigators. To develop adequate measures, the researcher must understand the nature of the inaccuracy in measurement so that he or she can avoid it as much as possible.

Errors in measurement are of two types: random error and systematic error. *Random error* refers to random influences that tend to make measurements differ from time to time or cause variations in performance from item to item on a single measure (Nunnally, 1978). Some sources of random error in measures are caused by chance elements with unknown causes, temporary circumstances such as fluctuations in memory or mood, momentary states such as irritability or tension, or fluctuating environmental conditions such as heat or noise that affect the object measured or the measuring instrument. Random errors of measurement are never completely eliminated, but efforts can be made to reduce errors as much as possible so that measures are consistent and stable. Random error affects the consistency of measurements—that is, their reliability. Because the reliability of a measure depends on its degree of consistency and repeatability, as the amount of random error in a measure increases, reliability is reduced (Zeller & Carmines, 1980). An important characteristic of random error is that it causes the measure to appear disorganized, with scores leaning one way at one time and another way at another time. Reliability is determined by the degree of nonrandom error, or true scores, in the instrument (Kerlinger, 1986).

Systematic error refers to systematic influences that distort the scale scores. This source of error has a biasing influence on measurement procedures and influences an instrument's validity. For example, if a thermometer yields exactly the same reading for an individual on 10 different occasions, it is reliable even if it is later discovered that the instrument provided a temperature of 103 degrees Fahrenheit for a patient whose actual temperature was 100. Thus the thermometer, as a measure, contains a systematic error, because repeated readings register three degrees higher than they should be. This systematic error clearly compromises the validity of the measurement instrument (Zeller & Carmines, 1980).

Systematic error is due to some characteristic that is regularly tapped by the measure other than that for which the instrument was constructed. If the instrument uniformly stimulates social desirability, encourages always positive or always negative responses, or includes items that measure knowledge skills or abilities irrelevant to the concept being measured, the instrument contains systematic error (Waltz et al., 1984; Zeller & Carmines, 1980). Other sources of systematic error are not associated with the instrument but with enduring aspects of the respondent. Such sources include characteristics that are likely to influence responses to the measure in a consistent manner, such as a consistently negative attitude, poor memory, or physical disability. Some of these sources of systemic error can also be implicated in random error. Another major source of systematic error is a situation in which the set of items in a measure index more than the intended theoretical concept or represent an entirely different concept (Carmines & Zeller, 1979).

Because systemic error has a consistent distorting effect on the scores of an instrument, it is difficult to detect. This source of bias causes a problem with validity because all results obtained with the instrument are contaminated and the accuracy with which the intended concept was indexed is open to question.

To formulate the idea of measurement error, it is necessary to understand the role of variance in measurement. Any set of measures has a total variance calculated after determining the mean and standard deviation. The total variance of a measure includes variance due to several causes. The total variance includes true variances, error variance, and systematic variance.

Reliability (r_{tt}) is the proportion of true variance to the total variance of the measure. Reliability also is the proportion of error variance to total variance subtracted from 1.00 (Kerlinger, 1986).

$$r_{tt} = \frac{V_{oo}}{V_t} \qquad r_{tt} = 1 - \frac{V_e}{V_t}$$

As seen in Figure 10.1, in a measure of anxiety, the reliability of the measure is 80, because of the total variance, 80% is true variance and 20% is error variance.

Validity is the proportion of total variance of a measure that is common variance, or the variance that the items have in common—that is, that which reflects the concept under measurement. Also included in the total variance of a measure are the random error and systematic

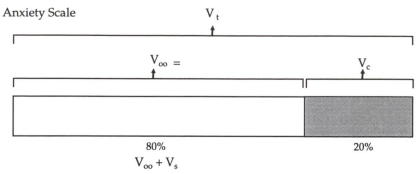

Anxiety Scale V_t

$V_{oo} =$

V_c

80%   20%
$V_{oo} + V_s$

V_t = Total variance
V_{oo} = True variance
V_e = Random error variance
V_s = Systematic error variance

Figure 10.1

variance. As explained earlier, systematic variance must be separated
from total variance to determine the validity of the instrument. Validity
(r_{xy}) can be viewed as that part of the total variance of a measure that is
neither systematic variance nor error variance (Kerlinger, 1986).

$$r_{xy} = \frac{V_t}{V_t} - \frac{V_s}{V_t} - \frac{V_e}{V_t}$$

where

V_t = total variance,
V_s = systematic error variance,
V_e = random error variance

Figure 10.2 represents the partitioning of error that must be removed
from total variance to obtain an estimate of the reliability and validity
of an instrument. A paradox exists between random error and systematic error. With systematic error, a measure will appear as more reliable
because all items will be similarly affected by the method artifact, yet
in such a case the measure will be less valid. With the opposite case, in
which items are differentially affected by a chance element—that is,
random error—reliability will be relatively lower, but the instrument
will perform with greater validity. However, because reliability always
exceeds validity, although it can be lowered in the case of random error,
its mathematical relationship with validity will be preserved. Thus,

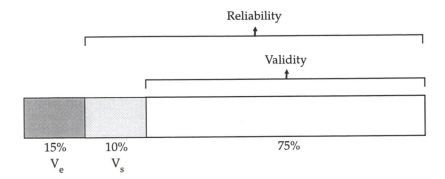

Figure 10.2

reliability and validity are inextricably bound, and both are influenced by the two types of measurement error (Bohrnstedt, 1970). Consistency among items does not indicate that the tool adequately measures the intended concept, only that whatever it does measure, it measures accurately. An instrument that has low reliability does not represent anything systematically; it cannot represent the concept as intended. Thus, for a measure to be valid, it must also be reliable. Reliability is a necessary, but not sufficient, condition for validity (Carmines & Zeller, 1979).

Measurement error, whether random or systematic, is problematic because it tends to attenuate the relationship between variables, thus weakening the study findings. Both types of error must be controlled to the greatest degree possible. There are well-known and -established methods to test for the presence of random and systematic error in reliability and validity testing procedures. Another approach is to attend to minimizing these error effects in the development of measures. Attention to instrumentation procedures can aid in ensuring that all possible steps are implemented to minimize error and to develop reliable and valid measures.

Concept Clarification

The term *concepts* will be used in this chapter to refer to highly abstract phenomena that can be considered concepts or constructs. The labels *concept* and *construct* will be considered interchangeable. The process of defining the structure of the concept must precede, and be separate from, the development of measurement techniques. The first step in the development of an instrument is to clarify the concept to be measured. This is initiated by developing the theoretical definition and then specifying the variables derived from that definition. Waltz et al. (1984) suggest that to formulate a theoretical definition for a concept, investigators must translate their informal working definition into a theoretical definition that is precise, understandable to others, and appropriate for the context in which the term will be used. Walker and Avant (1983) present three basic approaches to clarifying a concept for which an instrument will be developed: analysis, synthesis, and derivation. Each will be discussed, because each is useful in clarifying and defining a concept.

Concept analysis is a useful method for defining a concept when a body of theoretical literature exists. The researcher can carefully review the literature and attend to consistencies and inconsistencies in the use of the concept, the different sources of meaning given to the concept, and subtle differences in how the concept is defined. Before surveying the literature, it is useful to develop a preliminary definition using examples of the concept as it occurs in nursing situations. This helps to indicate the purpose for which the concept is being defined and operationalized.

At the conclusion of a concept analysis based primarily on a literature review, the researcher should be aware that knowledge of the concept is limited to what is available, tested, or found useful as a definition by others. Literature reviews do not facilitate the emergence of new, creative definitions. The use of concepts from other fields may not be applicable to nursing. Concepts may be defined differently in other areas of the social sciences and may have different dimensions and components than they would have in nursing. Sensitivity to this issue is necessary to prevent abstracting definitions from other fields without raising questions about the appropriateness of the definitions when moving concepts from one field to another.

Concept synthesis is a method for developing concepts based on clinical observation; thus it is data based (Walker & Avant, 1983). The process of concept synthesis is useful for building theory and permits the theorist to use clinical experience as a place to begin. Concept synthesis is based on the exploration of a phenomenon using qualitative methodologies. Data are gathered from clinical interviews and observations and are examined for similarities and differences.

Concept synthesis is a useful means for developing or clarifying a concept in the clinical field. Because the concept emerges from clinical data, there is no question as to its relevance in nursing. In this type of method, there is little question about whether the definition of the concept fits the phenomenon as it exists in nursing. Because this concept emerged from nursing practice and from nursing clinical data, it is grounded in clinical data and thus is a valid description of clinical phenomena (Glaser, 1978).

It is important to note that very few instrumentation studies in nursing have used qualitative methodologies to clarify concepts. It is suggested that qualitative methodologies be used more frequently as a means to generate concepts for measurement within nursing research.

Concept derivation consists of moving a concept from one field of interest to another. In the process of borrowing a concept, the concept must be redefined when moved to a new area of study. Creativity and imagination are necessary in redefining a concept; this is much more than simply assigning a slight modification to it. When a concept is placed into a new field, the definition of it must be innovative, relevant, and meaningful to the new field (Walker & Avant, 1983). When the nursing researcher is considering concept derivation, fields closely related to nursing are preferable and should be those initially explored (Walker & Avant, 1983). Disciplines such as medicine and social work may house relevant concepts, and because these disciplines are closely related to nursing, modification of the concept may be slight or even unnecessary. Because there are no rules governing where to search for concepts, the natural and behavioral sciences may also be considered as sources. The main advantage of concept derivation as a strategy is that the researcher need not start from scratch. The use of concepts from other fields often speeds the creative process.

THEORETICAL DEFINITION

After clarifying a concept, the researcher states the theoretical definition and specifies dimensions of the concept. On the basis of the literature review, the inductive qualitative study, or from deriving a concept from another field, the researcher is able to identify the dimensions of the concept, which are then specified in the theoretical definition.

Following the theoretical definition, the researcher generates relational statements from the literature or inductive work to provide explanations for the concept and embed it into a theoretical or conceptual framework. Relational statements indicate the association of the concepts. All concepts should be paired with relational statements because this provides a method for testing the construct validity of an instrument.

OPERATIONALIZATION

According to Waltz et al. (1984), the process of operationalizing a concept involves several related steps: (a) developing the theoretical definition, (b) specifying variables derived from the theoretical definition, (c) identifying observable indicators, and (d) developing a means for measuring the indicators.

Movement from the theoretical definition of the concept to the development of the measure happens through the process of operationalization. This is a process of determining and defining how the concept will be measured. In the process of operationalization, the researcher moves from the abstract, which is the concept, to the concrete, the specific observables or items that will index the concept. To operationalize the concept, the researcher specifies the empirical indicators and procedures used to measure it.

The process of moving from a theoretical to an operational definition involves a major component of the validity of the instrument. When the researcher moves from a conceptual variable to an operational variable, the attempt is to structure an operational variable that is isomorphic with the theoretical definition. Isomorphism indicates the degree to which the operational variable is equivalent to the conceptual variable. The term *operational variable* refers to the specific items that will be generated to address the specific aspects of the concept. Operational variables are the actual items developed for the concept. Because concepts are abstract, one never tests them directly but tests only the operational variables. The definitions of the conceptual variable are used as a guide for selecting the content of the operational variable. The relationship between the conceptual and the operational variable is called the *measurement assumption*.

MEASUREMENT ASSUMPTION

The measurement assumption is the supposition that the operational variable is a clear representation of the conceptual variable. This is the center of the validity issue. Validity testing is an attempt to support the measurement assumption. Validity is concerned with the extent to which one can have confidence in the operational variable as a replica of the conceptual variable. Until a measurement assumption is made and until the operational variable is defined as an indicator of the conceptual variable, the numbers indexed by the operational variable are relatively meaningless.

One test of the measurement assumption is concerned with the content validity of the instrument. Content validity depends on the extent to which an empirical measurement reflects a specific domain of content (Carmines & Zeller, 1979). Specific steps involved in attaining a content-valid measure will be addressed later in this section. At this point, it should be recognized that items should be developed to reflect isomorphism with the concept and should adequately tap the conceptual domain. Content validity is built into a scale from the initial steps through construction or selection of appropriate items (Anastasi, 1976). Items are designed with the goals of maintaining congruency with the concept definition and of adequately sampling the item universe. When items are inclusive of all dimensions of the conceptual domain, the likelihood of establishing a content-valid measure is enhanced.

A second test of the measurement assumption is concerned with the construct validity of the instrument. Construct validity depends on the degree to which the empirical measure performs according to theoretical predictions. To test the measurement assumption, the conceptual variable must be embedded in theory. A concept in itself has little explanatory value and becomes meaningful only when placed in a context. For example, a high or low level of anxiety is uninterpretable unless discussed as related to a certain outcome associated with another concept or influenced by another event.

By embedding the conceptual variable into a theoretical statement, a conceptual hypothesis can be formed. This conceptual hypothesis stipulates the relationship between two abstract variables but is never tested directly. Instead, there is indirect testing of the conceptual hypothesis through tests of its corresponding operational hypothesis. In later testing, support for the operational hypothesis provides evidence confirming the measurement assumption. Sustaining the operational hypothesis is evidence that each operational variable is a valid index of its conceptual variable because the operational hypothesis performs as was proposed by the theory—that is, the conceptual hypothesis.

Because the measurement assumption connects the conceptual and operational levels of a theory, the clarity of the theoretical definition will aid in specifying the domain of the operational variable. The specificity with which the domain of the operational variable is defined will mean less slippage when measuring the conceptual variable, thus increasing the probability of supporting the operational hypothesis. Accuracy in determining representative observables to index the concept is an important step in eventual support for the validity of the instrument. This information will be discussed again below, when construct validity is addressed. It is introduced at this point to give the researcher a clear understanding of the importance of defining operational variables so that they correspond with their respective conceptual variables. Ensuring isomorphism between the concept and the operation needs to occur early in the scale development process. Isomorphism should be a definite concern when moving from a theoretical to an operational definition, to minimize systematic error. This type of error can result when a lack of attention is paid to the domain of observables relevant to the concept and instead observables that index an irrelevant concept are included.

DEVELOPING ITEMS

Concepts vary widely in the extent to which the domain of the observable indicators is either large or small, specifically or loosely defined. If the domain of variables is small, it will be relatively easy to identify the specific indicators. At a higher level of complexity, typical of concepts that are investigated in nursing research, a large number of observables may be present, making it more difficult to define the concept and to determine which variables do or do not belong in the domain. The more abstract the concept, the greater the number of inferential steps that are necessary to translate observation into meaning (Waltz et al., 1984).

Items should be generated for each dimension of an instrument in such a way that items for each dimension are homogeneous. When all dimensions have item sets, they are combined to constitute the entire instrument. In later reliability testing, each dimension must be analyzed separately because consistency or homogeneity exists within but not across dimensions. Dimensions must, however, evidence a common theme by their intercorrelations.

Attending to the correspondence among items in the process of item development will minimize the degree of random error found in the instrument. When items are generated according to their similarity in thematic content, then each item is less likely to contain irregular characteristics that could stimulate inconsistent responses.

In developing items, the investigator can follow a variety of paths. He or she can use personal judgment concerning items, tap the clinical experience of colleagues, consult the relevant literature, or use more inductive methods, such as interviewing respondents about the concept and how it affects their lives. Regardless of the method used, the investigator must begin with some criteria for inclusion of individual items in the initial pool. It is important to include items that potentially apply to a wide variety of respondents and that are thought to remain stable over short periods of time (Kirshner & Guyatt, 1985). Major criteria for the generation of items include exemplars associated with the conceptual definition and affiliated with other items. These two points are usually considered for inclusion of items, because they address both reliability and validity issues.

A general method for generating items is to review the literature. Most nursing research instruments have been developed through review of published anecdotal studies, case studies, or reports of the experience of specific populations. Statements are identified from this material and converted into items. For examples of the use of this method from the nursing literature, see Baldree, Murphy, and Powers (1982); Jalowiec and Powers (1981); and Cox (1985). Another method for developing items is to use a combination of literature reviews, interviews with consultants or experts in the area, and patient interviews (see Wolf, Putnam, James, & Stiles, 1978). A third method involves selecting items from existing scales. Caution is advised with this method, however, because the investigator must determine whether the conceptual definition used as the basis for the original scale is consistent with the definition of the concept as stated by the present investigator. Items should not be borrowed from existing scales that are based on different definitions of the concept. A good example of a different approach to the use of items than has been presented is provided by Stevenson (1982). A second example by Hoskins (1981) presents good detail on expanding the original item domain.

The fourth approach to item generation is developing items for a scale from a qualitative investigation of the concept within the target population. This involves interviews with members of the target population to explore the concept. As examples of the concepts emerge, these examples or data bits are categorized according to similar themes. These themes then become the dimensions of the scale and the data bits are reworked into items. Examples of this approach to item development can be found in Mishel (1981) and in Benoliel, McCorkle, and Young (1980). Other examples of the use of qualitative interviews to generate items for a scale are provided by Hymovich (1983) and Cranley (1981).

In the process of developing items for a scale, the researcher must consider whether the scale will index a cognitive process or an attitude/personality variable, because the approach to item development differs based on the purpose of the scale (Carmines & Zeller, 1979). To ensure the content validity of a measure, the approach to the development of items will differ for a cognitive measure compared to an attitudinal or personality measure. According to Lynn (1986), the assessment of content validity should begin at the outset of instrument development. To attend to content validity concerns in the development of a cognitive measure, the researcher should develop the full content domain. For example, if one is attempting to index knowledge about diabetic care, all of the content concerning diabetic care would need to be identified and categorized. After identifying the content domain, a sample from the different areas of the content would be selected and items generated for each of these sample areas. The researcher need not address every specific area in depth but should have some items that refer to every major content area of the topic (Lynn, 1986). If instead an attitudinal or personality measure is being developed, the steps to ensure content validity would differ from those previously identified. The first step in developing an attitude or personality measure is to review the literature, as discussed previously, so that all dimensions and subdimensions of the topic are identified or to conduct interviews or qualitative work to identify the dimensions that arise inductively. Items are either generated from the literature or translated from the qualitative statements to reflect all of the dimensions. One should try to develop enough items to tap into each dimension fully (Lynn, 1986; Nunnally, 1978). The next step, the same as for cognitive and affective/personality instruments, is to assemble the items into a usable form. This will be discussed in more detail in the next section. The content validity efforts for the developmental stage of an index differ for cognitive and attitudinal/personality instruments (Lynn, 1986).

Developing items to support the content validity of an attitudinal/personality scale is more difficult than doing the same for a cognitive scale. It is easier to specify the domain relevant to a cognitive scale than it is for an affective scale because the cognitive scale will be based on a more specific and concrete domain, whereas the affective scale will be based on a more abstract domain.

ITEM CONSTRUCTION
AND RESPONSE CATEGORIES

The term *scale item construction* refers to the way in which the item is structured when it is given to the respondent. In this chapter, the focus is on scale items that can be summed to give a total index or measure of the specific concept. The total score is obtained by adding the scores on individual items. Summative scales have a number of advantages over all other methods: (a) They follow from an appealing model; (b) they are relatively easy to construct; (c) they are usually highly reliable; (d) they can be adapted to the measurement of different kinds of attitudes; and (e) they have produced meaningful results in many studies to date.

Considering the nature of the scale items used in summative models, these items can be affected by many problems that contribute to measurement error. Some of the major sources of error in the construction of scale items include the characteristics of the statement itself, such as imperfections, obscurities, and irrelevancies. Another problem is that items may be ambiguous in that they refer to two objects at once. Other types of problems stem from items that are obviously redundant, ambiguous, meaningless, or confusing.

Ware, Snyder, McClure, and Jarett (1972) report that Edwards summarized the work of several investigators and developed a list titled "Informal Criteria for Editing Statements to Be Used in the Construction of Attitude Scales." These informal criteria include 14 separate suggestions:

1. Avoid statements referring to the past rather than the present.
2. Avoid factual statements or those that could be interpreted as factual.
3. Avoid ambiguous statements (those that could be interpreted in more than one way).
4. Avoid statements irrelevant to the object under study.
5. Avoid statements likely to be endorsed by almost everyone or almost no one.
6. Keep language simple, clear, and direct.
7. Avoid item statements more than 20 words long.
8. Limit each statement to only one thought.
9. Avoid statements containing universals (*all, always, none, never*), because they often introduce ambiguity.
10. Use words such as *only, merely, just,* and others of a similar nature with care and moderation.
11. Use statements in the form of simple sentences rather than in the form of compound or complex sentences.
12. Avoid using words that might not be understood by those who are to be given the scale.
13. Avoid use of double negatives.
14. Select statements that are believed to cover the entire range of responses concerning the concept of interest.

In the process of developing items, an area of concern is the positive or negative phrasing of items. Nunnally (1978) notes that the purpose of each item on a summary scale is to obtain reliable variance with respect to the concept in question. Most of the items should be moderately positive or moderately negative. Neutral statements should not be used in summative scales. Statements that are very extreme in either direction tend to create less variance than less extreme statements. The pool of items should be about equally divided between positive and negative statements.

Another concern in item construction is the number of items that should be constructed for any scale. Because the major source of error within a test is the sampling of items, the more items in a measure, the less the error (Nunnally, 1978). One can never know for sure how many items should be constructed for a scale until after it is constructed and submitted to item analysis. Item analysis generally shows the number of items that will be needed to obtain an acceptable level of reliability. Nunnally (1978) suggests using the Spearman-Brown prophecy formula to estimate how much reliability would be increased if the number of items were increased by any factor. Nunnally (1978) notes that 30 dichotomous items are usually required to obtain an internal consistency reliability of .80. Fewer multipoint items than dichotomous items are required to obtain similar levels of reliability. It is not unusual to find, for example, a coefficient alpha level of .80 for a scale made up of 10 agree-disagree statements rated on a 7-point scale. To allow for item analysis to eliminate unsatisfactory items, Nunnally (1978) suggests that 60 items should be constructed initially. Another rule of thumb is that one should generate twice as many items as one would like the final scale to contain. If little is known about the homogeneity of items, it is wise to be conservative and initially construct more items than necessary.

RESPONSE CATEGORIES

Before study participants can use any scale, steps on the scale must be defined. Definitions of scale steps are referred to as anchors, and there are different types of anchors. Often, numbers are used in conjunction with anchors. On percentage scales, participants rate themselves or others on a continuum ranging from 0 to 100%. The scale is often divided into 10 steps, each corresponding to 10 percentage points, but one can increase the sensitivity of the instrument by employing more finely graded percentage steps.

A second type of anchor frequently used in rating scales is degrees of agreement and disagreement. These scales are easy to work with and are easily understood by study participants. Agreement/disagreement scales are of two types: numerical and graphic. A numerical scale has a set number of steps bounded by anchors such as *completely agree* and *completely disagree.* In graphic scales, numbers are followed by specific ratings, such as 1 (*completely agree*), 2 (*mostly agree*), 3 (*slightly agree*), 4 (*slightly disagree*), 5 (*mostly disagree*), and 6 (*completely disagree*). The graphic scale is generally considered preferable to the use of numbers alone. Because the graphic scale may remind people of a yardstick or degrees of phenomena, its presence helps to convey the idea of a rating continuum. Also, with the use of the graphic scale, there are fewer clerical errors in recording ratings.

Attitudes constitute the third type of anchor for rating scales. Scales often are anchored by two terms, such as *valuable-worthless* or *effective-ineffective.* Attitude scales using bipolar adjective pairs as anchors are easily constructed and can be applied to many types of attitudinal objects. A rating scale using bipolar adjective pairs as anchors is called a *semantic differential,* which is a type of scaling. The semantic differential will be discussed in the section on scaling.

Another concern in constructing items is the number of scale steps. There is always an advantage to using more rather than fewer steps. This is demonstrated by numerous studies showing that the reliability of a scale is a monotonically increasing function of the number of steps (Nunnally, 1978). As the number of scale steps increases from 2 up through 20, the increase in reliability is very rapid at first. It tends to level off at about 7, and after about 8 steps, there is little reliability by increasing the number of steps. Nunnally (1978) notes that as the number of scale points increases, error variance increases, but at the same time the true score increases at an even more rapid rate.

The question of the number of steps in a rating scale is very important if one is dealing with only one item, but it is less important if scores are summed over a number of items. When only one item is used to measure a concept (a practice that is not recommended) there should be at least 10 steps. If there are a limited number of items on the scale, the reliability of a dichotomous scale could be greatly increased by increasing the number of scale steps on the individual scales. On the other hand, when there are more than 20 items in a summated scale, the reliability is not greatly increased by the addition of scale steps to the individual scales. Nunnally (1978) recommends that in nearly all instances it is safer to have at least 5 or 6 steps than it is to have a dichotomous scale. Seldom are there practical advantages to having only 2 steps.

Another issue regarding the number of steps on rating scales concerns whether an even or an odd number of steps is preferable. Some argue for an odd number of steps to allow for a middle or neutral step, because they believe that participants are more comfortable making decisions if a neutral reaction is an option. On the other hand, some feel that having a neutral step induces response styles, with some respondents tending to use the neutral step more often than others. Nunnally (1978) concludes that the issue of whether to have a neutral step is not very important, particularly if scores are summed over a number of items.

To emphasize what was stated earlier, it is more important to do everything possible to prevent measurement error from occurring than to try to assess the effects of measurement error after it has occurred. In the area of item construction, measurement error can be reduced by writing items clearly, by making test instructions easily understood, by adhering closely to the prescribed condition for administering an instrument, and by increasing the length of the measure. Measurement error caused by subjectivity in scoring can be reduced when the rules for scoring are as explicit as possible.

SCALING

There are a number of methods available for distinguishing among objects or individuals in terms of the degree to which they possess a given characteristic. Each of these methods involves placing the person or object being rated at some point along a continuum or into one of an ordered series of categories and attaching a numerical value to that point or category. Scale types discussed here include differential, summated, and cumulative scales, as well as scales that are modifications of these basic forms. Because the object of scaling is to quantify accurately the most comprehensive, complete information for the least overall cost and with the least amount of measurement error, specific scale types are discussed in terms of their advantages and disadvantages.

In an effort to reduce error involved in rating others on the basis of observed behavior or responses to open-ended questions, standardized questionnaires have been developed based on expression of agreement or disagreement with a number of statements relevant to the dimension(s) of interest. In the process of standardizing the questionnaire, the investigator establishes a basis of interpreting agreement/disagreement response-assigned scores as indicating positions on the dimension. The separate items on such a scale are not of interest in themselves. Rather, researcher interest is in each individual's total score or in subscores that result from combinations of individual responses to various item subsets. The way a particular type of scale discriminates among individuals depends on how the scale is constructed and on the method of scoring. In the following discussion, the major types of scales used in nursing research will be presented. For further information on scale construction and scoring, see Kerlinger (1986).

Differential Scales

A differential scale consists of a number of ranked items, whereby the items themselves form a gradation. The individual will likely agree with only one or two items corresponding to the individual's position on the dimension being measured and will likely disagree with items at all other points on the dimension.

The Thurstone scale is the most common example of the differential scale type. Establishing the order of the items to approximate equal intervals is one of the major tasks in construction of a Thurstone scale. The various methods of providing accurate judgments of scale position include the method of paired comparisons (Thurstone, 1927, 1928), the method of equal-appearing intervals (Thurstone, 1929; Thurstone & Chave, 1929), and the method of successive intervals, which is most commonly selected.

This scale type allows for comparisons of changes in an individual's position on the dimension or for comparisons across individuals of differences relative to the dimension. Investigations have demonstrated that the procedure seeking to create equal-appearing intervals does provide an interval scale. The resulting data can be appropriately analyzed with parametric statistics.

Disadvantages include the amount of work and time necessary for securing the statements and judgments. Scale construction costs are significant. Item selection based on judged agreement tends to result in the elimination of items that less clearly manifest the dimension. Items included in the scale can be considered transparent, with participants easily able to discern the "socially acceptable" response pattern. Such scales may be more open to social desirability bias. Issues can also be raised regarding the scoring procedure. Because an individual's score is the mean (or median) of scale values assigned to items checked, different response patterns can be expressed by the same score. Two individuals could be rated as having the same degree of prejudice even though one person checked two moderately "anti" items and the other checked four items representing two "anti" positions and two "pro" positions. In general, the greatest disadvantage of this type of scale is its decreased reliability in comparison with some other types of scales due to reliance on choice between dichotomous responses for each item. The participant either agrees or disagrees with a given item and is not able to indicate more subtle responses that lie between the two extremes (Title & Hill, 1967).

Summative Scales

Like differential scales, the summative scale offers the respondent a set of items and requests a response to the items. Items that reflect divergent positions on the dimension are selected, and neutral or moderate (midline) and very extreme aspects of the dimension are omitted. Study participants respond to each item rather than only to those with which they agree. Each response is assigned a numerical score; it is part of instrument development to decide whether favorable or unfavorable responses will be scored positively. The sum of scores of the individual's responses to all items yields the total score and is interpreted as the respondent's position relative to the measured dimensions.

The most common type of summative scale is the Likert-type scale. This is the scale type most often selected as the scaling method for measurement of concepts of interest to nurses. In a Likert-type scale, participants respond to each item in terms of several degrees of agreement or disagreement. Five categories of response are common and are often stated as 1 (*strongly agree*), 2 (*agree*), 3 (*undecided*), 4 (*disagree*), and 5 (*strongly disagree*).

The Likert-type scale is "subject centered" (Torgerson, 1958), having as its purpose the scaling of respondents, not the scaling of the dimension. Any item found empirically to be consistent with the total score can be included. The Likert-type scale is practical in terms of construction costs. The assumptions relative to scoring the Likert-type scale are also lenient relative to measurement error. Because each item may contain considerable measurement error, no single item in summative scales is considered separately. Rather, each item is monotonically related to the underlying dimension continuum. This assumption does not imply that each item has exactly the same level of contribution to the dimension. It states only that the sum of the items is expected to contain all the important information relative to a single common factor (McIver & Carmines, 1978). Because the 5-point response format for each item allows more response alternatives, the reliability of the Likert-type scale is likely to be greater than that of a Thurstone scale having the same number of items. This range of responses also provides more precise information about the individual's position on the dimension as referred to by the given item.

Disadvantages of the Likert-type scale include the potential for introduction of response set bias due to inclusion of positively worded statements versus negatively worded statements. The inclusion of an approximately equal number of negatively worded and positively worded items partially controls for response set bias.

As in the Thurstone scale, the total score of the Likert-type scale can represent diverse response patterns. The safeguard against having a meaningless total score is careful item analysis, ensuring that only items that discriminate between high and low scorers are retained. In addition, a rigorous testing schedule is required to determine (a) whether responses remain stable over time; (b) if alternative tests are available, whether individuals receive the same score on different forms; and (c) whether different individuals achieving the same score in different ways react in the same way to particular stimuli, problems, and so on, with the ultimate question being concerned with estimating scale validity. The severest criticism of Likert-type scales has been that such scales can claim to provide only ordinal-level measurement. There has been much debate over the kind of statistical analysis that is appropriate for data provided through Likert-type scales (Armstrong, 1981; Burke, 1953; Labovitz, 1967; Nagel, 1974; Stevens, 1951).

Cumulative Scales

Cumulative scales, like differential and summative scales, offer the respondent a series of items requiring an agreement or disagreement response. But unlike the other scales, cumulative scales contain items that are related in an incremental fashion. Ideally, a respondent replying favorably to Item 2 would also reply favorably to Item 1; one who replies favorably to Item 3 would also reply favorably to Items 1 and 2. The individual's score is computed by counting the number of items answered favorably. The total score places the person on the scale of favorable-unfavorable attitude provided by the relationship of items to one another. Items can appear on the scale in order of favorableness or can be randomly arranged.

The Guttman scale is an example of a cumulative scale that also attempts to determine the unidimensionality of the scale. The Guttman technique, although providing a method for determining the unidimensionality of an item set, provides little guidance for selecting items that are likely to form a scale. The Guttman-type scale is useful when examining small changes or shifts in the dimension of interest. It has the potential to serve as a criterion-referenced instrument if items are selected relative to a set of predictable target behaviors.

Disadvantages of the Guttman scale include high costs of construction due to difficulty in initially selecting items likely to be scalable and to the fact that items may be scalable for one population but not for another. Scalability must be checked prior to use with a population other than that used in initial development. Scalogram analysis is usually performed on one or more samples of 100, with no certainty that a usable scale will emerge from the testing.

Other Scale Types

The scale discrimination technique advocated by Edwards and Kilpatrick (1948) borrows aspects of the construction of Thurstone's equal-appearing intervals, Likert's summated scales, and Guttman's scale analysis to develop a set of items that meet the requirements of unidimensional scales, possess equal-appearing intervals, and measure intensity. Although providing a scale with desired qualities of unidimensionality, interval-level measurement, and measurement of intensity, the construction procedure is very costly. And in the Guttman procedure for scaling, there is no certainty that a usable scale will emerge from the testing.

The semantic differential scale developed by Osgood, Suci, and Tannenbaum (1957) provides another method for measuring the meaning of an object to an individual. The semantic differential does not place individuals on an underlying scale representing some dimension of a concept; it instead provides a method for measuring the similarity or difference in how respondents view the dimension. Responses to scale subgroups can be summed to yield scores interpreted as the individual's position on three underlying dimensions of attitude: evaluation, potency, and activity. The actual analysis of a semantic differential scale includes a variety of measures that exceed the scope of this chapter. For an excellent discussion of these analyses, see Kerlinger (1986).

The visual analog scale is a type of graphic rating scale that can be used to bypass language limitations. It typically consists of a 100 mm horizontal or vertical line anchored at each end with a brief verbal description of a feeling (Bond & Lader, 1974), mood (Aitken & Zealley, 1970), or the like to be evaluated relative to the dimension being evaluated. This scale has been used most frequently to measure pain (Huskisson, 1974). The anchored endpoints represent opposing positions. The respondent places a mark on the line at the point best representing response to the item. Construction benefits of the visual analog scale are comparable to those discussed for summated scales. The visual analog scale provides a means for evaluating fine changes, and it has been shown to provide increased sensitivity and decreased divergent interpretations (Maxwell, 1978).

PRETESTING

Before an instrument is used in a structured investigation, pretesting of the instrument should occur to address many early questions in instrument development. Fox and Ventura (1983) note that pretesting is not frequently done and present two reasons this important step is often bypassed in the process of instrument development. The first relates to the organization of academic disciplines, in which there is a high demand placed on the individual to produce findings from research investigations and publish as soon as possible. The time and effort that pretesting entails is therefore not encouraged, often at the expense of quality results. The second reason focuses on the teacher-student relationship. Because pretesting is infrequently conducted, many mentoring relationships do not include role modeling regarding pretesting of instruments. Although Fox and Ventura (1983) note that pretesting can cover an assortment of activities that may include informal opinions from colleagues or more formal testing using small samples that resemble the population of interest, pretesting most correctly refers to formal testing with representative samples of persons.

Pretesting involves determining the feasibility of using a given instrument in a formal study. It provides an opportunity to try out the technique or the instructions that will be used with an instrument, especially if it has never been used with a specific population. Pretesting also allows the researcher an opportunity to simulate the conditions of the study and get some direct experience with what will happen. Through subsequent pretesting, data can be obtained from item analysis. Nunnally (1978) notes that the pretest population should be similar to the group with which the final instrument will be used. It is important that the data for item analysis be obtained under conditions very similar to those in which the final scale will be used. Consistency should be maintained between the type of instructions used in the pretest and those used with the final instrument.

Wolf et al. (1978) provide a fine example of the use of multiple field trials in the development of an instrument. Three pretests or field trials were conducted; each had a specific focus for instrument development. In the first pretest, items were presented to about 50 persons similar to the target population. The participants were asked to give feedback about the items in the scale in terms of the appropriateness and clarity of item wording. On the basis of this information, some of the items were reworded. A second pretest was aimed at item analysis. Similar participants were asked to complete the initial form of the scale. Two types of item analysis resulted from the data from the pretest, which then functioned to modify the scale. In the third pretest, the revised form of the scale was administered to about 50 persons who were the target population of a larger study. The data from the third pretest were again used for item analysis and for validity testing. This example demonstrates the continual evolvement in instrumentation that occurs as a result of well-planned pretests.

A pretest can be used to determine the base rate of the concept being measured. Derogatis and Spencer (1984) note that a problem exists with what they call "base rates," or the predictive value of a measuring instrument when the prevalence rates of the concept are particularly low. As the base rate or the occurrence of the concept becomes markedly low—that is, it pertains to less than 10% of the population—increasingly high sensitivity in the measuring instrument is required to achieve useful measurement. One advantage of pretesting is that it allows the researcher, if using a representative population, to get some index of the prevalence of the concept before further work is put into developing an instrument for a concept that may have a very low level of existence.

Fox and Ventura (1983) present a list of suggestions for conducting a pretest. Some of these are as follows:

- Allow sufficient time before the actual study to analyze the data and make changes in data collection procedures as necessary.
- Do not start the study until the pretest results have been analyzed for reliability and validity.
- Try out multiple methods of data collection to decide on a method.
- If major modifications must be made due to the results of the pretest, conduct another pretest before a major study is undertaken.
- Conduct several phases of the pretest, as discussed in the example by Wolf et al. (1978).
- After the pretest, ask participants to identify any problems they had completing the questionnaire and any suggestions they might have for improving the questions
- Perform item analysis on the pretest data.
- Pretest the questionnaire items on as many types of people as available who will be in the eventual study group.
- Use a sample size of 10 or 20 for a pretest, unless the instrument is complex or the sample is heterogeneous, in which case use a larger sample.

Although the participants in the pretest are similar to the participants who will use the final scale, they need not be exact representatives of the test population. Because the test will be used with many types of participants, it is important that, in the pretest, the sample group be highly representative of all the different groups with which the test will eventually be used. Although Fox and Ventura (1983) say that a pretest may have a small sample, Nunnally (1978) suggests that the scale should initially be administered to 10 times as many participants as there are items. Although Nunnally supports using a large sample for gathering data for item analysis, it is rarely possible to obtain such a large population in studies using clinical samples. Published instrumentation articles in the nursing research literature generally involve a smaller sample size than proposed. For examples of the use of pretests in nursing, see Cox (1985) and Stevenson (1982).

ITEM ANALYSIS

Item analysis is a procedure to estimate the reliability and determine the validity of a test by separately evaluating each item of the instrument to ascertain whether or not that item discriminates in the same way that the overall test is intended to discriminate and whether the item is of appropriate difficulty (Isaac & Michael, 1974). The content of the final instrument must depend on how the item performs in the setting in which the index will ultimately be used. Therefore, performance criterion must be established so that items that do not contribute to or actually detract from the total instrument can be detected and eliminated to strengthen the reliability and validity of the measure. Discriminative criteria are usually structured around two major performance criteria: (a) the discriminability of the item and (b) the accuracy/precision of the item. Discriminability of the item can be tested using three procedures: (a) the discrimination index, (b) split-group response, and (c) two-group response (Isaac & Michael, 1974; Waltz et al., 1984). These three methods assess an item's ability to discriminate—that is, to determine whether the performance of a given item is a good predictor of the performance of the overall measure.

In the discrimination index, to determine the discrimination or D value for a given item, Waltz et al. (1984) provide the following instructions:

1. Rank all participants' performance on the measure by using total scores from high to low.
2. Identify those individuals who ranked in the upper third.
3. Identify those individuals who ranked in the lower third.
4. Place the remaining scores aside.
5. Determine the proportion of respondents in the upper third who answered the item correctly (Pu).
6. Determine the proportion of respondents in the lower third who answered the item correctly (Pl).
7. Calculate D, $D = Pu - Pl$.
8. Repeat Steps 5 through 7 for each item on the measure.

D ranges from –1.00 to +1.00. It is desirable to obtain D values greater than +0.20. A positive D value is what is sought, and this indicates that the item discriminates in the same manner as the total test, which means that those who score high on the total test tend to respond the same way on the item. Conversely, those who score low on the item also tend to score low on the total test. Waltz et al. (1984) state that a negative D value indicates that the item does not discriminate like the total test and that respondents who score low on the total test tend to get the item correct and vice versa. Thus, a negative D value indicates that the item is not a good discriminator and possibly should be removed from the scale.

The split-group response is another procedure that functions like the discrimination index to identify how well an item discriminates relative to the way that the overall test is intended to discriminate. In the split group response method, respondents are ranked according to the upper and lower half following Steps 1 through 4 for determining D. Following this, a fourfold table is constructed based on two pairs of categories. The first pair is the category high scores versus the low scores, depending on how the ranks are divided. In the next step, the chi-square value of the resulting proportion is calculated using the standard shortcut formula for the chi-square. If the chi-square is significant, it can be concluded that a significant difference has been found in the proportion of high- and low-scoring respondents who gave correct answers. Items that meet this criterion should be retained, and items that fail to meet it should be discarded or modified to increase their discriminability.

The third method, the two-group response, is a technique used to discriminate between the responses of two groups given a series of items. For example, one might want to discriminate between medical patients and surgical patients in terms of a specific concept. In this procedure, a contingency table is established, with the two groups being compared constituting the rows and the item response options the columns. For each item, the frequency of each item response by group members is determined and subjected to a chi-square test. If the chi-square value is significant, it can be concluded that one group responded to the item differently than the other group. If the response is in the direction expected, the item would be discriminating as expected and would be retained. If the two groups fail to show any difference on an item, the item would not be discriminating and would either be removed from the scale or modified and retested to increase its discriminatory power (Isaac & Michael, 1974).

Another method for assessing the performance of an item is to determine its accuracy or precision. This method involves determining the item-total correlations, using the Pearson product-moment correlation (biserial correlations for dichotomous items) to derive an indication of how strongly an item reflects the total scale. Because the goal of norm referenced or discriminative scales is to discriminate between people according to the specific concept under investigation, item reduction methods that delete items not stressing the same theme function to improve the power of the scale to discriminate between two people on the specific variable. The precision of the index will increase based on the strength with which each individual item relates to the total scale.

In item analysis with item-total correlations, the first step is to determine the actual correlations. Then items are ordered based on the correlations, with the item with the highest correlation ranked first. Approximately 30 items is a common instrument length. The top 30 items, based on the item-total correlations, are selected to constitute the instrument. Even if all or almost all of the items in the original pool have high item-total correlations, they may or may not end up in the final instrument, depending on the reliability of the instrument.

Generally, the items having the highest item-total correlation are selected. Items with low item-total correlation are deleted. If the internal consistency of the scale is computed at this time, it can be determined whether adding items or deleting items raises or lowers the level of reliability. If reliability is sufficiently high with the items having the highest item-total correlation, little is to be gained by adding more items.

Nunnally (1978) advises that when one has multipoint items, it is wise to compute the internal consistency for the 10 items having the highest correlations with total scores and, if reliability is not high enough, to add several items until the desired reliability is obtained. Nunnally (1978) presents several reasons this method may fail to produce a homogeneous test. One of the most common is that the collection of items is factorally complex. Some items correlate strongly within themselves but have low correlations with other items, thereby preventing a homogeneous scale from being formed. If the researcher has hypothesized a number of factors, each of which relates to different attributes of the concept and there are sufficient participants with which to do so (n = 5-10 respondents per item), he or she should proceed to factor analyze the item pool initially rather than attempt the construction of a homogeneous scale. When a factor analysis is planned, the sample should be carefully selected to be representative of the kind of population to which the investigator will generalize the findings and must be large enough to give stable correlation coefficients.

Carmines and Zeller (1979) note that factor analysis is explicitly designed to address the situation in which the items in the scale are not unidimensional. This implies that the items as a group do not measure a single phenomenon but, rather, measure more than one phenomenon or aspects of a phenomenon. Factor analysis is a statistical method used to discover clusters of interrelated variables. When an instrument addresses several phenomena or aspects of a phenomenon, items tend to fall in clusters or factors. The items composing a factor are more highly correlated with each other than were the other items. Factor analysis is introduced here to explain that when factors have been incorporated into the construction of a scale, factor analysis should precede investigation of item-total correlations. After factor analysis has been computed, item-total correlations can then be meaningfully computed for each of the factors. Items that do not load heavily on a factor can be deleted. *Loading* refers to the extent to which each item is correlated with every other item on the factor. The higher the item loads on the factor, the more the particular item contributes to that factor. This is an alternative way to look at item-total correlations. Items that load heavily on a factor would then be retained and items with weak loadings on the factor would be deleted. For more information on traditional factor loadings considered appropriate during factor analysis, the reader is referred to texts on the topic. Some examples of the use of factor analysis as a basis for item deletion can be found in the work of Mishel (1981, 1983). Other examples of the use of criteria for item-total correlations can be found in the work of Stevenson (1982), Cox (1985), and Cranley (1981).

RELIABILITY

Reliability refers to the degree of consistency and repeatability of the scores on an instrument. A measure that is unreliable shows scores that are variable and fluctuating. Reliability is equal to the observed variance that is not random or fluctuating but is repeatable or true. Systematic error is not an issue in reliability because, since it is not random, it does not reduce consistency and repeatability. The culprit in reliability is random error. When random error is low, reliability is high. The reliability coefficient is the portion of test variance that is true or nonrandom variance. If, for example, a reliability coefficient is .70, then 70% of the variance in scores is due to variation in true differences between the participants on the concept under measurement. The remaining 30% of the variance is due to inaccuracy in the measurement (Isaac & Michael, 1974).

Types of Reliability

Test-Retest

The test-retest method is appropriate for determining the reliability of a measure when the concept being tested is thought to be relatively stable over the time period in which the testing will occur. Test-retest procedures are often used to determine the reliability of affective measures and attitudes. Because cognitive measures may change rapidly, this procedure is not usually used for such an instrument. With the test-retest procedure, the investigator is concerned with the consistency of measurement in the same group of participants from Time 1 to Time 2. Waltz et al. (1984) present the following three-step procedure to estimate test-retest reliability for a specific measure:

1. Under standardized conditions, give the measure to a single group of participants who represent the group for which the measure was developed.

2. Give the test again, 2 weeks later, to the same group of people under the same conditions (the time between tests may vary slightly). It is important to note whether any new activities occur between the first and second administration that may affect the consistency of the concept being measured.

3. Determine the extent to which the two sets of scores are correlated. If the data are considered interval level, Pearson product-moment correlation is customarily used as the estimate of reliability; if the data are at a nominal or ordinal level, a nonparametric measure of association is used.

The reliability coefficient from the test-retest procedure is called the *coefficient of stability* because it measures the extent to which participants perform at the same level on two separate occasions. The higher the coefficient of stability, the more stable the measuring device is assumed to be. For examples of the use of this method in nursing research, see Baldree et al. (1982); Jalowiec and Powers (1981); Hoskins (1981); and Norbeck, Lindsey, and Carrieri (1981).

Although test-retest may be an appealing procedure, it is not without serious problems. Zeller and Carmines (1980) note that researchers are often able to obtain a measure of a phenomenon at a single point in time, but it can be very expensive and impractical to obtain measures at various points in time. Even if test-retest correlations can be accomplished, their interpretation is often ambiguous. A low test-retest correlation may not indicate that reliability is low but instead indicate that the concept itself has changed. The longer the time interval between measures, the more likely it is that the concept has changed.

Knapp (1985) discusses some of the errors that frequently occur in nursing research concerning test-retest reliability. Test-retest reliability is meant to provide some evidence over a brief period of time regarding the short-term consistency of measures yielded by a particular test. It is not usually concerned with long-term consistency of the concept being measured. Often, the word *stability* is associated with reliability studies carried out over a brief period of time in which the investigator is concerned with the consistency of the concept instead of with the consistency of the scores. It is important to distinguish between a test-retest reliability study and the study of a particular concept. If scores change over the time period selected, presuming the interval between administration was appropriately selected for the concept studied, the instrument is assessed as not being stable (reliable) rather than the concept being noted as changed in those studied. Concept changes cannot reliably be identified using an unreliable instrument.

If the construct being measured is a trait, this will present different problems than if the concept is defined as a state. Traits are considered enduring, whereas states—emotions such as anxiety or depression—may be considered transitory. To use test-retest methods, the concept being measured should be conceptualized as a trait behavior and the level of the concept should not change over time. If an attitude or belief system is being measured, this is assumed to be relatively stable unless some unusual environmental event occurs and thus should remain stable over time. If the behavior exists in a transition state, test-retest methods can be used if an appropriate interval can be determined. Use of test-retest methods is based on the understanding that the ability of the instrument to produce the same score is being tested, not the ability of the concept to remain stable or fluctuate.

A second problem with the test-retest method is that it can lead to deflated reliability estimates due to reactivity. Reactivity is what happens when measuring a phenomenon induces change in the phenomenon itself. If a person's belief concerning a concept is measured at Time 1, he or she may become sensitized and may demonstrate a change at Time 2.

If the test-retest correlation is low, the alternate form correlation will be even lower. If the test does not correlate with itself when given on two separate occasions, it is less likely to correlate with another test measuring the same concept. Examples of the use of the test-retest method can be found in Hoskins (1981) and Norbeck et al. (1981).

Equivalence

The major method for achieving equivalence of a test involves using two different forms of an instrument to measure the same concept. In this form of reliability, one is attempting to determine whether there will be consistent performance on two different forms of a measure by the same participants during one specific testing period. The two different measures are considered alternative or parallel forms if they have some of the following characteristics: They were constructed using the same objective procedures, and based on the same conceptual definition, they have approximately equal means, they correlate about equally with any third variable, and they have equal standard deviations (Waltz et al., 1984). To conduct the alternate forms method, both instruments are given to the respondents on the same measurement occasion. The extent to which the two sets of scores are correlated is determined using an appropriate statistic for the level of measurement in both measures. If the measures correlate highly, they are seen as equivalent. If the correlation is above .80, this indicates that the forms may be used interchangeably. For examples of the use of alternate forms as a measure of reliability in nursing research, see Hoskins (1981, 1983).

Internal Consistency

The two methods subsumed under internal consistency are the most basic and popular ways of estimating reliability. This method for assessing reliability focuses on multiple indicators of a concept measured at a similar point in time. Each indicator, usually an item, is considered a separate but equal measure of the underlying concept. The early measure of internal consistency focused on split-half methods. In these methods, the total number of items was divided into two halves and the correlation between the two halves provided an estimate of the reliability of all of the items. The problem with this method is that the point at which each split occurs will produce a different correlation between the halves. This leads to differences in reliability estimates. Other problems with this method are that it applies mostly to cognitive measures, assumes that item content is evenly spread, and is not useful when the instrument is not fully completed by some respondents.

In response to some of the problems in estimating reliability by the use of the split-half method, other methods have been developed that do not require the splitting or repeating of items but still provide a measure of internal consistency. Of all of the methods to determine internal consistency, the method that is most popular and most generally applicable is Cronbach's coefficient alpha. Coefficient alpha is equal to the average of all possible split-half correlations for composite scales that are N items long (Zeller & Carmines, 1980). Alpha takes scores varying between 0 and +1, taking these extremes when the item correlations can be equal to 0 in unity or be perfect and equal to 1 (Zeller & Carmines, 1980). Generally, as the number of items on a scale increases, the average correlation among the items increases and alpha takes on a larger value. The criterion level for coefficient alpha with a new scale has been suggested to be at about .70 or above, and for a mature scale, .80 or above (Nunnally, 1978).

When considering intercorrelations between items in a scale, it is important that the correlations be high enough to index similarity between the items and yet not be so high that they index redundancy. Interitem correlations should average between .30 and .70. Correlations above .70 imply redundancy, and items at that point can be deleted (Gordon, 1968).

To measure internal consistency, two different estimates are used. Cronbach's alpha is applicable to scales with multiple responses, and the Kuder-Richardson 20 is applicable to cognitive scales with dichotomous items. KR-20 is the most useful reliability coefficient for dichotomous items because it makes no special assumptions regarding the distribution of items. Alpha measures the extent to which performance of any one item on an instrument is a good indicator of performance of any other item on the same instrument. Thus the addition of items to an instrument, if it does not result in a reduction in the average interitem correlation, will increase reliability.

A number of characteristics of the measurement situation can affect the alpha value that is obtained. Alpha is a function of test length; the longer the test, the higher the level of alpha. The second characteristic of coefficient alpha is that it increases with the spread of variance of scores. Perhaps the most important characteristic to remember concerning coefficient alpha is that alpha equals reliability only if the items are strictly parallel. Otherwise, the value of alpha merely sets a lower bound on the reliability; that is, the reliability of the scale cannot be less than the value noted for alpha. Alpha does not provide a very good estimate of reliability when the items making up the scale are heterogeneous in their relationship to each other or when their number is small. In each of these conditions, alpha will be smaller than the true internal consistency of the scale. When interitem correlations are low, the value given by alpha understates the true reliability. Zeller and Carmines (1980) note two conditions under which alpha may not provide a good estimate of reliability: (a) if the items measure a single concept unequally or (b) if the items measure more than one concept equally or unequally.

Although there are some limits to the conditions under which alpha can provide a good estimate of reliability, there are still many points in favor of using this measure of internal consistency. Kirshner and Guyatt (1985) note that coefficient alpha provides a good estimate of measurement error attributable to inappropriate or inadequate sampling of content domain. It is important to be able to determine what sources of error have been addressed by a specific reliability coefficient. Coefficient alpha is excellent for addressing sources of error due to inappropriate or inadequate sampling of items, which is the major source of error within a test. Nunnally (1978) goes further, noting that all of the types of errors that occur within a test can easily be handled by this measure of internal consistency. The general consensus is that coefficient alpha provides a good, albeit occasionally conservative, estimate of reliability in most situations.

It has also been shown that reliability estimates based on internal consistency also consider sources of error that are not, strictly speaking, due to the sampling of items but to the sampling of situational factors that accompany the administration of items. Many of these sampling decisions, noted by Isaac and Michael (1974), that can be potential sources of error are adequately handled by coefficient alpha. Coefficient alpha is frequently used as an estimate of reliability in nursing research. For examples of its use, see Hinshaw and Atwood (1982); Mishel (1983); and Murphy, Powers, and Jalowiec (1985).

Some conditions limit the usefulness of alpha as a reliability estimate. Alpha may underestimate the "true" reliability of an instrument composed of separate factors or subscales because there will be more consistency within these factors or subscales than when they are considered as a whole instrument. In such cases, reliability estimates should be obtained for each subscale as well as for the total scale.

When analyzing the reliability of scales that contain more than one dimension, the coefficients omega and theta represent the internal consistency of the items within each subscale. Coefficient theta and coefficient omega, the types of reliability coefficients used in factor analysis, have some important differences. Each coefficient is based on a different factor-analytic model. Theta is used with the principal components model, whereas omega is based on the common factor analysis model. Theta can be understood most simply as being a special case of coefficient alpha. Although theta and alpha are grounded in different factor analysis models, there are also some similarities between them. If the items constituting a scale are parallel measures, all three coefficients—alpha, theta, and omega—should be equal to one another and will equal the reliability of the scale. If the items are not parallel, omega will have the highest value, followed by theta and finally by alpha. Alpha is the lower limit for the reliability of a multi-item scale. Of all these three internal consistency coefficients, omega provides the highest estimate of reliability—that is, the closest to the true reliability of the instrument (Carmines & Zeller, 1979). There are assumptions about theta and omega that should be considered preceding their use. For information on these assumptions, the reader is referred to texts on factor analysis.

VALIDITY

Validity refers to the ability of an instrument to measure exactly what it is supposed to measure and nothing else. To determine the validity of an instrument, the researcher should consider the major reasons it was developed or the major functions it serves. Instruments serve three major functions: (a) to represent the universe of content related to a specific concept, (b) to establish a relationship with a particular variable, and (c) to measure attitudinal, affective behavior or cognitive variables (Nunnally, 1978). There are three types of validity; each represents a response to one of the three functions of an instrument: (a) Content validity relates to the representation of a specific universe of content; (b) criterion-related validity relates to establishing a relationship with a particular variable; and (c) construct validity relates to measurement of specific psychological variables.

A second approach to conceptualizing validity testing is in terms of two types of evidence: internal association and external association (Zeller & Carmines, 1980). *Internal association* refers to the pattern of interrelationships between the indicators designed to measure the concept. This can encompass the methods of determining content validity. *External association* refers to the pattern of relationships between items designed to measure a concept and other variables. External association can encompass criterion-related and construct validity methods.

Content Validity

The term *content validity* refers to an estimation of the adequacy with which a specific domain of content is sampled. It refers to the content representativeness of the concept—that is, the completeness with which items cover the important areas of the domain they are attempting to represent. To the degree that the items reflect the full domain of content, they can be said to be content valid.

Content validity has been criticized in the instrumentation literature due to the lack of agreed-on criteria for establishing whether a measure has obtained content validity. Nunnally (1978) notes that "inevitably content validity rests mainly on appeals to reason regarding the adequacy with which important content has been sampled and on the adequacy in which the content has been cast in the form of test items" (p. 93).

Other work has occurred in nursing that attempts to quantify the content validity process (see Lynn, 1986). Earlier in this chapter, the first step in assessing content validity was discussed for item development for either a cognitive or an affective/personality instrument. The second stage in assessing content validity is the judgment/quantification stage, which involves selecting experts to evaluate the content validity of each item and of the total scale (Lynn, 1986).

Lynn (1986) identifies the process for quantifying content validity as determining the number of experts needed to evaluate the items and the proportion who must agree for content validity to be established. It is recommended that specific guidelines be applied for the selection of experts. A minimum of three is recommended to obtain statistically justifiable results. For more than three available judges, Lynn provides a table for determining the proportion of experts who must agree in order to establish content validity of the item or scale beyond the .05 level of significance.

A structured procedure for the evaluation of the content validity of the instrument should be given to the experts. Experts selected must have specific criteria for deciding on the relevance of the content to the concept. If the concept includes multiple dimensions, criteria related to each dimension should also be supplied. According to the process defined by Lynn (1986), the content is quantified by use of the index of content validity. She notes that the authors of the index of content validity identify two limitations to the tool, but the method she proposes is presented as addressing these concerns. According to that procedure, a formula is applied to determine the number of experts needed and the proportion who must agree for content validity to be established. Each item, and the total scale, is quantified using the index of content validity. The experts identify areas that were omitted from the instrument, and items that do not achieve the required minimum agreement of the experts are eliminated or revised. Several items in the instrument may need to be evaluated more than once to establish sufficient content validity. In this case, the investigator, if using the same experts, waits for a period of 10 to 14 days between assessments. For further information on this process, see Lynn (1986). Content validity should not be an arbitrary decision; rather, it should include the application of rigorous criteria involving quantification.

Criterion-Related Validity

Criterion-related validity is at issue when an instrument is used to estimate some form of behavior that is external to the measuring instrument itself. The latter is often referred to as the *criterion*. There are two types of criterion-related validity: predictive validity and concurrent validity. *Predictive validity* refers to the extent to which an individual's future level of performance on the criterion can be predicted from his or her present performance on a specific measure. *Concurrent validity* refers to the extent to which a measure can be used to estimate an individual currently undergoing performance on the criterion.

The procedure for testing criterion-related validity is relatively straightforward. The researcher identifies the criterion variable and measures a sample of the population on both the predictor (the instrument) and criterion variables—a present criterion in concurrent validity and a future criterion in predictive validity. Scores of individuals' performance on the predictor and criterion variables are correlated, and this provides an index of the usefulness of the predictor variable in determining performance on the criterion for that specific population. The size of the correlation is a direct indicator of validity. Predictive validity is determined strictly by the degree of correlation between the two measures involved and not by any other form of evidence. Nunnally (1978) notes that in most criterion-related situations, one can achieve only modest correlations between the criterion and the predictor tests because people are too complex to permit a more accurate estimate of their performance from any test materials. Nunnally cautions that one should interpret a validity coefficient in terms of the degree of possible improvement in performance that might be expected given an individual's score on a specific instrument.

Criterion-related validity is important mostly for making decisions about certain types of applied problems in the social sciences. It is very important in the case of evaluating people for a training program, assigning people to different types of classes, or making decisions concerning the management of people. The results from criterion-related validity testing are generalizable only to the target population studied. Also, the validity coefficients are relevant only to one point in time or to some specified later point; they are not generalizable beyond that specified time period.

A major problem with criterion-related validity is difficulty in obtaining a good criterion. The more abstract the concept, the less likely it is that one will be able to discover appropriate criteria for assessing or measuring it. Also, in some situations external criteria are simply not available. Often, there are serious faults in the selection of a good criterion, and there may well be limitations on the reliability and validity of the criterion measure. The criterion that should be used against a test score should be logically derived from the same concept the test is trying to tap and not an operationalization of some other concept (Knapp, 1985). The use of criterion-related validity has been criticized in the nursing research literature because the criterion selected as the external criterion for an abstract concept has been inappropriate. Nurse researchers have used other variables as an external criterion of the predictor variable that are theoretically related but are not a higher level operationalization of the same concept as the predictor variable (Knapp, 1985). It has been noted that there has been some confusion between construct validity and criterion-related validity (Knapp, 1985). In construct validity, all the variables used in the testing are on equal footing, whereas in criterion-related validity studies, one of the variables has superior status (Knapp, 1985).

Construct Validity

Construct validity is concerned with the extent to which an instrument measures the concept or construct it was designed to measure (Kirshner & Guyatt, 1985). There are three major steps to testing construct validity. The first is the specification of the domain of observables related to the concept. The second is to support from research the extent to which the observables tend to measure the same concept, several different concepts, or many different concepts. The third is to subsequently perform studies of individual differences and/or controlled experiments to determine the extent to which the supposed measures of the concept produce results that are predictable from theory concerning the concept (Nunnally, 1978). The first two steps refer to the testing of validity by examining the internal association or pattern of interrelationships between the indicators designed to measure the concept. The third refers to validity testing by looking at the external association or the pattern of relationships between indicators designed to measure a concept and other variables.

Domain of Observables. This refers to the attempt to support validity that occurs during scale development. As noted earlier in this chapter, concern with defining the concept and embedding it in theory is an important aspect of ensuring validity of the measure. Nunnally (1978) notes that this area is often poorly attended to; perusal of recent studies in nursing research (1981-1985) supports Nunnally's criticism.

Relationships Between Observables. Nunnally (1978) notes that the way to test the adequacy of the identification of observables is to determine how well the measures of observables go together in empirical investigations. The quality of the work done in identifying the domain of observables will influence what occurs here. To determine the ships between the variables, the researcher obtains scores for a sample of individuals on the measure and then correlates different parts of the measure with other parts of the measure. An analysis of the correlations provides evidence on the extent to which all measures relate to the same concept.

Often, the concept has been conceptualized as containing attributes, and these attributes were seen as separate dimensions of the concept. These attributes were defined and items were developed for each at tribute or dimension. Factor analysis was then used to determine the relationship between the dimensions or the internal structure of the set of items. With the use of factor analysis, the researcher studies construct validity in terms of the internal consistency in which different aspects of a conceptual domain tend to correlate highly with one another and be similarly affected by experimental treatments.

Factor analysis as a construct validity technique is only as useful as the theory base on which the concepts have been developed. If factor analysis is used when dimensions of the concept have not been conceptualized, as Nunnally (1978) puts it, "shotgun empiricism" is occurring. Factor analysis is useful when the theoretical structure of the concept has been well developed. Although factor analysis is used frequently in nursing research as a validity technique, often the conceptual basis on which the factors have been proposed is poorly developed. Factor analysis functions as a construct validity technique only when the rotated factor structure produces factors consistent with those theoretically proposed in the conceptualization phase of instrument development.

If the factor analysis indicates that items cluster into multiple factors, which are interpretable according to the theoretically proposed dimensions, it can be concluded that the measure reflects the number of different dimensions consistent with the concept. It does not, by these statistical manipulations, support validity via external association.

As Heise (1973-74) notes, there are no purely mathematical procedures for identifying conceptual variables with guaranteed theoretical validity. Internal association is not adequate to determine the construct validity of an instrument. That variables can group together and appear to be isomorphic with conceptual variables is not sufficient evidence for determining construct validity. Because the proposed number of factors emerge from the factor rotation does not ensure isomorphism with the conceptual dimension. Zeller and Carmines (1980) note that there is an alternative interpretation of the factor solution. It may be that the dual dimensionality of the concept is a function of systematic measurement error and not a theoretically relevant dimension. A method artifact can systematically alter correlations among items and thus appear as a factor in a rotated factor solution. Therefore, factor analysis is not sufficient as a method of determining validity. To determine whether emerged factors are consistent with dimensions as theorized, the investigator must proceed from validity testing via internal association and proceed to testing validity via external association.

Relationships Between Constructs. In this test of construct validity, sufficient evidence is that the supposed measures of the concept behave as expected (Nunnally, 1978). Support for the construct validity of an instrument occurs by determining the extent to which the measures fit in a lawful way into a network of relationships that are expected on the basis of theory. Testing for relationships among constructs is a method for determining construct validity via external association.

Construct validity is assessed within a given theoretical context. The external association that occurs is the relationship between the measure under development and the measure of another external concept to which it is supposedly theoretically related. It is impossible to validate the measure of a concept and its relationship to another concept unless a theoretical network exists to support these two measures. The logic of construct validity can be supported whether the concept is embedded in a systematized or a loose theory or framework or is linked with other concepts by even a few simple propositions. All that is required is several theoretically derived hypotheses involving the particulate concept under measurement. Zeller and Carmines (1980) note that construct validity is never confirmed but is supported by predictions from multiple different studies. Construct validity requires a pattern of consistent findings involving multiple different studies across time performed by different researchers in regard to a variety of diverse theoretical variables.

Construct validity via external association is usually determined using three different methods: (a) discriminance approach, (b) causal inferences approach from experimental or nonexperimental data, and (c) the convergent/discriminant method.

Discriminance Approach. Construct validity estimation by discriminance requires hypothesizing, from theoretical relational statements, differences expected between two groups of participants hypothesized as extremely high and extremely low on the concept being measured by the instrument (Waltz et al., 1984). Determination of these groups and the rationale for why these groups should respond differently on the concept under measurement should be clearly supported by the theory surrounding the concept. The instrument is then administered to both groups and the differences in the scores are computed and examined. If the instrument performs as expected according to the theoretically proposed difference for these two groups, support for the validity of this instrument may be proposed. But because the two groups may differ on multiple characteristics other than that being measured, one must remain sensitive to this possibility when claiming support for the validity of the instrument using the contrasting groups approach (Waltz et al., 1984). For an example of the use of this approach, see Mishel (1981, 1983) and Stevenson (1982). If significant differences are not found between the two groups even though there was a conceptual basis for the expectation of these differences, three possibilities exist: (a) The test is unreliable or perhaps not sufficiently sensitive; (b) the test, although reliable, is not a valid measure of the concept; or (c) there is a need for the researcher to reconceptualize the concept in terms of this population (Waltz et al., 1984). For an example of this third possibility, see Mishel (1983).

Causal Inferences From Experimental or Nonexperimental Data. Construct validity testing by an experimental or nonexperimental approach involves generating hypotheses from a theoretical or conceptual framework. The conceptual basis should be well-developed, with a theoretical system that is as precise as possible. Operationalization of the other variables to be tested in the relational statements should be robust so as to reflect accurately the magnitude of the relationship. The researcher gathers data to test the hypotheses and then makes inferences on the basis of these findings as to whether or not the instrument under construction is adequate to explain the proposed relationships.

One of the ways to derive causal inferences is through use of experimental designs suitable for hypothesis testing. Nonexperimental methods for testing theoretical relationships between concepts include correlational descriptive studies and predictive modeling. Although predictive modeling uses a correlational descriptive design structure, not all correlational descriptive studies include predictive modeling. Predictive modeling involves theoretical model testing and requires a well-specified theoretical framework tested using multivariate data analysis methods (Hinshaw, 1984). On the other hand, correlational descriptive designs can be used to test relational statement from a looser theory or a few simple propositions. For an example of the use of predictive modeling for estimating construct validity, see Hinshaw, Gerber, Atwood, and Allen (1983).

Whichever method is used to test relational statements, a program of repeated testing should be planned to gauge the strength and generality of the relationships. One systematic procedure for investigating conceptual relationships is to begin testing in a tightly controlled setting, moving to progressively looser conditions to determine if the relationship persists. Specified relationships or a theoretical model of multiple relationships may behave differently under different conditions. Thus, populations and contextual variables can be systematically varied to test the viability of the relationship under diverse conditions.

If the evidence relevant to conceptual relationships is negative, four different interpretations are possible. The first is that the instrument does not measure the intended concept. A second alternative is that the theoretical framework on which the empirical prediction was based is incorrect. The third possibility is that the procedure used to test the empirical prediction was faulty. Finally, the negative evidence may be due to a lack of construct validity in some other variable in the analysis (Zeller & Carmines, 1980). Because there is no certain way to determine which of these explanations is correct, further programmatic testing is necessary. The determination of construct validity rests on the gradual accumulation of evidence.

Convergent/Discriminant Method. The multitrait, multimethod matrix method involves the concepts of convergence and discriminance. *Convergence* refers to measuring the same concept using different methods and obtaining similar results. *Discriminance* refers to measuring different concepts using the same method and obtaining different results. Obtaining convergence and discriminance supports the construct validity of the instrument. This approach estimates trait versus method variance. If the correlations between different concepts measured by the same method are higher than correlations between the same concept measured by different methods, a method artifact exists. Conversely, common trait variance exists if the correlation between measures of different concepts measured by the same method is lower than correlation between the same concept measured by different methods (Campbell & Fiske, 1959).

Because this approach requires measuring more than one concept as well as using more than one method to measure each concept, the several methods used to measure each concept must be appropriate to the conceptualization. Wherever possible, these methods should be completely independent of each other.

The correlations are cast into a matrix and examined to determine convergence and discriminance. The matrix consists of the reliability estimate for each measurement method used for each concept (reliability diagonal), correlations between two measures of each concept (validity diagonal), correlations between measures of two different concepts employing the same method (heterotrait-monomethod coefficients), and correlations between measures of different concepts measured by different methods (heterotrait-heteromethod coefficients). For further detail and an example of a matrix and its interpretation, see Campbell and Fiske (1959) or Waltz et al. (1984).

This approach has the advantage of using multiple operationalism in contrast to single operationalism. Multiple operationalism provides a means for distinguishing common trait variance from method variance. Although an extremely valuable means of reliability and validity testing, the cost in time and money may reduce the appeal of the approach. Another consideration is that of the demands placed on clinical populations who must complete multiple instruments at one point in time, which could potentially influence a person's willingness to participate (Waltz et al., 1984).

CONCLUSION

The process of instrument development continuously involves controlling measurement error, thus enhancing the reliability and validity of the measure. In this chapter, the steps in instrument development have been linked to measurement error issues. The intent has been to highlight how measurement error can be reduced at each step in the instrument development process. A central idea in instrumentation is that it is more important to do everything possible to prevent measurement error from occurring rather than to try to assess the effects of measurement error after it has occurred.

REFERENCES

Aitken, R. C. B., & Zealley, A. K. (1970, August). Measurement of moods. *British Journal of Hospital Medicine*, pp. 215-224.

Anastasi, A. (1976). *Psychological testing* (4th ed.). New York: Macmillan.

Armstrong, G. D. (1981). Parametric statistics and ordinal data: A pervasive misconception. *Nursing Research, 30*, 60-62.

Baldree, K. S., Murphy, S. P., & Powers, M. J. (1982). Stress identification and coping patterns in patients on hemodialysis. *Nursing Research, 31*(2), 107-112.

Benoliel, J. Q., McCorkle, R., & Young, K. (1980). Development of a social dependency scale. *Research in Nursing and Health, 3*, 3-10.

Bohrnstedt, G. W. (1970). Reliability and validity assessment in attitude measurement. In G. F. Sinamers (Ed.), *Attitude measurement* (pp. 80-99). Chicago: Rand McNally.

Bond, A., & Lader, M. (1974). The use of analogue scales in rating subjective feelings. *British Journal of Medical Psychology, 47*, 211-218.

Burke, C. J. (1953). Additive scales and statistics. *Psychology Review, 60*, 73-75.

Campbell, D. T., & Fiske, D. W. (1959). Convergent and discriminant validation by the multitrait-multimethod matrix. *Psychological Bulletin, 56*(2), 81-104.

Carmines, E. G., & Zeller, R. A. (1979). *Reliability and validity assessment.* Beverly Hills, CA: Sage.

Cox, C. L. (1985). The health self-determinism index. *Nursing Research, 34*(3), 177-183.

Cranley, M. S. (1981). Development of a tool for the measurement of maternal attachment during pregnancy. *Nursing Research, 30*(5), 281-284.

Derogatis, L. R., & Spencer, P. M. (1984, May 15). Psychometric issues in the assessment of the cancer patient. *Cancer* (Suppl.), pp. 2228-2234.

Edwards, A. L., & Kilpatrick, F. P. (1948). A technique for construction of attitude scales. *Journal of Applied Psychology, 32*, 374-384.

Fox, R. N., & Ventura, M. R. (1983). Small-scale administration of instruments and procedures. *Nursing Research, 32*(2), 122-125.

Glaser, B. (1978). *Theoretical sensitivity.* Mill Valley, CA: Sociology Press.

Gordon, R. A. (1968). Issues in multiple regression. *American Journal of Sociology, 73,* 592-616.

Guilford, J. P. (1936). *Psychometric methods.* New York: McGraw-Hill.

Hauser, P. (1969). Comments on Coleman's paper. in R. Bierstedt (Ed.), *A design for sociology: Scope, objectives, and methods* (pp. 122-136). Philadelphia: American Academy of Political and Social Science.

Heise, D. R. (1973-74). Some issues in sociological measurement. In H. Costner (Ed.), *Sociological methodology* (pp. 1-16). San Francisco: Jossey-Bass.

Hinshaw, A. S. (1984). Theoretical model testing: Full utilization of data. *Western Journal of Nursing Research, 6*(1), 5-10.

Hinshaw, A. S., & Atwood, J. R. (1982). A patient satisfaction instrument: Precision by replication. *Nursing Research, 31*(3), 170-175.

Hinshaw, A. S., Gerber, R. M., Atwood, J. R., & Allen, J. R. (1983). The use of predictive modeling to test nursing practice outcomes. *Nursing Research, 32*(1), 34-42.

Hoskins, C. N. (1981). Psychometrics in nursing research construction of an interpersonal conflict scale. *Research in Nursing and Health, 4,* 243-248.

Hoskins, C. N. (1983). Psychometrics in nursing research: Further development of the interpersonal conflict scale. *Research in Nursing and Health, 6,* 75-83.

Huskisson, E. C. (1974, November). Measurement of pain. *Lancet,* pp. 1127-1131.

Hymovich, D. P. (1983). The chronicity impact and coping instrument: Parent questionnaire. *Nursing Research, 32*(5), 275-281.

Isaac, S., & Michael, W. G. (1974). *Handbook in research and evaluation.* San Diego, CA: Knapp.

Jalowiec, A., & Powers, M. J. (1981). Stress and coping in hypertensive and emergency room patients. *Nursing Research, 30*(1), 10-16.

Kerlinger, F. N. (1986). *Foundations of behavioral research* (3rd ed.). New York: Holt, Rinehart & Winston.

Kirshner, B., & Guyatt, G. (1985). A methodological framework for assessing health indices. *Journal of Chronic Disease, 38*(1), 27-36.

Knapp, T. R. (1985). Validity, reliability, and neither. *Nursing Research, 34*(4), 254-256.

Labovitz, S. (1967). Some observations on measurement and statistics. *Social Forces, 46*(2), 151-160.

Lynn, M. R. (1986). The determination and quantification of content validity. *Nursing Research, 35,* 382-385.

Maxwell, C. (1978). Sensitivity and accuracy of the visual analogue scale: A psychophysical classroom experience. *British Journal of Clinical Pharmacology, 6,* 15-25.

McIver, J., & Carmines, E. (1978). *Unidimensional scaling.* Beverly Hills, CA: Sage.

Mishel, M. H. (1981). The measurement of uncertainty in illness. *Nursing Research, 30*(5), 258-263.

Mishel, M. H. (1983). Parents' perception of uncertainty concerning their hospitalized child. *Nursing Research, 32*(6), 324-330.

Murphy, S. P., Powers, M. J., & Jalowiec, A. (1985). Psychometric evaluation of the hemodialysis stressor scale. *Nursing Research, 34*(6), 368-371.

Nagel, E. (1974). Measurement Erkinnsnis 11 Bond, 1931. In G. Maranell (Ed.), *Scaling: A sourcebook for behavioral scientists.* Chicago: Aldine.

Norbeck, J. S., Lindsey, A. M., & Carrieri, V. L. (1981). The development of an instrument to measure social support. *Nursing Research, 30*(5), 264-269.

Nunnally, J. C. (1978). *Psychometric theory.* New York: McGraw-Hill.

Osgood, C. E., Suci, C. J., & Tannenbaum, P. H. (1957). *The measurement of meaning.* Urbana: University of Illinois Press.

Stevens, S. S. (1951). Mathematics, measurement and psychophysics. In S. S. Stevens (Ed.), *Handbook of experimental psychology.* New York: John Wiley.

Stevenson, J. S. (1982). Construction of a scale to measure load, power, and margin in life. *Nursing Research, 31*(4), 222-225.

Thurstone, L. L. (1927). The method of paired comparisons for social values. *Journal of Abnormal and Social Psychology, 21,* 384-400.

Thurstone, L. L. (1928). An experimental study of nationality preferences. *Journal of Genetic Psychology, 1,* 405-425.

Thurstone, L. L. (1929). Theory of attitude measurement. *Psychological Bulletin, 36,* 222-241.

Thurstone, L. L., & Chave, E. J. (1929). *The measurement of attitude.* Chicago: University of Chicago Press.

Title, C. R., & Hill, R. J. (1967). Attitude measurement and prediction of behavior: An evaluation of conditions and measurement techniques. *Sociometry, 30,* 199-213.

Torgerson, W. S. (1958). *Theory and methods of scaling.* New York: John Wiley.

Walker, L. O., & Avant, K. D. (1983). *Strategies for theory construction in nursing.* Norwalk, CT: Appleton-Century-Crofts.

Waltz, C. F., Strickland, O. L., & Lenz, E. R. (1984). *Measurement in nursing research.* Philadelphia: F. A. Davis.

Ware, J. E., Snyder, M. K., McClure, R. E., & Jarett, I. M. (1972). *The measurement of health concepts* (Tech. rep. No. HCP-72-5). Springfield, VA: U.S. Department of Commerce, National Technical Information Service.

Wolf, M. H., Putnam, S. M., James, S. A., & Stiles, W. B. (1978). The medical interview satisfaction scale: Development of a scale to measure patient perceptions of physician behavior. *Journal of Behavioral Medicine, 1*(4), 391-402.

Zeller, R. A., & Carmines, E. G. (1980). *Measurement in the social sciences.* London: Cambridge University Press.

PART IV

EXPLORATORY-DESCRIPTIVE
DESIGNS

Exploratory-descriptive designs, usually field studies in natural settings, provide the least control over variables. The data collected
either contribute to the development of theory or explain phenomena
from the perspective of the persons being studied.

There are two major types of *descriptive studies:* those that provide (a)
descriptions of a single broad variable in a single population or (b)
descriptions of population characteristics. These studies answer the
question, What are the X customs of Y population? or What are the
characteristics of X population? These questions result in description of
either the population characteristics or the variable. Lack of current
knowledge about either the variable or the population precludes the use
of a theoretical base for the study, because specific predictions of cause-
and-effect relationships cannot be made.

Studies of a single variable previously investigated in one population
but not in another are appropriately descriptive. Just because a variable
has been studied and described in one population does not necessarily
mean that it even exists in another population. Therefore, the first task
of a researcher is to find the variable itself, then describe how the

variable exists or acts in the new population. Previously studied variables usually form the basis for a theoretical explanation of their action. In this case, descriptive studies of single (previously studied) variables in unknown or understudied populations are usually based on theory derived from previous research.

A population survey, like the study of a single variable, is atheoretical, and no cause-and-effect relationship is sought and no predictions can be made other than the fact that population characteristics will exist. Such a statement is in fact a basic assumption of the study and therefore not a prediction or the basis of a hypothesis. Two reasons for doing population surveys might be that a similar study may have been done but a fresh perspective is being sought or that an update of an older study is needed to determine if there has been any change over time. In both cases, the studies are cross-sectional descriptions of a population.

Descriptive studies of populations take two perspectives. Population studies reflect the perspective of the investigator, using questionnaires and interviews as the primary data collection methods. In contrast, ethnographies, using multiple data collection methods (participant observation, census, available data, interviews, genealogies, life histories, and demographics) attempt to discover population characteristics from the perspective of the person being studied. Ethology, the minute observation and description of nonverbal behaviors of humans and animals, is purely descriptive. Ethnomethodology, through direct observation and film analysis, attempts to discover the cultural rules underlying everyday behavior and addresses the question, What are the informal rules underlying X behavior or X social interaction? Although descriptive studies attempt to discover the world of the research participant and describe it accurately, the analysis is usually from the perspective of the observer or researcher. Because the analysis is guided by the researcher, the study may be analyzed from the perspective of known theory as well as being purely descriptive in form.

Historical designs could have been discussed as descriptive designs that use content analysis of available data; however, historiography has been used by historians exclusively for a very long time. Our definition of descriptive studies has its antecedents in the social sciences rather than the humanities and so we felt it best to give the historical method its own chapter.

Exploratory studies, on the other hand, have three functions: (a) for in-depth exploration and description of a single variable, process, or phenomenon, to arrive at complete description and explication; (b) as a feasibility study (also known as a pilot project) to determine whether or not a study plan is feasible as designed (the pilot project will be dealt with separately in another chapter); and (c) as the first phase of a planned long-term research project.

Exploratory designs are commonly employed in an attempt to see the world as the participant or research participant sees it. These designs are often equated with qualitative designs, because they rely on qualitative data collection methods exclusively. Phenomenology, ethnoscience, and grounded theory are the major designs within qualitative research. Grounded theory always assumes process and aims for a theoretical explanation of how the process works. Ethnoscience uses linguistic analysis to define a situation or abstract concept. Phenomenology seeks to describe the experience of the phenomenon under study (e.g., What does it feel like to be a patient in a hospital?), although the goal is not to discover process as a grounded theory. Experience involves process; therefore, how one experiences a phenomenon constitutes a description of a process. Ethnoscience, more frequently called "ethnography" by some nurse-anthropologists (Aamodt, 1982), has rigid rules for data analysis based on repeated observation of natural behaviors, whereas phenomenology and grounded theory are more flexible and depend more on the creativity of the researcher in the analysis of data. They are also most likely to use nontraditional sources of data.[1]

The issue of control in exploratory designs is moot, because the situation not the investigator, controls the data. Rather, it is the flexibility of the investigator that is essential in these designs. The investigator must be able to "go with the flow," to abandon an area that is not fruitful or to go in depth into an area not previously planned. Descriptive studies, with their more structured data collection (instrumentation is available in many cases) and more specific samples, afford greater control over measurement than do exploratory studies. The least controlled, most flexible, and most creative study is the exploratory design. Critical to both studies are the step-by-step explication of the sample selection process, the data collection procedures used, and the techniques for data analysis. Because these designs often describe totally uncharted areas, validity and reliability depend on the meticulous use of detailed field notes, selection of field informants, and repeated observations and interviews of the same participant over time.

We conclude with a brief chapter on the pilot study by Nancy Lackey and Anita Wingate—a neglected subject in most research texts. Although authors have consistently placed pilot studies under the exploratory design heading, we feel the pilot study is not limited to the exploratory level. Indeed, if a pilot or feasibility is not planned at all levels of research, the final study is likely to be flawed. We heard this paper presented at the 1987 Midwest Nursing Research Society meeting and liked it. We hope you do too.

NOTE

1. We are indebted to Field and Morse (1985) for the clarity of their definitions and descriptions of qualitative research approaches in their text, and we are delighted that they frequently used the question approach to clarify the differences in these designs.

REFERENCES

Aamodt, A. M. (1982). Examining ethnography for nursing researchers. *Western Journal of Nursing Research, 4*(2), 209-222.

Field, P., & Morse, J. (1985). *Nursing research: The application of qualitative approaches.* London: Croom Helm.

11

Descriptive Designs

PAMELA J. BRINK
MARILYNN J. WOOD

Part of the development of a complete database for any science is the detailed description and classification of the various phenomena related to that science. Prior to the manipulation or disruption of any natural phenomena, the researcher spends years in the intimate study of a particular problem. The difficulty for any new science has been the establishment of the phenomena unique to that discipline. The fields of anatomy and physiology began with a painstaking description of gross anatomy based on detailed and repetitive observations of cadavers. Today, anatomy remains an essentially descriptive science, albeit at the microscopic level. Criminology is based on the intense study of criminals and their characteristics and on detailed study of the interactions between criminals and their victims. The sciences of astronomy, zoology, and botany are also based on painstaking description and classification. Nursing science similarly requires that any phenomenon first be explored at the qualitative level, then validated through the descriptive design. Thorough exploration and description of a phenomenon must precede the search for relationships between it and other phenomena.

Research studies using the descriptive design include anthropological ethnographies (descriptions of the social systems of single small societies or culture groups), census studies, and sociological demographics (demographic characteristics of particular populations). A number of descriptive studies in both the natural and social sciences have been featured on television. The work of Jane Goodall, Jacques Cousteau, and of the Leakey family (Louis, Mary, and Richard), and the story of Lucy are all descriptive field studies. A number of educational television series, including *The Disappearing World, Nova,* and *River Journeys,* provide ethnographic (descriptive) accounts of unfamiliar peoples and places. Descriptive designs are usually, but not always, cross-sectional and make use of both qualitative and quantitative data collection methods. The type of method chosen depends on the sample size and level of knowledge about the variable and the population. Descriptive research can be either inductive or deductive. For the most part, however, these terms are not useful, because valid description contributes to theory building as well as to theory testing.

BASIC OR CLASSICAL DESIGN

There are two major types of descriptive designs. The first is a simple population survey or demography whose purpose is to describe the total population or a representative sample of the population. These descriptive surveys are identifiable by the fact that the data are presented as frequencies. Frequently, data are presented in the form of descriptive statistics. Occasionally, correlations or differences between groups may be presented but this does not alter the type of design. To reiterate, a descriptive design does not *test* relationships between variables. When various characteristics of a particular population are either unknown or partially (incompletely) known, the design of choice is the descriptive design. Thus, the question, What are the characteristics of successful dieters? can be answered through a descriptive study. (Although some may respond, "Easy—they lose weight!" this response is, in reality, a definition of a successful dieter, not a description of their common characteristics—not the plural.) Even when there has been previous research about a variable, a descriptive design may be used if the researcher wishes to study that variable in a different population. Descriptions of the characteristics of men may or may not apply to women. But until the characteristics of women are also described for the same variables, knowledge of both sexes is limited. The critical point is that the variable in question either has not been studied (or reported) previously for a particular population or was reported long enough ago to warrant a new study. Thus, the descriptive survey design is used when we want to describe the incidence, prevalence or amount of particular characteristics present in a population. These might be demographics, health or illness indicators, social factors, or other such characteristics.

The second type of descriptive design involves the complete description of a single broad variable or concept within a given population. The variable should be either unstudied or understudied in that population. Examples of descriptive questions on single variables include, What are the health beliefs of the Amish of Iowa? What are the value orientations of the Annang of Nigeria? (Brink, 1984) and What types of birth defects occur among infants of teenage mothers? Complete description of specific phenomena within a population is critical to theory building (inductive) as well as to theory testing (deductive). Descriptive studies contribute to both purposes. For example, the work of Florence Kluckhohn served the purpose of contributing to anthropological knowledge about human nature and was inductive in its beginning stages. Florence Kluckhohn lived on or near a Navajo reservation for many summers, using participant observation. From her observations, she began to develop a concept of human nature as a series of societal decisions in relation to values. Kluckhohn felt that all human groups need to solve certain common problems and that the way a society solves its problems reflects what it values and believes. These values and beliefs are amenable to discovery through questioning. On the basis of her theory, Kluckhohn and Strodtbeck (1961) developed and tested the Value Orientation instrument on five cultural groups in the southwestern United States. The configuration of value orientations obtained by means of Kluckhohn's instrument constituted a description of a particular cultural group. Because Kluckhohn developed an instrument to test her theory, the resulting descriptive research was deductive. Several other authors also used the Value Orientation schedule (Brink, 1984; DeMay, 1982; Downing & Cobb, 1990; Edgecombe, 1994; Gushuliak, 1990) to describe the values in a specific culture group. All were descriptive studies. All contributed to the verification and validation of the instrument as well as to the underlying theory.

A purely descriptive study reported by McIver at the 1985 Council of Nurse Researchers meetings in San Diego was based on the question: "What are the symptoms reported by menopausal women?" She interviewed over 100 women, many of them several times, to discuss their experiences during and postmenopause and to discover their common symptomatology. Once the data had been analyzed and categories derived, McIver was able to report symptomatology (e.g., breast pain) very common among this population that had never been reported in the literature. She was not interested in building a theory about menopause; rather, she was concerned with a more complete description of this population.

BASIC ASSUMPTIONS UNDERLYING DESCRIPTIVE DESIGNS

The following assumptions are implicit in the use of descriptive designs:

1. The variable exists in the population under study, and it is a single variable amenable to description.
2. There is little or no literature that describes the current population (or variable) at the present time.
3. There may be no theoretical framework for the study, but a detailed rationale for the research based on a thorough literature review is necessary.
4. There may be a theoretical or conceptual framework underlying the study, as in the case of a known concept being studied in a new population. Previous research provides the rationale and framework for the present study.
5. When the population parameters are unknown and the basic criteria for external validity cannot be met through sample selection procedures, the findings cannot be generalized from the sample to the population.
6. When population parameters are known and the basic criteria for external validity can be met through sample selection procedures, population parameters can be estimated from sample measures.

A number of classic descriptive designs have emerged from different disciplines. These classic designs include demography, ethnography, ethnomethodology, content analysis, population census, opinion polls, ethology, ethnographic semantics or ethnoscience, descriptive linguistics, and archaeology. Each of these designs can be distinguished according to (a) whether a population (ethnography, demography, census) or a variable (ethnomethodology, ethnoscience, content analysis) is to be described and (b) whether the data collection method is observation (ethology, archaeology), questioning (ethnomethodology, ethnoscience, ethnographic semantics, descriptive linguistics), available data (content analysis, archaeology), or a combination of many methods (ethnography). All these designs appear to fit at least one of our two basic attributes of descriptive designs: a description of a single broad variable within a specific population (ethnoscience, ethology, archaeology) or a description of the characteristics of a population as a whole (ethnography, census, demography).

CONCEPTUAL FRAMEWORK

Descriptive studies frequently lack a conceptual framework; the rationale for the study therefore becomes critical. The investigator must explain, for example, how the research might promote the development of nursing knowledge and how the results might lead to further work. Without such rationales, descriptive studies tend to appear insignificant, are unlikely to be funded by granting agencies, and are unlikely to be published once completed. Only in this area does a descriptive design proposal differ from proposals using other designs.

CONTROL OVER DATA

Control over data is limited in descriptive designs. The setting is essentially uncontrolled or outside the control of the investigator. The investigator exerts some control over sample selection when drawing a representative sample from the population. Descriptive studies always examine the variable or sample as it exists, without investigator interference.

SAMPLING

The ideal sample for a descriptive design is either a total available population (particularly with small populations) or a sample drawn by means of probability sampling techniques from a target population. If the purpose of a study is to describe population characteristics, probability sampling techniques are necessary to ensure external validity. The U.S. census employs a descriptive design that uses both systematic sampling techniques (for in-depth data collection of 10% of the population) and total available population (for a comprehensive description of the population characteristics). Frequently, however, population parameters are not available and probability sampling cannot be used, thereby creating problems for external validity. When the purpose of the study is simply to describe the characteristics of a particular group of people using a sample from the target population, external validity is of importance to the design. If a total population is used, however, external validity is not relevant, because no generalization will be made. If the purpose is to describe an entire population, no predictions are being made or intended, so generalizations are not relevant. However, external validity can become an issue in a total population study if the rate of refusal to participate is high. Then the sample becomes a "volunteer" sample rather than a total population, and the results must be interpreted accordingly. For example, the University of Alberta conducts an exit survey of its graduates each year. Questionnaires are distributed with the diplomas received by the graduates. This attempt at a total population study typically results in a 30% response rate. The results are then subject to criticism because no data are available to distinguish respondents from nonrespondents. A random sample from the population using telephone interviews might result in a more representative sample. Most descriptive studies of this nature must be generalizable to the target population or interpretation of the results becomes impossible.

Even when a probability sample is planned, the nature of the population may be such that it is never achieved. This was a problem faced by Edgecombe (1994) in her study of the Copper Inuit. Although she had a list of the total population of the town of Coppermine, Northwest Territories, Canada, and she created a stratified random sample by gender, age, and years of schooling, she was unable to study all the participants in the predetermined sample. In this case, she was in Coppermine during the summer months, the time of caribou hunts. When she went to someone's home for the interview, often that person had left to go on a hunt (which lasted several days and sometimes weeks). What began as a probability sample deteriorated into a convenience sample of all those left who agreed to be interviewed within the time frame available (in other words before winter set in and transportation out became difficult). In this case, the research law (a corollary to Murphy's Law, which says that "if anything can go wrong, it will") of "as soon as you begin data collection, the sample disappears," went into effect. This is a common problem faced by researchers in other designs and is not limited to the descriptive design. For these reasons, internal validity is not an issue in descriptive designs because no attempts are made to examine causal relationships between variables.

METHODS OF DATA COLLECTION

The methods used in this design are primarily structured. Semistructured methods are used to enhance or to add information but are not the sole source of data. Data collection methods include observation, questioning, available data, projective techniques, physical assessment or physiological tests of humans, and chemical or physical tests on nonhumans or inanimate objects. Studies may use a single in-depth method, such as intensive interviewing, or combinations of structured and semistructured methods (structured interviews coupled with participant observation, collection of written and unwritten available data, oral histories, genograms and kinship charts, cartography, multiple physical specimens or measurements, still and moving photographs, recordings of music). Data in census studies are usually collected through interviews, questionnaires, or both (Fink & Kosecoff, 1985). Descriptive studies of single variables are usually grounded in ethnographic accounts of a single culture or group.

Ethnographies (e.g., Agar, 1980; Ellen, 1984; Field & Morse, 1985; Germain, 1986; Hammersley & Atkinson, 1983; Pelto & Pelto, 1978), also called fieldwork (Wax, 1971; Werner & Schoepfle, 1987; Whiting et al., 1966; Whyte, 1984), rely on a combination of data collection methods, usually including all of the following: participant observation (McCall & Simmons, 1969), available data (Pelto & Pelto, 1978; Stewart, 1984), intensive interviewing (Agar, 1986; Spradley, 1979), census, kinship charts (Crane & Angrosino, 1984), life histories, and photographic and audiotape evidence. Because ethnographies are assumed to be a description of a culture or specific group within a single culture, the purpose of the description is to be as comprehensive as possible. Different data collection methods are used to ensure that the description is valid. When only one method of data collection is used, whether it is interviewing or the use of questionnaires, there is no way to validate the self-reported information. Ethnographies rely on observations over time; available data, such as from newspapers and diaries; and cultural artifacts to support or to refute material gained from questioning. Many individuals make the error of assuming that if they use the ethnographic semantic method of interviewing (Spradley, 1979), they are *doing* ethnography. Ethnography demands participant observation and assumes the investigator will include a cultural description of the setting or context to support the interview material. When Spradley was talking about doing an ethnographic interview, he was referring to interviewing techniques useful in doing an ethnography. He did not intend for people to believe that using these techniques would yield an ethnography in the absence of other field methods. The book on interviewing was intended to be used in conjunction with his second book on participant observation (Spradley, 1980).

The data collection instruments used for ethnographies are predominantly structured and semistructured rather than unstructured, reflecting an important difference between descriptive and exploratory designs. In some instances, the variable under study can be found only in data such as in hospital charts or newspapers or in data collected for other purposes (including other research studies). These descriptive studies are thus based on available data, and the task of the researcher is to sort the data into some logical taxonomic form (see Hunter & Foley, 1976; Krippendorf, 1980). Animal field studies yield a great deal of photographic material on which secondary analysis can be based. Nurses' notes, nursing care plans, and published articles are all grist for the available data descriptive study.

A frequent method of data collection is questioning, in the form of either interviews or questionnaires (Spradley, 1979). The vignette technique used in the Kluckhohn and Strodtbeck (1961), Flaskerud (1980), and Brink (1984) studies to elicit culturally based belief systems is both a highly structured data collection device and a projective test of underlying values and beliefs. Hayter (1983) developed questionnaires based on sleep behaviors documented in younger populations, then modified the questionnaires to allow for differences that might be present in an older group. Archer's (1983) study of political participation, on the other hand, merely collected demographic data on the population using structured tools related to political behavior.

Observational techniques can also be used, particularly participant observation (McCall & Simmons, 1969; Spradley, 1980). Many descriptive studies of natural phenomena rely exclusively on direct but non-participant field observations, especially in fields such as archaeology, astronomy, and field primatology. Mixed methods are also used frequently. Because the knowledge base is so uncertain, the researcher may not be sure which method will be best or most efficient for data collection.

The relevance of the data collection method to the population must be considered. For example, interviewing individuals to ask them what they do in particular situations must be validated through the use of observational techniques to see if respondents actually do what they say they do in those situations. If, on the other hand, the sample is being asked about beliefs, personal history, or personal facts, observational techniques would not be useful. In this case, interviews with other knowledgeable people to support or refute participants' statements can be valuable.

In a descriptive study based entirely on questionnaire or interview data collection instruments, the questions and the order in which they are asked are completely planned before any interviewing takes place. In other words, the degree of flexibility needed in an exploratory study is not appropriate for a descriptive study. For example, in some exploratory studies, the investigator asks questions as they are conceived. The questions, as well as their order, may differ from participant to participant. In descriptive designs, this flexibility is not allowed. This structure gives the researcher control over the data insofar as questions are standardized and are asked in a standardized order.

The type of question asked can be either semistructured or structured. A semistructured question is one in which the question is standardized and the order in which the question is asked is preset, but answers are open and unstructured. Examples of semistructured questions include the following:

- *Grand tour questions* (Spradley & McCurdy, 1972) (setting the tone for the interview or questionnaire): "I would like you to tell me about the last time you gave birth. Just begin at the beginning, when you began to have labor pains, start from there."

- *Complete the sentence:* "People should abstain from alcohol and drugs because . . . "

- *Fill in:* "I believe nurses_____ every day."

- *Contrast or comparative questions:* "Tell me what you think are the differences between men and women in relation to their ability to successfully lose weight. In what way are they similar? In your opinion, who would have the most difficulty successfully losing weight?"

- *Inclusive questions:* "What kinds of people become drug addicts?" Or "If you were on the admissions committee of a school of nursing, what qualities would you insist applicants have?" Or "What are the qualities or characteristics of a *good* nurse?"

- *Exclusive questions:* "If you were to develop a new community program in eldercare, who would not be eligible?" Or "What kinds of research would you say are not nursing research?" Or "What kinds of problems are not health problems?"

The smaller the sample size, the larger the number of semistructured questions that can be included in an interview. One of the reasons for this is that semistructured questions (preset, open-ended questions) usually lead to large amounts of unstructured data that must be put into some sensible format. The purpose of many descriptive studies is to attempt to show contrasts or similarities among participants on a particular topic or series of topics. The more questions in the interview, the more pragmatic the data analysis. Rather than reading the entire interview for its content and flow, the analyst reads each participant's answers to each question. The question and its answer becomes the data set, not the interview in its entirety. The intent is to describe similarities and differences in answering the particular question, not to explore holistically an entire transcript.

If one person is asked to tell a life history in 1 or 2 hours, the amount of data to be transcribed and analyzed will be enormous. Two people answering the same question with the same amount of data will yield twice the complexity of analysis—three even more so, and so on.

Investigators find that large amounts of unstructured data can be unwieldy and that some mechanism for analysis through the use of computers becomes necessary. Even though computer programs that can handle this type of data are now available, investigators limit the number of people in the sample rather than the amount of data from each person.

The opposite is equally true: The larger the sample, the more structured the questions need to be and the fewer the unstructured questions allowable. This results partially from computer-assisted analysis of data, in which numerical answers can be entered easily into a computer and statistically manipulated. The more numerical answers in a questionnaire or observational checklist, the more easily the data can be prepared for computer analysis.

Examples of structured questions on an ordinal scale include the following:

- *Multiple choice:* Which of the following best represents your family income level? Select only one answer.
  a. $ 0-4,999 per year
  b. $ 5,000-9,999 per year
  c. $10,000-19,999 per year
  d. $20,000-29,999 per year
  e. $30,000 or more per year

- *Likert-type scale:* Check the one response that best describes how you feel about this statement: "Alcoholism is basically a character disorder."

  |———— |———— |———— |———— |———— |

  strongly   strongly
  disagree   agree

  Please rate how well the following statement fits your belief about abortion: "Abortion is an act of murder."

  |———— |———— |———— |———— |———— |

  strongly   strongly
  disagree   agree

- *Ranking:* Which three of the following life events have been most difficult for you? Please rank your three choices in order, from the most difficult (1) to the least difficult (3).

  _____ Childhood

  _____ Marriage

  _____ Retirement

  _____ Illness of self or spouse

  _____ Death of spouse or other close relative

  _____ Children leaving home

  _____ Parenthood

  _____ Other (please specify)

Some seemingly open-ended fill-in questions are, in reality, highly structured, metric-scale questions. For example, when you ask an individual, "How old are you?" and provide a fill-in blank, the answer will be given in numerical years. Numbers or numerical answers of this kind are considered structured questions, as are fill-in answers requiring blood pressure readings, temperature, and pulse, despite the fact that a fill-in blank is provided. In this case only a number is expected.

Whether questions are structured or semistructured, the purpose is to be as standardized as possible at this stage of the research in order to analyze the answers to each individual question as a unit in and of itself using descriptive statistics. Later analysis (using tests of association or correlation depending on the type of question) might attempt to show an association between the answers from one question and one or more other questions or the demographic data.

RELIABILITY AND VALIDITY

Issues of reliability and validity in studies using qualitative data collection methods can be treated as a different order of phenomena than quantitative data (see Lincoln & Guba, 1985) or as similar (Brink, 1989). Instruments developed in one population may prove unreliable or invalid in another. For example, the variable may not exist in a population other than the one in which it was previously described; or it may not exist in the same form, causing the measurement to miss critical elements of the variable in the new population. Reliability and validity of the source of the data are also important. Lack of knowledge about the population can lead an investigator to make serious errors in designing the study. This possibility makes pretesting of all tools essential. *Acquiescent response set* (in which certain individuals always tend to agree with the interviewer) and *social desirability* (in which people tend to answer according to what they think is the socially correct answer rather than the actual answer, which may make them look silly or stupid) are validity issues that need to be addressed. These traits may be more prominent in an unknown culture than the investigator expects. Depending on who else is present in an interview session, social desirability can be a confounding factor in any culture. When the investigator is seen as having high social status or when the interviewer is thought to be connected with the police or other law enforcement, as in the case of interviewing illegal aliens, social desirability becomes especially problematic.

There are two standard methods of ensuring the reliability and validity of data in descriptive studies: (a) the use of repeated interviews over time on the same participant and (b) the use of observations in conjunction with interviews. In the first instance the researcher tests the stability of the informants' statements. Because it is difficult to tell an untruth over and over again on a variety of topics, repeated interviews with a single informant yield reliable data in the end. While interviewing the informant in a natural setting, the researcher usually asks for interpretations, explanations, or both of what is going on in that setting at the time of the interview. The researcher observes the social scene, then asks the informant for an explanation. The researcher can also ask informants what they do in particular situations and then observe them in those situations to see if, indeed, their reports were accurate. Such validation procedures are a necessary requisite to descriptive designs using either interviewing or observation. When a descriptive design uses available data, the researcher can return to the data again and again to make certain that the database elicited from the written material is correct. Such repeated readings may also yield new insights into the material that were not immediately apparent on the first reading. To validate these new insights, the researcher can ask a second person to review the materials, given this new definition; that person can tell the researcher if the material supports the new conclusions.

DATA ANALYSIS

Methods of analysis will differ according to the type of study, the sampling procedures, and the degree of complexity of data collection methods. The least complex study would involve one type of data collection method and one level of measurement in a predominantly structured data collection instrument supplemented with a few semi-structured items most usual in surveys. A more complex study would involve a combination of data collection methods and a combination of levels of measurement within and across methods, resulting in a mixture of structured and unstructured data, a mixture of nominal, ordinal, and metric-scale data, and a mixture of informational sources. This is the case in ethnographic research.

When data are semistructured or unstructured, data analysis begins with content analysis (Krippendorf, 1980; Miles & Huberman, 1994; Wilson, 1985, chap. 14), separating the answers to each question into mutually exclusive categories of similar content. The first step in content analysis is to read all answers to each question several times to establish a "feel" for the answers. As each answer is read, a "general sense" of the implication of the answers is established, producing a beginning formulation of possible contrasting categories of content. An initial attempt is made to separate all content into these initial categories. During this process, subcategories of content within each of the original categories become apparent, and a second analysis is begun based on the new categorization of mutually exclusive contrast material. At each step, the decisions or rules guiding separation of content are written down. Eventually, all the data will be accounted for in some category. The number of responses within each category and subcategory can be tabulated, and frequencies can be reported on that tabulation.

Also basic to this design are descriptive statistics (frequencies, percentages, means, medians, and modes), including standard deviations, quartiles, and ranges. If the collected data already exist in numerical form, the first step in analysis is to summarize the responses to each question. For nominal data, this will include simple frequencies and modes; for ordinal data, it includes frequencies, ranges, and medians; and for interval and ratio data, frequencies, variances, and means.

Interval and ratio data can also be described in relation to ranges, standard deviations, and quartiles.

In studies of population characteristics, sample statistics are used to predict population parameters. It is possible, therefore, to estimate the incidence of disease or other health problems in the population from data collected from a random sample.

When the study calls for nonprobability sampling and/or when measurement is at the nominal or ordinal level, nonparametric statistics are used. Whether the study is of a single variable or of a population as a whole, simple tests of association are helpful as an aid to discovering whether or not there are any indicators for further research on the same or other populations. The question to be answered is, Is there any association between the answers to any of the individual questions and any of the population characteristics? When the study is of a single variable, these tests are usually done between the variable under study and the demographic characteristics of the sample. If all data are nominal or if the major variable is nominal and all other variables are run against a nominal variable, the chi-square test is useful. If ordinal variables are used as the base variable against ordinal or metric data, Spearman's rho is helpful. Otherwise, the Pearson is used to test for relationships between metric variables. When the study is of population characteristics as a whole, all population variables are run against one another (using tests appropriate for the level of measurement) to determine whether there are any associations worth following up in another study.

HUMAN SUBJECTS ISSUES

Human subjects issues vary widely. In ethnographic studies, the participants' lack of understanding of the research process may present problems. In this case, issues of *informed consent* are very important, because explanation of the research in terms the participant can understand is critical. In participant observation studies, the issues are the same as those in qualitative research. In census studies, the major ethical concerns include confidentiality of the data and anonymity of the study participants.

EXAMPLES OF DESCRIPTIVE DESIGNS

Archer (1983) designed a study to provide baseline data on nursing administrators' participation in policy-making processes. A random sample of 1,086 nurse administrators from community health agencies, home health agencies, hospitals, and schools of nursing was drawn for the study, according to the following proportionate design:

1. All directors of public health nursing services of state and territorial health departments
2. Five directors of local public health nursing services, randomly selected from each state and territory
3. Five directors of home health agencies, randomly selected from each state's list of member agencies in the NLN Council of Home Health Agencies and Community Health Services
4. Seven directors of hospital nursing services, randomly selected from each state's and territory's list of Joint Commission Accredited Hospitals with more than 200 beds
5. Three deans, randomly selected from NLN-accredited baccalaureate and higher degree programs in each state and territory

The rationale for sampling was to have each type of institution represented in approximate proportion to its representation in the national agency or institutional population. The instrument for data collection was a self-administered, mailed, anonymous questionnaire developed specifically for this study and extensively pretested to develop face and content validity. Overall political participation for the sample of nursing administrators was relatively high and is described in detail in the report in the form of a typology of activities. Archer explains that the results may have been influenced by the fact that data collection occurred during a successful campaign to overturn the Nurse Training Act veto. The most common reason given for lack of political participation was deficient understanding and skill in the political process.

This report provides a good example of a descriptive study based on a survey of population characteristics. The author uses a proportionate random sample from carefully defined nursing administration groups that can be generalized to this population of administrators. There is no conceptual framework for the study, but the author explains that political participation in issues related to public policy affecting nursing is part of the professional responsibility of the nurse.

Hayter (1983) studied sleep behaviors of older persons. This study exemplifies how a variable (sleep behaviors) that is well-documented in different populations can be studied in a population in which it has not been examined before (older persons). Because of lack of norms for the elderly population, older persons' sleep had been evaluated on the basis of sleep norms for younger adults. The purpose of this study was to determine the nature of sleep behaviors in older persons of different ages.

Two instruments were devised for the study, both based on previous literature on sleep behaviors. The first was a questionnaire designed to supply information about typical sleep behaviors, demographic variables, and daily activities that might affect sleep. The second was a modified version of another researcher's sleep chart, on which participants marked each 30-minute period they were asleep during each 24-hour period for 2 weeks. Both instruments were pretested with healthy older persons. A pilot study was conducted to test reliability and validity of the instrument on 22 residents without major health problems at a home for the aged.

The investigator drew a random sample of 325 older persons from a pool of over 1,000 who had given their permission to be contacted as potential study participants for research through a gerontology center. The instruments were mailed to the participants, along with instructions; 212 people returned complete responses.

The findings clearly document a pattern of gradually increasing need for both rest and sleep with advancing age, with the need for increased rest occurring earlier than the need for increased sleep. These data show that certain changes are expected in sleep behaviors with increasing age and that sleep patterns differ markedly from those of younger people. These findings emphasize the need for documentation of known concepts in unknown populations and support the idea that patterns that are valid in one population may not be so in another.

In a different type of descriptive design, Flaskerud (1980) compared perceptions of problematic behavior in three different populations. Three groups of respondents (Appalachian laypersons, non-Appalachian laypersons, and mental health professionals) were interviewed using eight vignettes that described various problematic behaviors. The vignettes were developed from actual case histories of Appalachians diagnosed as mentally ill and hospitalized with that diagnosis. Each respondent was asked to label the behavior and suggest appropriate methods of management.

A metropolitan neighborhood that served as an entry point for Appalachian migrants was selected as the available population of lay Appalachians. A sample of 75 households was drawn from a list of 250 houses. To ensure an equal number of men and women in the sample, the sex of the participant selected differed in alternate households. Other criteria for sample selection included age and area from which respondents migrated. A total of 50 households were eligible for inclusion in the study. Mental health professionals were selected from all agencies serving the Appalachian migrant or located within the target neighborhood. The total population of professionals making diagnostic judgments in these agencies were asked to participate, and 54 agreed. Lay non-Appalachians were selected from a random sampling of names from a telephone book listing persons living in an area contiguous to the Appalachian neighborhood. The phone book page, column, and line were all randomly selected. To account for individuals who did not have telephones, the household next to the one selected from the book was included. In the case of multiple units, all units were listed and one selected at random. Of the persons selected by this process, 51 agreed to participate.

Content analysis was used to categorize all labels as mental illness (MI) or non-mental illness (NMI), and all treatments as psychiatric treatment (PT) or as nonpsychiatric treatment (NPT). The composition of the resulting categories was then compared both within and across groups using a one-way analysis of variance. No significant differences were found between mental health professionals and the lay group of non-Appalachians, but significant differences were found between these two groups and the lay Appalachians.

This report provides a good example of a descriptive design that examines a known variable (diagnosis of mental illness) in three different populations, looking for similarities and differences among the three. The findings show that the Appalachian population did not see the behavior described in the vignettes as abnormal, indicating a significant cultural gap. This study differs from a comparative design in its lack of theoretical framework and hypotheses and in the manner in which the concept of diagnosis of mental illness was measured. The study uses random sampling from two of the populations and the total population for the third, thus producing generalizable results. However, because the purpose of this study was to describe the population, we can only speculate about reasons for the findings. The study, therefore, leads to the development of hypotheses for further study.

SUMMARY

Essential features of the descriptive design include the following:

1. Breadth of data—comprehensive data collection from every conceivable source, using every available method from every available knowledgeable participant—should result in a *complete* description of the variable or the population.
2. Reliability and validity of the measurements is crucial. When instruments are used for the first time with a population, they must be pretested to establish their reliability and validity. If the data collection instruments are completely unstructured, perhaps the choice of design is incorrect and the study belongs in the qualitative arena.
3. The sample should be either a total population or a representative sample from a larger population.

Suitable Nursing Problems

The descriptive design is useful for documenting various characteristics in populations of interest to nurses to gather baseline data on those populations. Variables such as uncertainty, nutritional status, and depression, for example, could be measured on populations of patients with different diagnoses. In the development of nursing science, patient resources can be described and reported in taxonomies.

REFERENCES

Agar, M. H. (1980). *The professional stranger: An informal introduction to ethnography.* New York: Academic Press.
Agar, M. H. (1986). *Speaking of ethnography.* Beverly Hills, CA: Sage.
Archer, S. E. (1983). A study of nurse administrators' political participation. *Western Journal of Nursing Research, 5*(1), 65-75.

Brink, P. J. (1984). Value orientations as an assessment tool in cultural diversity. *Nursing Research, 33*(4), 198-203.

Brink, P. J. (1989). Issues in reliability and validity. In J. M. Morse (Ed.), *Qualitative nursing research: A contemporary dialogue* (pp. 139-154). Rockville, MD: Aspen.

Crane, J. G., & Angrosino, M. V. (1984). *Field projects in anthropology: A student hand book.* Prospect Heights, IL: Waveland.

DeMay, D. A. (1982). *Health care professional value orientation: A comparative study.* Unpublished master's thesis, University of California, Los Angeles.

Downing, C. K., & Cobb, A. K. (1990). Value orientations of homeless men. *Western Journal of Nursing Research, 12*(5), 619-628.

Edgecombe, N. (1994). *Value orientations of the Copper Inuit.* Unpublished master's thesis, University of Alberta, Edmonton.

Ellen, R. F. (1984). *Ethnographic research: A guide to general conduct.* London: Academic Press.

Field, P. A., & Morse, J. M. (1985). *Nursing research: The application of qualitative approaches.* London: Croom Helm.

Fink, A., & Kosecoff, J. (1985). *How to conduct surveys: A step-by-step guide.* Beverly Hills, CA: Sage.

Flaskerud, J. H. (1980). Perceptions of problematic behavior by Appalachians, mental health professionals and lay non-Appalachians. *Nursing Research, 29*(3), 140-149.

Germain, C. (1986). Ethnography: The method. In P. L. Munhall & C. J. Oiler (Eds.), *Nursing research: A qualitative perspective* (pp. 147-162). Norwalk, CT: Appleton-Century-Crofts.

Gushuliak, E. T. (1990). *Value orientations of Hutterian women.* Unpublished master's thesis, University of Alberta, Edmonton.

Hammersley, M., & Atkinson, P. (1983). *Ethnography: Principles in practice.* New York: Tavistock.

Hayter, J. (1983). Sleep behaviors in older persons. *Nursing Research, 32*(4), 242-246.

Hunter, D. E., & Foley, M. B. (1976). *Doing anthropology: A student centered approach to cultural anthropology.* New York: Harper & Row.

Kluckhohn, F., & Strodtbeck, F. L. (1961). *Variations in value orientations.* Elmsford, NY: Row, Peterson.

Krippendorf, K. (1980). *Content analysis: An introduction to its methodology.* Beverly Hills, CA: Sage.

Lincoln, Y. S., & Guba, E. G. (1985). *Naturalistic inquiry.* Beverly Hills, CA: Sage.

McCall, G. J., & Simmons, J. L. (Eds.). (1969). *Issues in participant observation: A text and reader.* Reading, MA: Addison-Wesley.

Miles, M. B., & Huberman, A. M. (1994). *Qualitative data analysis: A sourcebook of new methods* (2nd ed.). Thousand Oaks, CA: Sage.

Pelto, P. J., & Pelto, G. H. (1978). *Anthropological research: The structure of inquiry* (2nd ed.). Cambridge, UK: Cambridge University Press.

Spradley, J. P. (1979). *The ethnographic interview.* New York: Holt, Rinehart & Winston.

Spradley, J. P. (1980). *Participant observation.* New York: Holt, Rinehart & Winston.

Spradley, J. P., & McCurdy, D. W. (1972). *The cultural experience: Ethnography in complex society.* Chicago: Science Research Associates.

Stewart, D. W. (1984). *Secondary research: Information sources and methods.* Beverly Hills, CA: Sage.

Wax, R. (1971). *Doing fieldwork: Warnings and advice.* Chicago: University of Chicago Press.

Werner, O., & Schoepfle, G. M. (1987). *Systematic fieldwork* (2 vols.). Newbury Park, CA: Sage.

Whiting, J. W. M., Child, I. L., Lambert, W. W., Fischer, A. M., Fischer, J. L., Nudegger, C., Nudegger, W., Maretzki, H., Maretzki, T., Minturn, L., Romney, A. K., & Romney, R. (1966). *Field guide for a study of socialization.* New York. John Wiley.

Whyte, W. F. (1984). *Learning from the field: A guide from experience.* Beverly Hills, CA. Sage.

Wilson, H. (1985). *Research in nursing.* Menlo Park, CA: Addison-Wesley.

12

Exploratory Designs

PAMELA J. BRINK

Only recently have exploratory designs (synonymous with qualitative research) taken their place alongside descriptive and experimental designs as valid means for gaining knowledge and building theory in nursing. Beginning with Jeanne Quint Benoliel, the first graduate of the doctoral program in nursing at the University of California, San Francisco, several nurses conducting doctoral research began to use grounded theory as developed by Glaser and Strauss (1967). Their studies were presented at a series of annual western research conferences beginning in 1968. Simultaneously, in the East, particularly at Boston University, phenomenology was being introduced as a valid research approach. For many years, these exploratory designs were considered suspect by the scientific/academic community and suffered the ridicule typically encountered by new ideas. They have, however, been demonstrated to be essential designs for developing nursing knowledge. This book presents them as the first level of research design, for exploration of new research questions.

Exploratory designs have two major goals. The first is problem discovery—identifying and describing a problem area never previously studied or known. The second goal is problem definition—exploring a concept in depth in as loose and as free ranging a way as possible to arrive at a description of an experience or its meaning. Indeed, an exploratory design is also the design of choice when a problem has been identified but no literature exists on the topic. *Ethnomethodology, ethnoscience, grounded theory, qualitative research,* and *phenomenology* are all labels for designs or approaches that meet the requirements of exploratory research designs. Each type of design was developed by researchers in a different discipline to describe how they go about exploring phenomena of particular interest to them. Consequently, each differs somewhat from the others in purpose, sampling, data collection, and data analysis.

Exploratory designs use qualitative data collection methods based on unstructured interviewing techniques, unstructured observations, unstructured available data, small samples, and a variety of forms of content analysis. They are purposefully flexible, allowing researchers to discover new phenomena or to gain new insights into known phenomena. They are also insightful, allowing for the development of new ideas, theory, and concepts. These designs enable the researcher to intuitively rearrange and make sense of the known universe, opening up an entirely new field of research in the process.

Goffman (1961a, 1961b, 1963) was one of the first sociologists in the United States to use the exploratory design in studying American culture; his books are now classics. Goffman made qualitative research meaningful for certain kinds of sociological questions. For example, his work on role distance resulted from watching children at play on a merry-go-round (Goffman, 1961b). His perceptive observations of their behaviors led him to propose that people distance themselves from roles that they are forced to enact but that conflict with their perceptions of themselves. This concept of role distance incorporated the notion of a "situated activity system" whereby a repetitive series of interactions is confined to a particular ongoing situation, with roles evolving that are completely separate and distinct from other roles in other situations. It was these "situated" roles from which persons became dissociated or distanced themselves.

Goffman's work on role distance was based on nonparticipant observation over time and on an intuitive analysis of what was occurring in the situation. These activities are the hallmark of exploratory studies: observing or asking about previously unexamined, everyday occurrences, trying to "tease out" the essence of what is going on. The result is an examination and subsequent explanation of the processes and procedures or rules underlying human behavior and interactions. The explanation or theory not only makes sense to anyone who has experienced something similar but also appears to have application in settings other than the one described. For example, Brink (1972) was able to use Goffman's theoretical formulation on role distance quite successfully in analyzing nurses' behaviors during daily ward rounds on a psychiatric unit in a large midwestern teaching hospital. The nurses' seemingly irrational and unprofessional behavior was interpreted as a statement of role distance for the role assigned them in that "situated activity system."

Glaser and Strauss (1967) disapproved of Goffman's published works, claiming that he focused on his incredible findings and failed to explicate his methods of collecting and analyzing data. They set about to fill this gap by describing in precise terms how to use what they termed "grounded theory." Glaser and Strauss, of course, were themselves subsequently criticized for their imprecision and accused by "hard" scientists of practicing "soft" science. The same kind of criticism has been leveled against such renowned scientists as Zborowski (1952), who made health professionals aware of cultural differences in the expression of pain; William Foote Whyte (1955), who increased knowledge with his seminal work *Street Corner Society*; and Howard Becker et al. (1961), who continued Whyte's tradition in studying medical students in *Boys in White*. Yet none of these studies has ever been seriously challenged. Quite the contrary, the insights the authors brought to their explorations have formed the groundwork for a great deal of social science theory.

The decision to use an exploratory design is frequently made when the researcher has no specific problem to study but is interested in a particular population or experience. In this situation, the exploratory design is the first step in a longitudinal research program, usually descriptive in focus. This type of exploratory research within a particular culture is common in anthropology. The research design, termed *ethnography*, encompasses both exploratory and descriptive designs, due to the longitudinal nature of the research and its emphasis on participant observation as the basic method of data collection. In the past, anthropologists traditionally have lived in the field for at least 2 years to learn a language, find a problem, and study it in its cultural context. The works of Malinowski (with Trobriand Islanders in 1922; Malinowski, 1961) and Radcliffe-Brown (with Andaman Islanders in 1922; Radcliffe-Brown, 1964) made many persons aware of cultural relativity for the first time and created the climate for greater international understanding and respect. Current anthropologists more often enter the field with a well-defined problem and very specific objectives. Consequently, ethnography has evolved from its initial conceptualization as an exploratory-descriptive design into more of a descriptive science. This outcome may reflect our increased knowledge base of other peoples and cultures.

Different types of exploratory designs are selected to achieve different outcomes. To document an experience from the perspective of the person who has lived that experience, to put into words how an experience is lived and how it feels, the design of choice is phenomenology. If the goal is to explain the antecedents, consequences, or process involved in a particular problem, then grounded theory is appropriate. Ethnomethodology or ethnographic semantics can be used to understand the cultural rules underlying a particular custom or practice. And if a clear definition of all the components of a particular phenomenon is desired, ethnoscience should be chosen. For each design, the procedures of data collection and analysis are firm and unvarying. Therefore, to choose the type of qualitative design best suited to answer the question, the researcher needs to know the desired outcome of the research.

The underlying premise in grounded theory is that every human interaction involves a problem and a process to solve that problem (Hutchinson, 1986, personal communication, 1987). The problem is defined through interviewing and/or participant observation, with the questions initially exploring the stages and phases of the problem. Initial interview questions might take the following form: Tell me what happened. What happened next? And then what happened? Once the problem has been isolated, questions are directed toward discovering the conditions under which the problem occurred, the precursors, the context, and the consequences.

THE BASIC EXPLORATORY DESIGN

The purpose of an exploratory design is to study that which has not been previously studied. The exploratory researcher is looking for new knowledge, new insights, new understanding, and new meaning. The intent is to be holistic in the approach to whatever is being studied. The exploratory researcher "explores" the phenomena or variable or population of interest. The exploration is as broad or as narrow as the researcher and encompasses every conceivable idea or notion that may affect a thorough perusal of the topic. The researcher must be flexible enough to follow the meandering of the respondent but sufficiently controlled to pull back from the data, ask questions of the data (Miles & Huberman, 1994), and set a new direction or new course of exploration. The exploratory researcher must be sufficiently creative to analyze the growing body of data and derive new insights or new meanings previously out of awareness and return to the informants for validation or verification. Exploratory research is "discovery" research in which the researcher discovers, frequently with the informant, new meaning or new understanding. The exploratory researcher is what Munhall (1989, p. 164) calls "theory suspended."

An exploratory study frequently results from an examination of the literature in which the researcher can't find the answer to the question. What is it like to have, or to live with, Crohn's disease, even after the disease has been "controlled" by medical treatment? How does a young woman feel while she watches her features change because of a disease or its treatment? How does it "feel" to be a handicapped person and have to live in a nonhandicapped society that does not see, perhaps not even care about, the barriers it places in the way of the handicapped? What is it like to live in a society that stigmatizes you and discriminates against you for a single trait or quality over which you have no control, as is the case for ethnic minorities, the disfigured, or the disabled? What is it like to live as a person who is seen as "morally defective" in some way, whether it be because of a sexually transmitted disease, sexual preference, or through some lack of control such as obesity, alcoholism, drug addiction, or smoking? These are exploratory studies of personal experiences that may be common to groups that share those stigmata and are the "devalued" of society.

These "lived experiences" have a tremendous impact on the rest of the individual, which may result in a stronger person, psychologically, or may create emotional problems for which one seeks professional advice. If the health professional has no idea what life has been like for these clients, he or she may inadvertently treat the client exactly the same way, reinforcing a negative valuation of self-worth. A study that enumerates the costs of mental health treatment does not generate an understanding of, or an empathic response to, the chronic daily pain of the socially stigmatized. Only the exploratory researcher can provide those insights and can make individual pain a shared reality.

Cultural perspectives influence the direction of the research and color the insights and understanding available from the research. All researchers are bound by their own culture and are frequently unaware of their own biases. One way of handling cultural or personal biases is through the mechanism of "bracketing." Bracketing, in the Spiegelberg (1976) sense of the methodology, is for the researcher to first write out, fully, everything she or he has ever experienced or thought about the particular topic to date. This constitutes a full and complete exploratory interview of the researcher by the researcher. This "bracket" is then set aside as part of the data and is used to refer to later as a possible bias or direction that has influenced the "intuitive" process.

"Memoing" data, on the other hand, highlights for the researcher portions of the data that reflect possible bias or are ideas (intuitions) that arise in reading the transcribed notes. In this instance, a memo is written out and set aside for later review. The point is not to lose the idea that the data generated but to honor the intuitive process and acknowledge the idea. At the same time, the idea may have come from personal bias or experience that does not reflect what the informant is saying. The memo, and laying aside of the memo, allows the researcher to continue with the current task at hand and later examine the memo in context of the material recorded in the bracket. If the memo material cannot be found in the bracket, it may be a "valid" intuitive response to what the informant has said and can be taken back to the informant for further clarification and discussion.

Memos and bracketed material are expected to be explored later or held in "suspension" until a more appropriate time. Nevertheless, bracketing and memoing make the researcher more aware of possible skewness. These methods are useful only to the extent that the researcher can see his or her own biases. Usually, a bias is unconscious. Another way of bringing biases to conscious awareness is to have another person read the transcripts or listen to the tapes with the intent of seeking out those biases.

Yet another way of becoming aware of a cultural bias in directing the research or in analyzing the collected data is to deliberately include different cultural groups as part of the informant pool and compare the stories and experiences across these cultural boundaries. Allan (1993) has done this in her work with women who manage their weight. She found that middle-class black women were more like white women (both middle-class and lower-socioeconomic class) than they were like lower-socioeconomic-class black women in their beliefs and attitudes toward body weight and self-care strategies. She found (Allan, 1988, 1989, 1994, personal communication) in looking over her interviews with African American, Mexican American, and Anglo American women, that none of the African American women used pejorative terms for obesity, whereas the white women and the Hispanic women did. The black sample simply had no negative belief systems about obesity for either men or women. Therefore, the "lived experience" of an obese black woman would have no negative connotations for the obesity, in complete contrast to the Anglo American woman who must live with constant "belittlement" or negativity specifically due to the obesity. Allan's unreported finding is supported by a study by Kumanyika, Wilson, and Guilford-Davenport (1993) in which they state that there is an absence of strong negative social pressures toward obesity in combination with a relatively positive body image in the black women of their study. Attitudes and belief systems are colored by life experiences that may affect the findings of any exploratory study. The selection of the sample to include or exclude cultural differences must be part of the rationale for the study and the definition of the sample.

The aim of the phenomenologist is to capture the essence of the experience in such a way that others who have lived similar experiences can recognize themselves. This "recognition" is the "validation" of the research. (This recognition process is part of the fourth and fifth transformations described by Sauer, 1985, in the Utrecht Phenomenological Method.) If there is no "instant recognition," the researcher has got it wrong. Because phenomenology, as an exploratory design, has few rules to follow in either the data collection or analysis of the data, there are few ways for an outsider (someone who has not had the experience) to read the final report and say it is true. The reader can say, "it hangs together," or "it makes sense," but the reader has no other way of validating (Brink, 1989) the report or of knowing (or even of feeling) that the report is trustworthy (Lincoln & Guba, 1985), that it accurately reflects the experiences of the participants or informants.

Munhall and Oiler (1986) and Oiler (1982) contend that phenomenological research is possible with existing data such as that used by Oiler (1982, 1983) in her analysis of nurses' poems. Other phenomenologists (Omery, 1983; Van Manen, 1984) believe that the method is to be used with "live" informants in an interactive dialogue. Van Manen (1984), specifically, describes phenomenology as a method that will yield a "grand" experience that should encompass all other experiences. He believes the phenomenologist's task is to construct an experience, from all the other experiences, that is inclusive of all the others, and that the final report will be a composite experience, identifiable to all who have had the experience as reflecting their own experience.

Because phenomenology as a research method was developed from phenomenology as a philosophy, the method can have several perspectives, depending on the school of thought or philosophy espoused by the researcher.

The exploratory design requires the personal involvement of the investigator with a small number of people (usually fewer than 25), a small geographical or circumscribed setting (such as a hospital ward, a village, or a small interest group), repeated unstructured or semistructured interviews (usually accompanied by observations of the same participants over time), data recorded in the form of field notes, ongoing content analysis yielding categories of mutually exclusive content, negative cases to explore further with the sample, and insights and hunches to pursue the following day.

Because the purpose of exploratory studies is to uncover something that has never been examined before, there is minimal investigator control over data. In fact, it is just the reverse: The data control the investigator. Basically, the only control the investigator has is over what is asked and what is observed. What is found then directs further questions and observations. The investigator needs to have the flexibility to "go with the flow," to challenge accepted reality and explore it for its own reality, to accept other people's rules and judgments as basic premises, to set aside prejudices and prejudgments as far as possible, and to record phenomena as they are, rather than as the researcher would like them to be.

Assumptions Underlying the Design

The following assumptions are implicit in the use of the exploratory design:

1. The topic has not previously been studied or explored or has not been studied from the point of view of the participant or informant.
2. The sample has personal experience in, or knowledge about, the topic.

USE OF THE EXPLORATORY DESIGN IN NURSING

The types of studies done using this design assume the perspective of the person being interviewed or observed. The researcher is not interested in finding examples that fit an existing theory but, rather, in finding examples from persons' lives that have not been heard of or imagined before. Exploratory studies examine the patient's perspective, the view from the hospital bed, the horizontal viewpoint (Taylor, 1970). What is it like to face surgery? What does infant pain look like? What does privacy mean? What does health mean? What do you mean when you talked about a "good" nurse? What kinds of things have to happen to you before you seek health care? What do you expect will happen to you when you are admitted to the hospital? What will happen when you reach menopause? Puberty? What are people's expectations, in their own words; what do they think about health professionals, in their own words; and what have their experiences been in the health care system, again in their own words? What has been asked of prospective patients or clients can be asked of health professionals, of laypersons or other professionals, and of teachers and students. If you, as a researcher, want to know about any particular group, go talk to them. Ask them, from their perspective, what life is like for them. Each exploration into a particular client group adds information about the range of behaviors, beliefs, and practices of the people we nurse. We need information about people in both the healthy and the ill or traumatized state because we need to know what they want (or need) from us.

The second group of people we need to do exploratory studies on are nurses. Our major need is to document nursing interventions associated with (as well as independent of) nursing diagnosis. We need to observe nursing behaviors in interaction with patients and clients to document what nurses do with and for patients. We need to interview nurses to ask them to explain their rationale for what we observe. We need to interview nurses and ask them to describe the patients they have known and what they have done with and for them while on the job. From these experiences, we can tease out nursing action, nursing rationale, and nursing process. All of this remains exploratory.

Even if a study has previously been done that has taken the perspective of the researcher or the theorist, the same population can be studied from its own perspective. The point is to come up with new ideas, new insights, new "grounded" theories, and not to try to "fit" the data into previously delineated areas.

Long-term or longitudinal studies take an enormous amount of time, often spanning several years. In the past, many exploratory studies were not funded. They were conducted by the primary investigator with as many informants as possible, given the constraints of time and money. For example, Anderson (1987) worked as a nurse practitioner with adolescent girls at a juvenile facility. From her clinical work, she developed an interest in this population, wondering in particular what issues the girls were concerned about. Her contacts with these girls continued over a period of 6 years and culminated in her doctoral dissertation. Saunders (1981) interviewed newly bereaved women monthly for 13 months postloss to explore bereavement as it was being experienced by widows whose husbands had died from different causes. Saunders obtained her participants by searching weekly death records of the Los Angeles coroner's office. Only recently has the enormous value of studies like these been recognized by granting agencies to the extent that they have received funding.

STRENGTHS AND WEAKNESSES OF THE DESIGN

A strength of exploratory designs is the constant return to informants to verify information. Anthropological field research is usually longitudinal, with a minimum of 6 months spent living with the population. Phenomenology and grounded theory require a constant return to the same informants, to the same material, to continue interviewing in increasing depth. In grounded theory, for example, the investigator interviews a single informant on the selected topic, returns home, and reviews the interview, seeking gaps or missing information. The interviewer then returns to the informant and asks about the missing information. This process is repeated until the informant can provide no new information on the topic. The investigator then selects a second informant to interview and covers the same information with the second informant as has been elicited from the first. Generally, new information is gained from the second informant that must be explored in subsequent interviews. Any new information is taken back to the first informant to find out what he or she knows about it. Discrepancies in information from the two informants are noted. When no new information is obtained from the second informant, a third informant is deliberately selected and the same process is continued until no new information is elicited. This repeated return to the original informants provides verification of the information obtained, because most humans are unable to lie consistently over time. They simply cannot remember a lie as well as the truth they know, which is consistent over time.

Exploratory clinical research, or case study research, is also longitudinal, demanding a return to the same participants again and again to ask what is happening at the moment in relation to X. The repetitive nature of the interviews and observations, over time, and on the same participants, lends strength and credence to the exploratory study. At the same time, it discourages many individuals from conducting such research.

One weakness of this design is its lack of replicability. No single researcher can return to the same participants, ask the same questions, and receive the same answers. Persons change their minds, their beliefs, and their positions as a result of new experiences. Therefore, the same researcher will not achieve perfect reproducibility from the same informants over time. More problematic, no other researcher can enter the same field site, find the same individuals to interview or observe, and achieve the same results. All researchers are selective in what they observe and what they report. No two humans "see" the same phenomena identically unless trained to do so, nor do they record and report identical sorts of things.

In addition, informants chosen by one researcher may not be there when the next researcher comes to study. An alternate informant may not express beliefs and values identical to those of an earlier informant. Ironically, longitudinal research mandates a relationship between researcher and informant that cannot be duplicated by another researcher, even when he or she is interviewing the same informant. The quality of that relationship makes or breaks a study, yet it is rarely reproducible.

SAMPLES

When population parameters are unknown, some form of nonprobability sampling technique is chosen to reflect the population or the variable being studied. In this case, snowball or network sampling is frequently employed. The purpose is to have as homogeneous a sample as possible on one central characteristic. Snowball sampling is based on the assumption that people who are interested in the same things will know each other. Because not all people interested in the same topic belong to groups, the snowball technique will also reach hard-to-find informants. The snowball technique is also used in conjunction with advertisements in newspapers, on radio, or through social clubs to elicit the friends of the people who read newspapers, listen to the radio, or join clubs.

The purposive sample is used when specific members of the population are desired as study participants. The criteria for sample selection are listed, and study participants are sought to meet those criteria from whatever source is available. All methods of soliciting participants are used, but the screening is rigorous. The study by Gushuliak (1990) had to do with a Hutterian sample. Among the Hutterites there are three different "Leuts" or historically different groups who have descended from the original immigrants. Each Leut is descended from a different male head. Each Leut has a number of colonies. She deliberately chose to select one colony from each Leut. She visited four Hutterite colonies (one colony was part of her pilot study) and asked permission of the elders (men) to study all the women in the colony. Her interest was to see if there were differences across the Leuts or if the Hutterite women were similar despite their Leut affiliation.

The concept of the target population is very useful in exploratory studies. The researcher strives to interview anyone who has had the experience under study. For example, if one were looking at the experience of birthing, the obvious target population would be women who have given birth. However, several details regarding the birth experience would also have to be specified. Should the sample be restricted to women who have had uneventful full-term pregnancies? Should it include women who have had spontaneous abortions, multiple births, C-sections, anomalies, or stillbirths? Should a woman's description of her experience be elicited during the event, soon after the event, or does it matter how long after the event she is queried? These questions about the target population are answered depending on the experience under study.

A second-order question regarding the target population involves the degree to which contrasting views of the same phenomena are desired. In the birthing example, does the researcher want the experience of birthing solely from the perspective of the laboring woman, or is the perspective of her husband, birth attendant, friend, or mother also sought? Each is valuable and valid, but is it what the investigator wants? An exploratory study of birthing from the woman's perspective alone is just as valid as one eliciting all contrasting perspectives. Specification of the desired perspective is critical to all definitions of the target population.

Exploratory design calls for small samples that are chosen through a deliberative process to represent the desired perspective. For this reason, samples are usually purposive. The rationale for selection of informants depends on the purpose of the research. If the purpose is to discover a problem, the target population is frequently selected on the basis of personal interest of the researcher. Aamodt (1982) selected a Norwegian community in the Midwest because her relatives lived there; Ragucci (1981) selected an Italian neighborhood in Boston because she was living in Boston and was herself Italian-American. Personal relationships also frequently provide entry to the field site or the target population. An acquaintance can introduce the researcher around, making access to the population easier and allaying suspicions about the researcher's intentions.

The concept of *theoretical sampling* is used differently by different authors. Strauss and Corbin (1990, pp. 176-193) use theoretical sampling as an integral part of the emerging theory. One samples incidents in the data that are of direct relevance to the theory and that are useful in developing coding schema. They stress that *concepts* rather than people are at the base of grounded theory; therefore, "theoretical sample" does not refer to the people from whom the data were gathered.

Grounded theory uses the approach of an initial target or available population from which to obtain informants. From this beginning, one collects data from the people, incidents, or both that will yield the greatest amount of relevant information on the topic. Initially, the choice of individuals or incidents is "indiscriminate." As the researcher gathers data, the sampling technique may become targeted to certain categories of data that have emerged from initial analysis or that can be systematized through following some sort of listing, while at the same time making comparisons; or the sampling may simply arise "fortuitously." As data are collected, they are analyzed. The analysis and its emerging themes or categories then direct further sampling to attempt to support the emerging theory or to refute it. For Strauss and Corbin, therefore, theoretical sampling cannot happen in the planning stages of grounded theory research.

Another way of viewing theoretical sampling at the outset of a qualitative study is to determine beforehand what is wanted from the study and who or what can best provide that information. Having read all the literature about the topic, the researcher has a sense of where to go to find the answers. In fact, the literature review assists the researcher to establish the criteria for sample selection. The clearer the research question, the clearer the direction for sample selection. The sample, therefore, should *theoretically* represent the known population.

If, for example, the study is about what it is like to be a hospital administrator, the initial thinking about the sample should include all possible types of hospital administrators. The question in selecting a representative sample is, Who needs to be represented? Sampling only from male administrators would yield only a male model. Theoretically, one would need both men and women represented in the sample to give a "human" perspective to the answer. Would length of experience affect an administrator's response? Should length of experience be "represented" in the sample? Those who are in their first year as an administrator may have a different view of the job than more experienced individuals. Another possible difference in administrators would be the type of hospital they administer. Whether the hospital is small or large, acute care or hospice, may affect the administrative experience—and again, may not. But theoretically, you believe it may have an effect. We now have a grid of individuals to select from to represent other individuals within the same category. From this grid, we develop our theoretical sample and the number of individuals needed to interview to represent our pool.

METHODS OF DATA COLLECTION

Exploratory designs call for either unstructured or semistructured data collection methods, but *not* structured methods—usually participant observation with interviewing. Many quantitative researchers have difficulty with exploratory studies because of their flexible data collection procedures and lack of specificity. Because the point of the research is to get at the desired information in the best or most efficient way possible, a trial-and-error approach to what works, with whom, and when, is required. Because not every human understands a question in exactly the same way, a flexible approach helps the researcher to find the best question for a given individual to understand and answer. Here are some examples based on Spradley and McCurdy (1972):

- *Grand tour questions* (setting the tone for the interview or questionnaire): "I would like you to tell me about the last experience you had with a person you thought was a 'problem patient.' "
- *Contrast or comparative questions:* "Tell me what you think are the differences between men and women in relation to their ability to successfully lose weight. In what way do you think they are similar?"
- *Inclusive questions:* "What kinds of studies are research studies?" Or "If you were to define and give examples of qualitative nursing research, what studies would you cite?"
- *Exclusive questions:* "If you were to develop a new community program in eldercare, who would not be eligible?" Or "What kinds of research would you say are not examples of qualitative nursing research?"

One of the errors exploratory researchers make is in the lack of precision or lack of attention to detail in data collection and analysis. Simply because the researcher is expected to be flexible does not mean the researcher is also "loose." A meticulous research log is as important in this type of research as it is in any chemistry experiment. The researcher keeps a running series of notes of what was done, when it was done, why it was done, and what was learned in the process. This is the research journal, critical in fieldwork but just as important in qualitative designs. The notes are written *as the researcher goes along in the process*. These are not post hoc or recall notes, months later, but a daily diary. In this way, there is no need to rely on inconsistent, spotty, or faulty recall to reconstruct decisions. Memoing, discussed in most works on qualitative data analysis, is part of the same process, although it occurs during analysis of data. It is a means of annotating the decisions made during the analytic process. The same "memoing" is necessary during the rest of the process.

Perhaps the most important element of exploratory research is not the questions that are asked per se but the interview itself. Because analysis is based on the interview in its entirety and not on each specific question, the interviewer's approach to the interview is of paramount importance. In their book on the cultural experience, Spradley and McCurdy (1972) talk about the "grand tour question," an opening gambit for finding out "what's going on here." The grand tour question sets the tone, opens the discussion, and lets everyone know what the interview is about. Because not everyone would know how to answer the question, What's going on here? without some preliminary information, it is necessary for the investigator to explain about the topic of the research. Simply approaching an informant abruptly and asking "Tell me all about your birthing experience," might elicit some very odd answers. Instead, the investigator tells the informants what is being studied and why, what aroused the investigator's interest in the topic or area, and so on. In this way, the investigator "primes the pump," so to speak. Informants may be cued in by a simple statement, such as "Ever since I gave birth to my first child, I have wondered if other women have gone through the same feelings I have had. So I decided I'd like to ask other women about their experiences with birth."

Some investigators begin not by asking questions but by "entering the field" and "getting a feel for" the area. Anderson (1987) would not have succeeded with the girls at the juvenile facility if she had begun by asking direct questions, because they would not have trusted her. Being an employee in the facility, however, she had a legitimate reason to interact with the girls, and she spent a great deal of time with them on the unit prior to developing her research questions. Anderson's approach was not unlike the approach of anthropologists who enter a

Pacific island community or an African village for an extended period of time, getting a feel for the place, meeting people, finding the post office and grocery store, and generally watching everyone to find out who's who and what's going on. Only later, when widespread familiarity has been established, does the investigator begin asking direct, but unstructured, questions in formal interviews. Prior to that time, all interviews could be considered informal conversations, which nevertheless provide a great deal of data about the field site and the population.

Two other, perhaps more familiar, examples of the semistructured interview are the clinical interview and the mental status examination. The goal of these interviews is to assess the level of functioning of the client. Although the clinician has in mind an outline of the facts needed to achieve the goal, in neither case does he or she rely on a predetermined set of questions or a predetermined ordering of questions. Although these interviews are completely unstructured, the inherent validity or reliability of the obtained data are not questioned in clinical practice. Although errors can occur in eliciting information from an informant, these errors are just as possible with a standardized or structured questionnaire.

DATA ANALYSIS

Data analysis in exploratory research, like data collection, requires a fluid, flexible, somewhat intuitive interaction, this time between the investigator and the data. Essentially, the investigator "lives with" the data, reading and rereading field notes or transcripts of interviews on a daily or frequent basis and deciding what has been learned so far, what is puzzling, what is unanswered, and what does not fit. The investigator takes notes, writes self-reminders about what is wanted (a technique called "memoing"; see Chapter 13), and prepares for the next interaction with informants. New questions may be written out in advance, old questions may be asked again, or an observation might be planned. This material provides the basis for new areas of exploration in subsequent interviews or for new field observations and subsequent field notes, which themselves are analyzed in exactly the same way. This process of interaction between data collection and analysis continues throughout the research experience or the periods of data collection.

Because analysis, including the development of hunches and insights, requires the personal involvement of the investigator with the data, it is difficult for anyone else but the investigator to be involved in the process. There is simply no room for a research assistant at this stage of analysis. If, on the other hand, a research team is involved in the data analysis, regular and frequent discussions, involving the whole team, about the analysis process must be planned in advance. The analysis itself is a holistic examination of all collected data at the same time. Exploratory analysis thus contrasts with descriptive analysis, in which each individual's responses to questions are examined separately.

Several analytic methods can be used in exploratory studies, depending on the specific type of design: Constant comparison and saturation of categories, yielding a theoretical model, is used in grounded theory (Glaser & Strauss, 1967); componential analysis, yielding a taxonomy of terms, is used in ethnomethodology (Spradley & McCurdy, 1972); thematic analysis, yielding the essence of the lived experience is used in phenomenology (Van Manen, 1984); and reading participant observation field notes over and over in their totality to derive a descriptive distillation of the meaning of the material is used in analytic induction (Wilson, 1985). The analysis process sifts through the information, within context, to arrive at a description that makes sense to both those who have lived the experience and those who have no prior knowledge of the concept or content. The most comprehensive work on the analysis of qualitative data can be found in the second edition of Miles and Huberman's (1994) book. Every exploratory researcher should have a copy of this book as a reference during the analysis phase of the research.

Because all data take the form of words, sentences, and paragraphs, the smallest unit of analysis is the single word or concept, which can be treated as a nominal scale item. As in semantic analysis, however, it is possible to categorize all terms into mutually exclusive saturated categories that, taken together, describe the concept in its entirety. Content analysis therefore involves making decisions about the categories of content and assigning code numbers or code labels to those categories. The entire text of data is then completely coded. Every bit of collected information can be coded, using as many categories as needed. Consider, for example, an interview in which an informant describes a series of steps involved in making pasta. Each sentence may include material on the recipe, the carbohydrate content, and the color, texture, weight, density, or taste of the pasta and, consequently, may be coded under more than one category. These codes are a simple means of differentiating content for filing or retrieval purposes and are immensely useful in computer analysis of data using a search feature. If any form of structured analysis is wanted, such as the number of times an item was mentioned or the number of people who mentioned the item, availability of a computer search is important. When the accumulated data are extensive, this form of analysis becomes critical.

HUMAN SUBJECTS ISSUES

As with any other research, the principal investigator must be aware of the need for informed consent, confidentiality, and anonymity. However, the three major problems involving ethics in human research (invasion of privacy, withholding benefits, and coercion to participate) are not all problematic in exploratory research. Invasion of privacy can be a concern in exploratory studies, particularly when the participants are patients or clients and the researcher is a professional within the system. Withholding benefits, associated primarily with experimental research, does not concern the exploratory researcher, who may not know what the benefits might be until the study is over. Institutional review panels, however, being particularly concerned with cost-benefit ratios, sometimes question exploratory research precisely because the investigator cannot specify the possible benefit of the research in advance or predict the outcome prior to data collection. Whenever benefits cannot be specified, they are considered to be outweighed by the risks. This is one reason the "expedited review" has been developed for social science research. If an investigator can document that the informants will be able to understand the research and can discontinue participation at any time, then just talking to the investigator is not considered a major risk.

The investigator also needs to document the means by which confidentiality and anonymity will be established and maintained. How the investigator explains to informants what will happen to their stories or interviews and whether or not their names, stories, and location will be made public is critical. If audio- or videotapes are to be made of the participants, what will happen to these tapes? Because much exploratory research yields new information, handling of data, particularly from fieldwork in foreign countries, can have political implications. Protection of the study participant is paramount, even to the extent of destroying research records if necessary.

THE RESEARCH PROPOSAL

Exploratory research studies are not funded as frequently as other types of designs, because they do not lend themselves to detailed proposals. (See Tripp-Reimer & Cohen, 1989, for a more detailed description of grant proposal writing.) The major budgetary items in exploratory studies involve travel for interviews, transcription of taped or filmed interviews, and salaries. Nevertheless, investigators submitting grant proposals need to recognize several problems they are likely to encounter.

First, exploratory research is often conducted by the investigator alone simply because exploratory researchers prefer to interact with the data and answer the questions themselves. Consequently, few exploratory researchers have research assistants to help them with data collection. Research assistance, whether for data collection, data analysis, or computer analysis, increases the size of a grant proposal budget. More recently, among grounded theorists particularly, teams of researchers are working together to study a single problem area. Field research in foreign countries or well-demarcated communities is usually conducted using field teams, but again, the predominant form is the single researcher going to the field and hiring informants there.

An even more difficult problem encountered in grant writing is how to justify funding a proposal that has no question or hypothesis. How does a review panel determine the importance of a project if the investigator cannot specify what is being studied? Therefore, the first task of the researcher is to "declare" a problem area within which exploration will be conducted. This problem area will of necessity be a broad one, to allow the latitude necessary for later formulation of a valid question. But granting agencies usually require a defined problem that is tied to a literature base and, usually, to some rationale. Because most exploratory researchers cannot specify the problem this neatly at the outset, they often cannot obtain grants at this stage of the research. The Center for Nursing Research now has more qualitative researchers as members of a scientific panel who understand the problems of grant writing for qualitative methods. They recommend that the researcher "walk" the review committee through the proposed steps in the process, talk about the literature that was reviewed and what was found, provide the panel with an understanding of why this research is different from the current literature (other than in its method), and finally, give the panel an idea of the kind of outcome desired, whether in the form of a table, a short descriptive paragraph, or a concept.

The third area that causes major problems in proposal writing is the sample. Frequently, exploratory researchers have no idea what the size of the sample will be at the beginning of the study, because the size of the sample is dictated by the comprehensiveness of the data to be collected. Exploratory researchers frequently find more and more persons to interview, until they have "saturated their categories" (Glaser & Strauss, 1967; Hutchinson, 1986) or until nothing new is being added to the database. For this reason, specifying sample size at the outset is problematic. Review panels, which generally need specificity and closure, require investigators to make an educated guess at the sample size. Is it possible to complete the task with 10 persons or 25? Might it take 50? The researcher must pick a reasonable number or specify a time frame for data collection to be devoted to the project. For instance, "the data will be collected on a minimum of 10 persons over a period of 6 months." Or "a maximum of 25 persons will be interviewed over a period of 6 months."

Most exploratory designs pose problems for reliability. The standard methods of establishing reliability would require something like test-retest reliability of the research participants or having another researcher interview the same or similar informants and achieve the same results. As explained earlier, neither of these is likely to be possible. Therefore, the research proposal should address those forms of reliability that can be used in qualitative data collection (see Brink, 1989).

Reliability is primarily determined by the investigator's use of alternate-form questions while interviewing informants or by the use of two observers (interrater reliability) during initial observations. In observational studies, filming the interaction and capturing the conversation in context is the usual form of reliability check. Tapes of interviews and their subsequent transcriptions also aid in the reliability of interview data. (In this case the second observer is not a member of a research team but is called in on an ad hoc basis to provide a reliability check.) Exploratory researchers frequently ask the same questions in a variety of ways to ensure that the answers given by the informants are indeed similar. Because many exploratory researchers also interview the same informant several times on the same topic, alternate-form questions become built into the method of data collection. In other words, repeating questions to the same participant on the same topic over time provides a form of test-retest reliability. The questions used to monitor test-retest reliability are critical. If the question reflects changes over time, test-retest is not possible. If the question used is a point of past fact, the answer should be the same each time. How alternate-form reliability will be used should be described in detail. Brink (1989), Brink and Wood (1988), Polit and Hungler (1987), and Selltiz, Wrightsman, and Cook (1981) can be cited as references.

Unelaborated descriptions of methodology are also problematic in proposals for exploratory studies. Because there are no standardized instruments, the procedures for data collection need to be specified in as much detail as possible. The review panel needs to know precisely how data will be collected from each informant and what will be done if enough information is not obtained from that person. The researcher should try to give the review panel members all the information they need to make a clear recommendation. This information might include an example of an interview, a description of what will be looked for, a chart depicting use of available data, a poem, a letter, an oral history— whatever will be used.

Although exploratory studies are inherently nonreplicable, few qualitative researchers question their validity (Pelto & Pelto, 1978); review panels, however, usually do. The type of validation sought is very important to the success of a grant proposal. Most exploratory research studies have pragmatic or concurrent validation (Brink, 1989; Brink & Wood, 1988; Polit & Hungler, 1987; Selltiz et al., 1981) "built into the design," because they use more than one method of data collection. Usually, interviewing is accompanied by observation or available data or both. In this way data are "triangulated" (Sohier, 1989) or validated by alternate methods, just as the informant is deemed reliable through the use of alternate forms of questions. Unlike quantitative studies, in which concurrent validation is achieved through the use of another, previously validated, instrument, no previously validated instrument exists in exploratory studies. Therefore, using different methods of data collection is extremely important in establishing the validity of the data. For example, Dean and Whyte (1969) discuss the interesting issue of how a researcher knows if the informant is telling the truth.

During a participant observation study on an Indian reservation, Brink (1969) interviewed mothers about their child-rearing habits. When one mother was asked, "What do you do when your baby cries?" she replied, "I pick him up." However, as the interviewer sat with this mother in her front room, her toddler crawled over, pulled himself up on her knee and hit his head on a table. Although he began to scream and cry, the mother ignored him. She did not pick him up and hold him in her lap until he tugged at her clothing. Had the investigator not observed this incident, the answer to her question would have been recorded as the mother gave it. This example demonstrates the difficulty of obtaining valid self-report data without some form of alternative or substantiating information.

Finally, the fluid nature of sample selection and methodology make the data analysis section of a proposal difficult. Review panels understand content analysis (Krippendorf, 1980), but they may not understand "musing," or "thematic analysis," or a "lived experience" (see Chapter 14). Again, the researcher must try to describe for the panel what he or she would do with an interview, an observation, or a poem. If the analysis and data collection plans allow it, the researcher can label a single section of the proposal "Methods and Analysis" and can discuss them simultaneously. This is particularly useful for grounded theory and phenomenology. The use of constant comparison requires analysis of each interview as it compares with preceding interviews in order for the researcher to decide how to interview the next informant. Such approaches must be described in detail.

A major problem with exploratory research proposals is the mixing of qualitative design strategies. If the researcher uses grounded theory in data collection and sampling, constant comparison should be used in data analysis. Grounded theory resources should be referenced for grounded theory approaches. A phenomenological study is at a disadvantage when mixed with grounded theory approaches. *Thematic analysis, musings,* and *bracketing* are all phenomenological terms, and their use should be limited to proposals for studies using that approach. Again, because each approach is very different, documentation is very important.

CRITIQUE OF EXPLORATORY DESIGNS

When critiquing an exploratory study, one should look for the name of the design somewhere in the paper. If a design is named, then the paper must meet the design criteria. For example, if an author states that the design is grounded theory, one should look for theoretical sampling, constant comparisons, and the delineation of a core variable underlying the theory. The final theoretical outcome should be some type of basic psychological or interactional process that forms the central theme of the paper (Hutchinson, 1986, p. 119). If these criteria are not met, the paper may be critiqued as a generic exploratory study. The author should also be informed of the error.

An article based on phenomenology will not include much explication of the method. Like historical research, the findings are considered to be more important than the techniques and procedures used to derive the description. The report may be written in a variety of ways, and it is up to the reader to decide whether it is complete and comprehensive according to the method of presentation. Because phenomenology is essentially an example composed of other examples, the number of questions remaining after reading the example gives an indication of the author's success in describing the phenomena or the lived experience. Van Manen (1984, pp. 26-27) has stated that a phenomenological report can be written thematically, analytically, exemplicatively, existentially, or exegetically (organized in the form of a dialogue with another phenomenological writer). Any of these approaches is acceptable in a phenomenological study.

If an author uses qualitative methods in a generic exploratory design, the reader should look for the development of the problem; a literature review that supports the question, the methods, and the sample; evidence of the reliability and validity of the researcher as the research instrument; and content analysis yielding a basic listing of the components of the report. These elements are frequently more brief than they would be in an experimental design, because the bulk of the report will focus on the findings. No section should be missing, however, and all sections should be relevant to the findings. The reader should look for any missing or mismatched parts, such as failure to describe the sample, use of structured data collection instruments, or attempts at enumeration. The findings should always describe a process, a phenomenon, or a new theoretical formulation. Again, the reader should have little sense of incompleteness or unanswered questions. If this exists, the article needs rewriting.

Particular caution is necessary when evaluating a researcher's sample. In Rosenhahn's (1976) classic paper, "On Being Sane in Insane Places," it is difficult to determine if the eight field-workers were the sample or if the eight hospital wards were the intended sample. In reality, however, it makes no difference. The outcome of the research remains the same—namely, the staff were unable to differentiate between "planted pseudopatients" and regular patients. Rosenhahn was, on the basis of this study, able to propose a theory of "labeling" to describe how health professionals (like others) often interact with labels and stereotypes rather than with individuals.

SUMMARY

Essential features of the exploratory design are as follows:

1. Problem discovery or problem definition as the research goal
2. Small purposive or theoretical samples of 25 or fewer
3. Longitudinal rather than cross-sectional data collection
4. Multiple interviews over time on the same participant as opposed to one-shot interviews
5. Repeated measures on the same participant
6. Unstructured data collection techniques and procedures
7. Continuous analysis of data, with return to participants for verification
8. Formulation of a new concept, definition, explanation, or theory, or description of a process or experience

REFERENCES

Aamodt, A. M. (1982). Examining ethnography for nursing researchers. *Western Journal of Nursing Research, 4*(2), 209-222.
Allan, J. D. (1988). Knowing what to weigh: Women's self-care activities related to weight. *Advances in Nursing Science, 11*(1), 47-60.

Allan, J. D. (1989). Women who successfully manage their weight: A naturalistic study. *Western Journal of Nursing Research, 11*(6), 657-675.

Allan, J. D. (1993). Body size values of white and black women. *Research in Nursing and Health, 15*(5), 323-333.

Anderson, N. L. (1987). *Doing time and making choices: The anthropology of pregnancy resolution decisions in juvenile detention.* Unpublished doctoral dissertation, University of California, Los Angeles.

Becker, H. S., et al. (1961). *Boys in white.* Chicago: University of Chicago Press.

Brink, P. J. (1969). *The northern Paiute.* Unpublished doctoral dissertation, Boston University.

Brink, P. J. (1972). Role distance: A maneuver in nursing. *Nursing Forum, 11(3),* 323-332.

Brink, P. J. (1989). Issues in reliability and validity. In J. M. Morse (Ed.), *Qualitative nursing research: A contemporary dialogue* (pp. 139-154). Rockville, MD: Aspen.

Brink, P. J., & Wood, M. J. (1988). *Basic steps in planning nursing research: From question to proposal* (3rd ed.). Boston: Jones & Bartlett.

Dean, J. P., & Whyte, W. F. (1969). How do you know if the informant is telling the truth? In G. J. McCall & J. L. Simmons (Eds.), *Issues in participation observation: A text and reader* (pp. 105-115). Reading, MA: Addison-Wesley.

Glaser, B. G., & Strauss, A. (1967). *The discovery of grounded theory: Strategies for qualitative research.* New York: Aldine-Atherton.

Goffman, E. (1961a). *Asylums.* Garden City, NY: Doubleday.

Goffman, E. (1961b). *Encounters: Two studies in the sociology of interaction.* Indianapolis, IN: Bobbs-Merrill.

Goffman, E. (1963). *Stigma: Notes on the management of spoiled identity.* Englewood Cliffs, NJ: Prentice Hall.

Gushuliak, E. T. (1990). *Values orientations of Hutterian women.* Unpublished master's thesis, University of Alberta, Edmonton.

Hutchinson, S. (1986). Grounded theory: The method. In P. L. Munhall & C. J. Oiler (Eds.), *Nursing research: A qualitative perspective* (pp. 111-130). Norwalk, CT: Appleton-Century-Crofts.

Krippendorf, K. (1980). *Content analysis: An introduction to its methodology.* Beverly Hills, CA: Sage.

Kumanyika, S., Wilson, J. F., & Guilford-Davenport, M. (1993). Weight-related attitudes and behaviors of black women. *Journal of the American Dietetic Association, 93*(4), 416-422.

Lincoln, Y. S., & Guba, E. G. (1985). *Naturalistic inquiry.* Beverly Hills, CA: Sage.

Malinowski, B. (1961). *Argonauts of the Western Pacific.* New York: E. P. Dutton.

Miles, M. B., & Huberman, A. M. (1994). *Qualitative data analysis.* Thousand Oaks, CA: Sage.

Munhall, P. (1989). Qualitative designs. In P. J. Brink & M. J. Wood (Eds.), *Advanced design in nursing research* (pp. 161-179). Newbury Park, CA: Sage.

Munhall, P. L., & Oiler, C. J. (Eds.). (1986). *Nursing research: A qualitative perspective.* Norwalk, CT: Appleton-Century-Crofts.

Oiler, C. (1982). The phenomenological approach in nursing research. *Nursing Research, 31,* 118-131.

Oiler, C. (1983). Nursing reality as reflected in nurses' poetry. *Perspectives in Psychiatric Care, 21,* 81-89.

Omery, A. (1983). Phenomenology: A method for nursing research. *Advances in Nursing Science, 5*(2), 49-63.

Pelto, P. J., & Pelto, G. H. (1978). *Anthropological research: The structure of inquiry* (2nd ed.). Cambridge, UK: Cambridge University Press.

Polit, D. F., & Hungler, B. P. (1987). *Nursing research.* Philadelphia: J. B. Lippincott.

Radcliffe-Brown, A. R. (1964). *The Andaman Islanders.* New York: Free Press.

Ragucci, A. (1981). Italian Americans. In A. Harwood (Ed.), *Ethnicity and medical care* (pp. 211-263). Cambridge, MA: Harvard University Press.

Rosenhahn, D. L. (1976). On being sane in insane places. In P. J. Brink (Ed.), *Transcultural nursing: A book of readings* (pp. 175-197). Englewood Cliffs, NJ: Prentice Hall.

Sauer, J. (1985). Using a phenomenological method to study nursing phenomena. In M. Leininger (Ed.), *Qualitative research methods in nursing* (pp. 93-107). New York: Grune & Stratton.

Saunders, J. (1981). A process of bereavement resolution: Uncoupled identity. *Western Journal of Nursing Research, 3,* 319-336.

Selltiz, C., Wrightsman, L. S., & Cook, S. W. (1981). *Research methods in social relations* (4th ed.). New York: Holt, Rinehart & Winston.

Sohier, R. (1989). Multiple triangulation and contemporary nursing research. *Western Journal of Nursing Research, 10,* 732-742.

Spiegelberg, W. (1976). *The phenomenological movement* (2 vols.). The Hague: Martinus Nijhoff.

Spradley, J. P., & McCurdy, D. W. (1972). *The cultural experience: Ethnography in complex society.* Chicago: Science Research Associates.

Strauss, A., & Corbin, J. (1990). *Basics of qualitative research: Grounded theory procedures and techniques.* Newbury Park, CA: Sage.

Taylor, C. (1970). *In horizontal orbit: Hospitals and the cult of efficiency.* New York: Holt, Rinehart & Winston.

Tripp-Reimer, T., & Cohen, M. Z. (1989). Funding strategies for qualitative research. In J. M. Morse (Ed.), *Qualitative nursing research: A contemporary dialogue* (pp. 209-220). Rockville, MD: Aspen.

Van Manen, M. (1984). *"Doing" phenomenological research and writing: An introduction* (Monograph No. 7). Alberta: University of Alberta, Faculty of Education, Department of Secondary Education.

Whyte, W. F. (1955). *Street corner society: The social structure of an Italian slum.* Chicago: University of Chicago Press.

Wilson, H. (1985). *Research in nursing.* Menlo Park, CA: Addison-Wesley.

Zborowski, M. (1952). Cultural components in response to pain. *Journal of Social Issues, 8,* 16-30.

13

Qualitative Research

PATRICIA L. MUNHALL

A growing enthusiasm and interest in qualitative research designs has broadened the research perspective of nurse researchers today. Lively discussions and enlightening critiques are a part of the evolving research paradigm for nursing (see Morse, 1989). The prevalent qualitative research methods that nurse researchers seem most interested in are phenomenology, grounded theory, ethnography, history, case studies, and analytic philosophy. Discussions of these methods can be found in texts by Leininger (1985); Field and Morse (1985); Munhall and Oiler (1986); Parse, Coyne, and Smith (1985); Swanson and Chenitz (1986); and Morse (1989).

Qualitative research methods have been explained by Benoliel (1984) "as modes of systematic inquiry concerned with understanding human beings and the nature of their transactions with themselves and with their surroundings" (p. 3). She further states, "Qualitative approaches in science are distinct modes of inquiry oriented toward understanding the unique nature of human thoughts, behaviors, negotiations and institutions under different sets of historical and environmental circum-stances" (p. 7). Field and Morse (1985) write,

> Qualitative methods should be used when there is little known about
> a domain, when the investigator suspects that the present knowledge
> or theories may be biased or when the research question pertains to
> understanding or describing a particular phenomenon or event about
> which little is known. (p. 11)

Wilson (1985) points to the nonqualitative aspects of qualitative re-search: "Qualitative analysis is the nonnumerical organization and interpretation of data in order to discover patterns, themes, forms and qualities found in field notes, interview transcripts, open-ended ques-tionnaires, journals and diaries" (p. 397). And Leininger (1985) offers this conception: "The qualitative type of research refers to the methods and techniques of observing, documenting, analyzing and interpreting attributes, patterns, characteristics and meanings of specific, contextual or gestaltic features of phenomena under study" (p. 5).

This chapter focuses on two qualitative designs or the methods of phenomenology and grounded theory. The intention is to introduce the nurse researcher to some of the underlying ideas and assumptions of qualitative research. The chapter is an overview and as such does not answer as many questions as it raises. In that spirit, references are provided for those readers who may find their nursing research inter-ests philosophically compatible with qualitative research methods and who are spurred on to further discovery.

QUALITATIVE DESIGN: A BEGINNING[1]

A person or situation presents interests, problems, or questions, and we can often respond in one of two ways. We can respond from extrapo-lation and hunches about what is known or assumed about the phe-nomenon, or we can suspend preconceptions or inferences and say, "I'm not sure about that," "I don't know about that," or "There's virtually nothing known about that." The first approach leads to deduction, the latter to induction. The first response lends itself to traditional hypothe-sis testing and deduction from existing theory; the second response lends itself to going out and finding out what's going on and leads to theory development.

For example, consider the question, What's it like being divorced? A deductive approach to this question would be to arrive at some hunches from the literature on divorce and the family, from existing role theory, from developmental theory, from psychology, and so on. The hunches would become hypotheses, linking some variables found in the literature to, in this instance, divorce. They would be, as called for, directional, and might have as dependent variables increased role stress, role conflict, or role ambiguity. There may be increased life satisfaction, increased sense of generativity, or decreased interaction with old friends. The variables deduced from the literature could be endless. Regardless, the researcher would test hypotheses using, say, a quasi-experimental or correlational design to support or refute hypotheses based on a statistical level of significance. The answer to the question, then, is based primarily on what can be deduced from what is already known.

In contrast, the answer to the question can be approached from a qualitative perspective. This is particularly appropriate when there have been rapid sociological changes, so that if theory does exist, it may be outdated and no longer relevant. With a qualitative design, the answer may be obtained by asking people the question in a direct way or by spending time observing and interacting with people who are divorced. Interviewing people, observing people, and, perhaps, in this case, asking people to keep diaries or other written records would all yield fresh authentic data. Questions that lend themselves to qualitative approaches might start with "What's going on here?" "How does it feel to be . . . ?" "What does the experience mean?" or "What's it like to be . . . ?"

With a qualitative design, we are seeking to discover knowledge, to develop or reformulate theory from the authentic source. We are looking at the whole within context.

The interest in qualitative designs is directed toward discovering or uncovering new insights, meanings, and understandings. The research is often serendipitous, often leads to wonderment, and requires from the researcher an ability to remain flexible. Other assumptions that should be considered concerning qualitative designs include the following:

1. There may be a current theory about the subject we wish to investigate, but what is known may now be out of contemporary context. Answers to the question, What's it like being divorced? differ dramatically from one generation to another. Theories need to be revised in light of societal changes, other new discoveries, and human evolution. Theory is culturally and time bounded. As culture "advances" and time progresses, different descriptions and explanations are critical to accurate understanding.

2. Nursing has advanced a philosophy that embraces the whole of the human condition. We profess to values that include respect for all individuals and their cultural interpretations of meaning in experience and events. Following from this is an emphasis on self-determination and autonomy. A qualitative perspective then becomes essential from the philosophical perspective of nursing not only as a research design but for actual implementation of a holistic, empathic, individualized delivery of nursing care. In the discussion below of phenomenology as a design for research, we will see that a broad question could be asked, such as, What is the lived experience of being divorced about? An exploratory, open, theory-suspended approach actualizes the belief that the individual interprets his or her own experiences and gives meaning to them.

3. With many qualitative designs, there is an attempted suspension or bracketing out of what we have already come to believe, suspect, or assume. Qualitative designs yield new understanding and insights.

4. Qualitative designs are needed in current theory formulation and reformulation to assess the extent to which gender biases have influenced our view of the world and have established norms and standards that may be inappropriately generalized. Sex bias research results in asymmetry of findings, role stereotyping (parent = mother), failure to address sex as a variable whether a subject variable or a stimulus variable, and a general devaluation of women's interpretation modes and epistemological interests. There is a growing recognition of the need to reexamine and perhaps reconstruct theories so that gender, class, and ethnic background are recognized outright. Qualitative designs are critical to this pursuit.

When to Use Qualitative Designs

Qualitative designs are appropriate

1. when virtually nothing seems known about a topic or phenomenon;
2. when what seems to be known or believed somehow does not seem accurate (intuiting), prompting
   a. hunches about inconsistencies,
   b. hunches about biases,
   c. hunches that time has changed what is believed,
   d. hunches about ineffective approaches;
3. when feelings arise such as
   a. "something doesn't ring true"
   b. "that's not real life,"
   c. "something's going on here and I'm not quite sure what it is";
4. when the researcher wonders what it would feel like to experience something he or she knows nothing about.

As mentioned, a researcher might want to explore the design itself, taking on the question, What's the lived experience of doing a qualitative design like? (Hutchinson, 1985, gives a good description of that process.) An important dimension to the process is to become comfortable with the philosophical and ethical underpinnings of qualitative designs (see Field & Morse, 1985; Leininger, 1985; Munhall & Oiler, 1986; Parse et al., 1985; Swanson & Chenitz, 1986).

PHENOMENOLOGY AS METHOD

Omery (1983) notes that "most researchers in the social sciences who have advocated or implemented the phenomenological method have been inspired by it, rather than directly apply steps" (p. 53). This is a critical point to remember when defending a departure from some lockstep designs. The point here illustrates the philosophy-design juncture. The philosophy is open, interpretive, and individualistic. Designs with prescribed steps in themselves are prescriptive and give direction to the lived experience of doing phenomenology as interpreted by a phenomenological philosopher or researcher. In this sense, they contradict the philosophy. The researcher should recognize that such contradictions are part of the lived experience of doing phenomenology and, accepting that, move on, remembering the theme of "being inspired" rather than of strictly applying steps.

Regardless, for most of us, a "where to begin" and a "how to do it" frame our thinking and help us actualize the concepts and beliefs underpinning the method. The question of how to gain access to lived experience then is answered by many philosophers and social scientists. Among those who have advanced a particular method are Giorgi, VanKaam, Spiegelberg, Colaizzi, Merleau-Ponty, and the Utrecht school (method) as practiced by Martinus Langveld. The researcher contemplating a particular phenomenological method should consult the work of these authors and look at various studies using these methods; however, he or she also should remember that to be faithfully phenomenological, a study should not necessarily be structured by a linear design. The experience itself will often provide the direction. In the discussions of the two studies that follow, we can see how two nurse researchers have been inspired by phenomenological philosophy. Oiler (1982, 1983) uses Spiegelberg's phenomenological method to guide her through the task of exploring a phenomenological perspective in nursing, and Sauer's (1985) study advances her own interpretation of a phenomenological method. Both demonstrate qualitative designs in that both ask questions concerning phenomena about which virtually nothing is known in nursing—Oiler asks what a phenomenological perspective in nursing is like, and Sauer asks about what it is like having a child later in life than is the cultural norm.

Oiler and Spiegelberg

In Oiler's (1982) "The Phenomenological Approach in Nursing Research," nurses' expression in the art form of poetry are used to examine nursing reality. The "lived experience" of the nurse is a critical dimension in nursing practice, in that nurses' ideas about that reality continuously inform and direct nursing practice, education, and reality. Oiler notes,

> Nurse poets help us to see nursing reality by disrupting our customary way of referring to it with technical language. In the poetic form, the nursing situation is seen from a different vantage point. Poetic expres-

sion enlarges our view, giving us an opportunity to know about nursing experience in a different way. (p. 121)

The aims of the study were (a) to examine the concept of subjectivity in the nursing literature, (b) to describe a phenomenological perspective in nursing, and (c) to contribute to a clarification of lived experience. Spiegelberg's method of phenomenology inspired Oiler's exploration into phenomenology and demonstrates the underlying concepts of this philosophical perspective on reality.

One Phenomenological Method

Spiegelberg's (1976) method of doing phenomenology was used as a guideline. The essential operations are briefly described here, and the same steps are presented in a second format.

1. *Bracketing:* This is a process by which the researcher attempts to be, to the extent possible, free of bias, working to recognize bias and "control" for it. To see lived experience, one must suspend and lay aside what one thinks one already knows about it. Because the researcher wishes to recognize what it is, he or she thinks about an experience and then brackets or suspends it—a literature review at this point would only give the researcher more to bracket out. The more unknown the subject is, the less bracketing is necessary. The researcher might write a description of everything he or she knows or believes about the topic of exploration and then set it aside.

2. *Intuiting:* Here, the researcher becomes absorbed in the phenomenon, looking at it fresh, without layering it with what he or she has bracketed out. Concentration is very important here, because the involvement is very intense.

3. *Analyzing:* At this point the researcher compares and contrasts descriptions of the phenomenon under study. This allows for identification of recurring themes and interrelationships.

4. *Describing:* This is the final step for the researcher: communicating to others what he or she has found. This is the actual communication of phenomenological seeing.

For Spiegelberg, these steps are for the purpose of investigating particular phenomena, investigating general essences, and apprehending essential relationships among essences.

Procedures in Oiler's Study

Nursing journals published over the previous 10 years were reviewed for poems authored by nurses. During a 3-month period, 58 poems were read and reread. This was a "dwelling with" period, in which the researcher attempted to lay aside what she might write in poetry or another aesthetic form, instead imaginatively and intuitively assuming another's point of view. This allowed for the emergence of recurring themes, which then enabled description of particular phenomena, general essences, and essential relationships between essences. The value and opportunities of aesthetic expressions for understanding lived experience cannot be overstated.

With qualitative designs in particular, every avenue of access to awareness should be looked at and dwelled with. In the process of dwelling with the language of poetry, Oiler (1983) gained access to nurses' lived realities, and because she attempted to bracket out what she knew about the world, she allowed different awarenesses to surface. The researcher attempted to suspend her preconceptions and/or conceptions and look at experience fresh. From such newly gleaned awarenesses descriptive theory can emerge.

Descriptions

In the examination of selected poems, Oiler (1983) discovered the intensity of nurses' emotional responses to nurse-client situations. We learn of this part of nurse valuing—the determination to explicate the meaning of caring in the nursing situation. We learn that such human expression brings meaning to existence. Oiler moves beyond technical language and meanings that objectify the world, which, as Zbilut (1977) notes, leave much of nursing experience in silence.

Returning to Spiegelberg's (1976) three purposes (investigating phenomena, general essences, and essential relationships between essences), let us review what has been described.

Themes, Essences, and Interrelationships

Oiler's (1983) work reveals many themes, essences, and interrelationships:

1. Nurses feeling angry and frustrated; awareness of obstructed pursuit; interrelationship with feminist theory development

2. Nurses as nurturers and as surrogate and real mothers; interrelationships of dependence and independence; letting go, ambivalence, and changing roles

3. Nurses struggling with the risks of closeness, pain of separation, tensions between person and role, and a need to integrate personal history more adequately through the role

4. Nurses' awareness of the meaning of patients' circumstances in the context of the life cycle

Thus, this study reveals themes, essences, and interrelationships that should command our attention. The use of a qualitative design in this instance allows us to come closer to the experience of nursing. Implications from the descriptions are critical to the nursing profession, to nurses as individuals, and to the recipients of nursing care. One can imagine the consequences, or perhaps we already know the consequences, of not attending to these responses. A qualitative design such as this enables us to answer the question, What's going on here? when perhaps the consequences are already being felt as problems. Such consequences of the above essences and theories might include attrition, low morale, burnout, and the like. The findings from this study enable an enlightened view of the experience and thus enable knowledgeable and relevant intervention. Thus, Oiler has accomplished her aims of examining the concept of subjectivity in nursing literature, describing a phenomenological perspective, and contributing to the clarification of lived experience.

Sauer and Her Own Phenomenological Method

Sauer (1985) related that the phenomenological method with which she is most familiar is the Utrecht school method as taught and practiced by Martinus Langveld of the Netherlands. In this interpretation of method, the concept of transformation is critical and is referred to as the "validity of their (phenomenologists') claims to knowledge." Sauer then goes on to use Reinharz's (1983) five steps of phenomenological transformation to underpin the advancement of her "own" method. Sauer's personal interpretation concurs with Omery's (1983) statement that this phenomenological method is often interpreted within the philosophy rather than by applying a specific set of steps.

- *First transformation:* A person's experience is transformed into actions and language that become available to him or her by special interaction with the phenomenological researcher.
- *Second transformation:* The researcher transforms what is heard into an understanding of the original experience.
- *Third transformation:* The researcher attempts to capture the essence of the original experience by clarifying conceptual categories.
- *Fourth transformation:* These conceptual categories are transformed into some type of written or visual description that attempts to capture the experience the person has spoken about.
- *Fifth transformation:* This written or visual description clarifies for the recipients of the description the phenomenon under investigation.

The Aim of the Study

Sauer (1985) states that the aim of her study was to "clearly understand a poorly delineated phase in the life cycle of a modern woman, that is, the timing of childbearing" (p. 98). Specifically, the study focused on couples planning to have their first child later in life than is usual in their culture. The phenomenological method, as interpreted by Sauer, was carried out in the following steps:

1. Interviews were conducted with three couples as they lived through the last 3 months of a delayed pregnancy and the first 3 months of parenthood. Two additional women were interviewed during the last month of pregnancy. Sauer also used literature, in the form of Phyllis Chesler's book (1979), *With Child: A Diary of Motherhood.* In the spirit of bracketing, Sauer delayed using some of her own and her husband's experience when, toward the end of this study, she herself became pregnant.

2. *First transformation:* Interviews took place in the informants' homes, with the goal of creating a setting that would make possible near-natural conversation. Sauer recorded notes, and in an effort to ensure accuracy of her recordings, gave informants transcriptions of their interviews. Thus, the informants had the opportunity to validate that the materials expressed what they meant to say.

3. *Classification of conceptual categories:* Sauer describes the overwhelming process of analyzing the dialogues and separating out

themes for each informant. With themes identified for each informant, variations in themes could be selected out. In reporting the data, the headings "Forms" (themes) and "Variations" were used so that ground structure or clarifying conceptual categories could be identified. For example, the identification of a conceptual category of "planned, orderly lives" was advanced as one of the ground structures of the lived experiences of delayed parenthood for women.

4. *Description and essences:* The meaningfulness of transition to delayed parenthood becomes more comprehensible when viewed from this conceptual framework of "planned, orderly lives." Sauer expands our understanding of this experience and its ramifications when she reminds us that with planning comes a sense of control. She notes that these individuals actually "planned" their pregnancies and then revealed "shock, surprise, and disbelief" at what they found to be an uncontrollable situation.

The foregoing is an excerpt from a broader description, but it represents an attempt to provide a sample of what "knowing about what's going on here" in the form of descriptions of lived experience has to offer nurses. Understanding and interventions in patient support, teaching, and planning for the "unplanned" when we encounter parents who may be bearing children in later years needs to be founded on the answer to the question, What's it like for couples who have delayed pregnancy? In a larger context, our interventions need to be based on answers to the question, What's it like to be pregnant at different phases in the life cycle? The humanistic themes of context and individuality become apparent when we articulate clearly that differences may exist in the lived experience of pregnancy according to when pregnancy occurs in the life cycle. This may sound fundamental, but qualitative designs for studying specific phenomena like Sauer's clearly bring to awareness some of the essences and interrelationships of lived experiences.

In Summary

Both Oiler and Sauer have presented nurse researchers with descriptions that reflect the influence of a phenomenological perspective. The descriptions as presented here are, of course, encapsulated; to appreciate the richness and the significance of the contributions, the reader will want to study the primary sources.

Oiler and Sauer explored lived experiences as described by those who experienced them through their articulated perceptions. As we move on now to grounded theory, we will see many of the same philosophical underpinnings permeating this qualitative design but with an emphasis on formulating concepts and theory.

GROUNDED THEORY

The grounded theory method of research goes beyond describing an event or situation to conceptualizing it. Stern (1980) states that grounded theory "aims to generate theoretical constructs which explain the action in the social context under study" (p. 21). The intent of this method is to develop concepts that are abstractions grounded in the data and set off with specific definitions (Diers, 1979). Glaser and Strauss developed the grounded theory method in the 1960s. These two sociologists, whose works have significantly influenced their own field and many nurse researchers (Benoliel, Hutchinson, Swanson & Chenitz, Stern, Wilson), have provided the method to go about formulating theories at the first level of theory development. Examples of their work include *Awareness of Dying* (1965) and *Time for Dying* (1968), as well as in a book on the method itself, *Discovery of Grounded Theory* (1967).

Like phenomenology, the grounded theory method is most useful when little is known about a topic and few theories, if any, exist to explain a phenomenon. Hutchinson (1986), in a description of grounded theory, states:

> Grounded theory utilizes an inductive, from the ground-up approach using everyday behaviors or organizational patterns to generate theory. Such a theory is inherently relevant to the world from which it emerges whereas the relevance of verification research (second level inquiry) varies widely. (p. 113)

Norris (1982), who also uses the terms *comparative analysis* and *idea testing* for grounded theory methodology, says that this design "proves useful not only for the discovery of substantive theory but also for the clarification of theoretical building blocks, or nursing concepts" (p. 41). Stern (1985) places this design within context:

> Nurse scientists who use grounded theory find it ideal for teaching nursing problems. . . . Because the scientist generates constructs (or theory) from the data rather than applying a theory constructed by someone else from another data source, the generated theory remains connected to or grounded in the data. (p. 149)

One of the basic assumptions in grounded theory is that there are unidentified concepts or constructs that, if identified, will enable understanding and problem solving. As with the preceding methods, language varies. What we generally refer to as concepts or constructs are referred to in the grounded theory literature as core variables or basic social processes (BSPs). Wilson (1985) states, "Despite the diversity that characterizes qualitative data, the grounded theory approach presumes the possibility of discovering fundamental patterns in all of social life" (p. 416).

These patterns are called basic social processes, and because they are not as yet articulated, they are not accessible for problem solving or theory development. For example, Hutchinson (1986) identified a basic social process she called "creating meaning" in response to an unarticulated problem that she assumed existed in neonatal intensive care units. The social psychological problem for nurses of dealing with what Hutchinson termed "horror" resulting from dealing repeatedly with deformities and deaths among newborns was solved by the BSP of "creating meaning." This will be discussed further in the description of her study, below. Wilson's study (1982, 1986) identified the BSP of "infracontrolling" to describe how social order is maintained among schizophrenics living under conditions of freedom. She further developed concepts of "presencing," "farring," and "limiting intrusion" to enable the process of developing propositions and theories.

The Grounded Theory Method

Again, it is beyond the intent of this chapter to provide in detail the actual steps of the grounded theory method. Rather, a general idea as to the process is provided and, as with all methods, the reader is referred to additional references and to a "grounded theorist." The steps listed below represent a compilation of Stern's (1985), Wilson's (1985), and Hutchinson's (1986) grounded theory procedures:

1. *The research problem:* The purpose of the study is to *identify* problems; therefore, the researcher does not start with a research problem. The question could be, What are the basic social and psychological processes that explain interaction in a particular setting or under certain conditions?

2. *Literature search:* This is considered disadvantageous, because it can lead to premature closure of ideas, prejudgments, and an inaccurate aim when participating in the social process.

3. *Data gathering:* Data collection generally follows the pattern of field research, with the researcher finding himself or herself on the study participant's "home ground." As in ethnographic research, the researcher immerses himself or herself in the social environment. The form this takes varies according to what is necessary and possible and to what fulfills necessary requirements for meaningful interaction. "Bracketing," described in the discussion of phenomenology, is also used in grounded theory, so that "objectivity" in the form of an open mind is possible.

4. *Data recording:* Whether field notes or recordings are used, the data are eventually coded and categorized as the researcher searches for clarification of the phenomenon and a way to describe it. Coding—applying labels to what is going on—usually uses verb forms. Stern (1985) gives these examples: "side-stepping, tuning in, tuning out, labelling, selling, teaching" (p. 155). The coded data are compared until patterns and categories emerge. Placing data within categories is a hypothetical process, but when performed correctly, it leads to concept development. Coding in words expresses "what is going on" and develops terms to describe dimensions, properties, conditions, strategies, and consequences. Glaser (1978) identifies "families of theoretical codes"; this work is essential reading for a grounded theorist. "Memoing" is a spontaneous activity in which the researcher records his or her ideas in order to capture elusive and shifting connections. A memo in this sense is a recording of a spontaneous thought process, not a formal, filed note of description.

5. *Discovering the overriding analytic theme:* Within this process, categories are reduced, sorting takes place so that coherence can generate ideas, and a core category is identified. The researcher searches through the data, codes, and memos for what seems central, what recurs, and what makes sense to the people in the setting. Many researchers diagram a set of interrelationships when writing up their final analysis. (We will see this below for the BSP of "creating meaning.")

6. *The research report:* The BSP serves as the central focus of the proposed descriptive theory that seeks to describe the basic social processes occurring in a given context. When reworking and writing the theory, the researcher can incorporate relevant literature. Many nurse researchers, when reporting grounded theory, do so by identifying the problem they uncovered within the situation and the BSP that was discovered in operation. Hypotheses can then be generated from these findings. Examples of this include Stern's studies on stepfather families, Pyler and Stern's discovery of "nursing gestalt," Wilson's (1982) previously mentioned study, and Benoliel's (1967) study on the dying patient.

Glaser/Strauss and Hutchinson

Using Glaser and Strauss's steps from grounded theory method, Hutchinson has conducted many studies. The one briefly described here is titled "Creating Meaning Out of Horror" (Hutchinson, 1984). An outline of the study is presented here.

1. *Question:* "What is going on in the neonatal intensive care unit?" was the question asked by administrators concerned with NICU nurses' low morale and high turnover rates. Hutchinson agreed to study the situation.

2. *Method:* Over a period of 3 months, Hutchinson spent 20 hours a week as a participant observer in a 16-bed NICU.

3. *Findings:* After implementing the procedures of data collection developed by Glaser and Strauss, Hutchinson found that nurses had to cope with the social psychological problem of facing the stress that comes with caring for newborns with extreme deformities, who were subjected to extreme treatments, and who died. The core variable, or BSP, that she

described in her theory was called "creating meaning." When nurses failed to create meaning in their work, they experienced burnout, depression, and low morale. If they were able to create meaning, nurses obtained a satisfaction that enabled them to continue in the face of what was described as "horror." Implications of this study come from the recognition that finding ways to assist nurses in creating meaning would indeed be a worthwhile goal to pursue.

4. *Diagram of the major theoretical codes for NICU research:* The following diagram illustrates the interrelationships and integration of the concepts. It is a model of the theory.

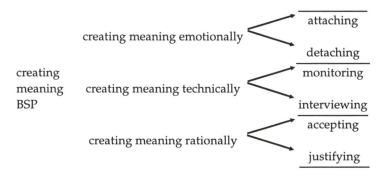

Objectivity, Reliability, and Validity

Objectivity is the essential basis of all good research, including qualitative designs. In the scientific world, however, the assumption seems to exist that we all use the word *objectivity* in the same way, as though it has a fixed universal definition (i.e., the definition associated with positivistic science). Kirk and Miller (1986) offer this contrasting definition:

> Objectivity is the simultaneous realization of as much reliability and validity as possible. Reliability is the degree to which the finding is independent of accidental circumstances of the research, and validity is the degree to which the finding is interpreted in a correct way. (p. 20)

Refocusing our perspective somewhat from the traditional view of objectivity, where the researcher is separate from his or her research or at least not contaminating it, is important in understanding the concepts of objectivity in qualitative designs. Although the researcher is a primary "instrument" in qualitative designs, this presence is aimed at coming as close as possible to a reality or lived experience as it occurs in its natural unfolding. The steps for the two qualitative designs described include measures for acknowledging, dealing with, and laying aside the researcher's values, biases, and preconceptions. They are laid out at the beginning of the study, as part of a good design. The literature review is postponed to further this effort. The researcher makes every effort to clear his or her perceptual field so that he or she can absorb experience as fresh, new, and unbiased. To do this completely, of course, is impossible, but the attempt is aimed at the "realization of as much reliability and validity as possible."

"Instruments" other than humans are also filled with values, biases, preconceptions, and other hindrances to objectivity. More important to theory development in nursing—and to the questions of objectivity, reliability, and validity is the use of instruments developed in one context or environment to test hypotheses with populations in other cultures or contexts.

With the two qualitative designs presented here, a researcher could have instead chosen from a number of life or work satisfaction scales to reach some conclusion about nurses' experiences or about having a child later in life. But (and here is my bias) would this produce the richness in data and detail, the authenticity, the "real-life" dimensions that qualitative designs offer us?

The question of reliability and validity remains even when the researcher reports "unbiased" perceptions. We can all view or participate in the same event and each tell the story of what occurred very differently. That is why the steps in a qualitative design ask the researcher to reflect on personal foundations and intuitions. But what about different versions of the same event? Qualitative researchers see this as part of the context, part of the "objective" world. Differing perceptions, for example, about any lived experience play an essential part in any study. What we are seeking is a faithful representation of what is happening, and that, of course, may be different for different individuals; *that* then becomes part of what is happening in a lived experience.

If we dispense with using the word *objectivity* with the meaning that the positivists assign it, our ideas for validity and reliability can be reinterpreted. Currently, the same criteria used to evaluate the scientific method, as we commonly call the positivist view of the world, are used to evaluate qualitative methods that are based on an entirely different worldview (see Brink, 1989). Leininger (1985) presents a good argument for applying different criteria when evaluating the reliability and validity of qualitative research. She contends that *validity* in qualitative research refers to "gaining knowledge and understanding of the true nature, essence, meaning, attributes, and characteristics of a particular phenomenon under study. Measurement is not the goal" (p. 68).

Sampling

With a qualitative design, the sample is considered that part of reality that is observed and recorded. There is a research focus or research question, and the researcher proceeds to sample until satisfied that the richness of the data is accurate and meaningful to report. Because there are no statistical requirements mandating a specific number of subjects, the goals of reliability and validity guide the sampling process. A case study with an N of 1 may provide the seed of an important theory. A sample of one NICU, as in Hutchinson's report discussed above, provides a basis for further comparison and exploration. One guideline that may be helpful (if not always practical) in determining sample size is to continue to collect data within the research focus until no new information is obtained (see Morse, 1989).

HUMAN SUBJECTS ISSUES

Informed consent, type of participation by the researcher, differentiating roles, "off-the-record" remarks, and "unwelcome results" must be attended to in qualitative methods. Methods textbooks for each qualitative design give suggestions and guidelines for handling these problems. There are special ethical considerations to be taken into account when using qualitative designs (see Munhall, 1988, 1989a; Punch, 1986).

CONCLUDING REMARKS

The challenges of qualitative research can be metaphorically likened to the challenges facing any explorer: the unknown, the unforeseen, the unpredictable. The whole idea of discovery involves not knowing what you are about to come on, unveil, and bring to consciousness. In this chapter, the opportunities to explore phenomena through the qualitative designs of phenomenology and grounded theory are presented to stimulate and guide the reader through uncharted waters. The aim of this chapter has not been to provide a definitive methods map but, rather, to generate enthusiasm and interest in qualitative designs as additional ways of studying nursing phenomena. These designs can enrich our understanding and descriptions of human responses and human experiences in a humanistic scientific dialect. I have found these qualitative designs to be enormously meaningful, lending an authentic type of insight, enriching me and enabling me to know people in ways I never thought possible.

NOTE

1. This section is reprinted from Munhall, P. L. (1989b). Philosophical ponderings on qualitative research methods in nursing. *Nursing Science Quarterly*, 2(1), 20-28. Copyright by William & Wilkins, 1989. Reprinted by permission.

REFERENCES

Benoliel, J. (1967). *The nurse and the dying patient.* New York: Macmillan.

Benoliel, J. (1984). Advancing nursing science: Qualitative approaches. *Western Journal of Nursing Research,* 7(1), 1-8.

Brink, P. (1989). Issues in reliability and validity. In J. Morse (Ed.), *Qualitative nursing research.* Rockville, MD: Aspen.

Chesler, P. (1979). *With child: A diary of motherhood.* New York: Thomas Crowell.

Diers, D. (1979). *Research in nursing practice.* Philadelphia: J. B. Lippincott.

Field, P., & Morse, J. (1985). *Nursing research: The application of qualitative approaches.* Rockville, MD: Aspen.

Glaser, B., & Strauss, A. (1965). *Awareness of dying.* Chicago: Aldine.

Glaser, B., & Strauss, A. (1967). *The discovery of grounded theory.* Chicago: Aldine.

Glaser, B., & Strauss, A. (1968). *Time for dying.* Chicago: Aldine.

Hutchinson, S. (1984). Creating meaning out of horror. *Nursing Outlook,* 32(2), 86-90.

Hutchinson, S. (1985). Perspective: Field research in a neonatal intensive care unit. *Topics in Clinical Nursing,* 7(2), 24-28.

Hutchinson, S. (1986). Grounded theory: The method. In P. Munhall & C. Oiler (Eds.), *Nursing research: A qualitative perspective* (pp. 111-129). Norwalk, CT: Appleton-Century-Crofts.

Kirk, J., & Miller, M. L. (1986). *Reliability and validity in qualitative research.* Beverly Hills, CA: Sage.

Leininger, M. (Ed.). (1985). *Qualitative research methods in nursing.* New York: Grune & Stratton.

Morse, J. (Ed.). (1989). *Qualitative nursing research: A contemporary dialogue.* Rockville, MD: Aspen.

Munhall, P. (1988). Ethical considerations in qualitative research. *Western Journal of Nursing Research, 10*(2), 150-162.

Munhall, P. (1989a). Institutional review: A task of no small consequence. In J. Morse (Ed.), *Qualitative nursing research: A contemporary dialogue.* Rockville, MD: Aspen.

Munhall, P. (1989b). Philosophical ponderings on qualitative research methods in nursing. *Nursing Science Quarterly, 2*(1), 20-28.

Munhall, P., & Oiler, C. (Eds.). (1986). *Nursing research: A qualitative perspective.* Norwalk, CT: Appleton-Century-Crofts.

Norris, C. (1982). *Concept clarification in nursing.* Rockville, MD: Aspen.

Oiler, C. (1982). The phenomenological approach in nursing research. *Nursing Research, 31*, 118-131.

Oiler, C. (1983). Nursing reality as reflected in nurses' poetry. *Perspectives in Psychiatric Care, 21*, 81-89.

Omery, A. (1983). Phenomenology: A method for nursing research. *Advances in Nursing Science, 5*(2), 49-63.

Parse, R., Coyne, A., & Smith, M. J. (1985). *Nursing research: Qualitative methods.* Bowie, MD: Brady.

Punch, M. (1986). *The politics and ethics of fieldwork.* Beverly Hills, CA: Sage.

Reinharz, S. (1983). Phenomenology as a dynamic process. *Phenomenology and Pedagogy, 1*, 77-79.

Sauer, J. (1985). Using a phenomenological method to study nursing phenomena. In M. Leininger (Ed.), *Qualitative research methods in nursing* (pp. 93-107). New York: Grune & Stratton.

Spiegelberg, W. (1976). *The phenomenological movement* (2 vols.). The Hague: Martinus Nijhoff.

Stern, P. (1980). Grounded theory methodology: Its use and processes. *Image, 12*, 20-23.

Stern, P. (1985). Using grounded theory method in nursing research. In M. Leininger (Ed.), *Qualitative research methods in nursing* (pp. 149-160). New York: Grune & Stratton.

Swanson, J. M., & Chenitz, W. C. (1986). *From practice to grounded theory: Qualitative research.* Menlo Park, CA: Addison-Wesley.

Wilson, H. S. (1982). *Deinstitutionalized residential approaches for the severely mentally disordered patient: The Soteria House approach.* New York: Grune & Stratton.

Wilson, H. S. (1985). *Research in nursing.* Menlo Park, CA: Addison-Wesley.

Wilson, H. S. (1986). Presencing: Doing grounded theory. In P. Munhall & C. Oiler (Eds.), *Nursing research: A qualitative perspective* (pp. 131-144). Norwalk, CT: Appleton-Century-Crofts.

Zbilut, J. P. (1977). Linguistic constraints in nursing practice. *Forum, 16,* 339-342.

14

Historical Research

LAURIE K. GLASS

The historical method of research is the process of critically examining and analyzing records of the past. Historiography is the imaginative reconstruction of the past from the data derived by this process. Although historical research is a respected method of inquiry, it has not always been popular in nursing. However, there has been a resurgence of interest in this area in the past few years.

According to Notter (1972), "Historical research is not merely a collection of incidents, facts, dates, or figures; it is a study of the relationships of facts and incidents, of themes or currents of social and professional issues that have influenced past events and continue to influence the present and future" (p. 483). Specifically, historical research is conducted for one of the following reasons: to discover the unknown; to answer the question, Why?; to look for implications or relationships to the present; and to communicate the past accomplishments of individuals as well as the profession. This last reason to study history serves the secondary purpose of instilling pride and esprit de corps in the members of the profession.

One basic assumption underlying the use of this method is that the study of the past is valuable and provides useful information for the present. Without a belief in retrospective analysis, it is difficult to justify the use of the historical method. An additional assumption is that data are available. Unlike other methods, historical research relies strictly on data created by someone other than the researcher. If records (data) have not been generated and retained, no information exists on which to base an investigation. In the historical method, the researcher acts as the instrument, in that the data are all filtered through the investigator before being identified as significant or insignificant. The strength of the results hinges on the belief that a researcher will be guided by the research questions and maintain an objective view of the data. While plowing through mountains of data, the researcher must remain conscious of the need to retrieve all relevant data and not just the data that answer research questions to the researcher's liking. Historical research should be a clear, unbiased quest for answers.

THE BASIC DESIGN

The basic method for historical analysis involves locating and examining documents, interpreting the evidence, and explaining the response. Seven steps are identifiable:

1. Think about and define a question.
2. Identify the secondary sources.
3. Locate and read the secondary sources.
4. Frame and focus the research questions.
5. Identify and locate the primary sources.
6. Use the primary sources.
7. Conduct analysis, synthesis, and exposition.

The initial question is usually broad. It may reflect an area of interest; for example, Why did this school give so many different kinds of degrees? Or, Who was Laura Logan? The investigator then needs to identify the secondary sources, which implies finding what has been written on the area of interest. Secondary sources include books, monographs, articles, and similar items written about the subject. With historical topics, this often means paging through journals of the era looking for news items or examining history books about institutions and organizations with which an individual or issue was associated. The investigator reads as much as can be found on the subject and related organizations, events, and people. As the investigator learns more about the subject, he or she can identify specific questions to be answered.

The questions so formulated are specifically focused and provide a framework for the research. The breadth and depth of the project will determine the number of questions to be answered. These questions also guide the researcher in examining the primary sources because data are sought from these sources to answer the questions.

Identifying primary sources involves discovering and locating manuscript collections that include pertinent historical documents. Primary sources are those that contain the words of a witness to or first recorder of an event. Examples include minutes, diaries, correspondence, manuscripts, and speeches. Primary sources can be located using published indexes to manuscript collections or by communicating with agencies and organizations about the location of their historical records. Established archival agencies usually have inventories for each collection, which facilitates the location of specific items or files.

Gathering information from primary sources is considered the actual "data collection." Volumes of data are examined in the search for answers to the focused questions. Significant data are recognized by their relationship to or fit with the whole picture or by repeated findings that identify trends or patterns. Each document is judged using external and internal criticism (validity and reliability). This means that all documents must be judged for authenticity and credibility. Notes are meticulously kept, not only on the content of the document but on the document itself and its location.

During the analysis, synthesis, and exposition phase of the historical research process, the data are interpreted. The researcher reviews the data thoroughly, categorizing it according to topic or theme and then reconstructing the results into a response that answers the questions. Interpretation is based in the time period of the events discussed. Supplementary data on events, organizations, or people that surface during the use of both secondary and primary sources are sought and used to further explain situations. If an argument is proposed, the support or refutation of that argument lies in the strength of the data. The analysis and synthesis of the data are largely intellectual tasks grounded in the researcher's knowledge and experience with the topic. Exposition involves writing the narrative story that results from the interpretation (analysis and synthesis) of the data. Footnotes are used to document sources, explain statements, or to provide verification and make possible additional research by an interested reader. The exposition of the research is considered the "art" of history. The report may be written as a story that is pleasant to read yet based on sound research.

Degree of Control Over the Data

In historical research, the degree of control over the data can be discussed both from the vantage point of the creation and existence of the data and from that of the use of the data. The investigator has no control over the creation of the data or the environment in which it was created. The data either exist or do not exist. If the information sought was not recorded and saved, there are no data. It is possible for some historical research questions to go unanswered because data do not exist. The saving and storage of the data also lie outside the control of the investigator. Documents may be discarded as useless or may be stored in conditions that hasten their deterioration. The investigator is thus dependent on the actions of others for the data.

To use the data, the investigator must travel to the data. The data are under the control of the agency where they are stored. For nursing history, this may be an archive, a historical society, or a hospital. The investigator has access to the data only under the conditions defined by the controlling agency. Brooks's (1969) review of the most common regulations and rules concerning historical data should be required reading for every neophyte historical researcher. The most overriding condition is that most of these agencies are open, and thus the data are available, Monday through Friday, 8:00 a.m. to 4:30 p.m. If the investigator must travel some distance to the data and the amount of time that can be spent with the data is limited, the pursuit of the research can become expensive, in both time and money. At this point, the data almost control the investigator, because data access is controlled by the owners of the data. The investigator must work within the structure provided by the agency housing the data and must alter his or her schedule and design the work to ensure the most efficient quest for data.

While using the data, the researcher does have control over the process of defining what constitutes significant information. As records and manuscripts are perused, information most significant to the problem at hand is retrieved. As information is selected from the volumes of documents examined, these items become the data that will be used for the analysis and synthesis. The investigator has complete control here by defining what is important and selecting from the records what he or she deems significant. As mounds of notes are carried away, the situation becomes one in which the investigator has complete control over the data and their interpretation.

To summarize, the investigator has no control over the creation and storage of the documents that become data. However, he or she has total control over the selection of what information in the documents will become data for the research project.

NURSING PROBLEMS SUITED
TO HISTORICAL METHODS

The historical method has been used in nursing research to reconstruct events, to analyze the rationale behind decisions, to trace activities and influences leading to current events, to analyze the scientific base and origin of procedures, to discover the impetus and sequencing of events, to analyze a person's ideas, to interpret the influence of a leader, and to understand nursing within the realm of the social, economic, political, and cultural setting of the time. Although many readers may think of history as a chronology of dates and places, historical research relies heavily on the analytical and interpretive skill of the investigator.

In their research on the experience of nurses as prisoners of war, Kalisch and Kalisch (1976) not only reconstructed a series of events, they placed them within the setting and cultural scene that existed at the time. By describing the situation that existed before the occurrence of the main event (nurses taken prisoner), they provide the reader with a sense of the "normal" situation and introduce the key factors in that situation. Using a chronological framework, they then describe and interpret the events that subsequently occurred, and the reactions of the nurses. For data, they relied on newspaper and journal articles by nurses and correspondents at the scene, books (primarily diaries and biographies) published after the war, and government reports. The writing style of their report gives the reader a sense of being in the situation with those unfortunate nurses. In the end, Kalisch and Kalisch accomplished their task of discovering what the experience was and reconstructing it so that others might learn from it. Knowledge has been gained in the areas of military nursing, ingenuity and creativity in times of stress, the needs of wartime nursing, and World War II.

My own work on Katharine Densford Dreves illustrates the importance of studying the people who have contributed to the nursing profession (Glass, 1984). As a nursing leader, Dreves's (1890-1978) professional life spans a time of great importance for nursing. The original purpose of the research was to discover who Katharine Densford Dreves was and what her influence had been on the profession. The final analysis yielded relevant data on professional organizations, nursing research in the 1930s, the profession's response to the need for nurses during World War II, and an individual's professional commitment. The basic data for the research were located in the Katharine Densford Dreves Papers at the University of Minnesota Archives. Available sources included diaries, extensive private and professional correspondence, speeches, manuscripts, and photographs. These data were supplemented with additional primary data from institutional and organizational records (such as the university president's papers and the School of Medicine's records). Secondary sources (books, journal articles) provided additional information related to the events and concerns of the era. This project required 3 years of source use and analysis. The results not only reconstruct the past but also contribute new knowledge in a number of areas.

During the analysis of Dreves's life from early childhood until her entry into nursing, it was possible to identify factors that contributed to her ability to become a leader. In addition, the analysis of her later life as a nursing leader led to the identification of distinct characteristics of her leadership style. This study has contributed to knowledge of leadership behaviors and women as leaders. An analysis of Dreves's status as an educated single woman during a time when women were expected to be in the home also provides insight into the struggles of someone breaking ground in uncharted territory. A contribution also has been made to documenting the history of women. A large project such as this can be partitioned into smaller topics to ensure a more in-depth analysis or to stimulate additional related research.

Dreves's work on a specific project over a 4-year time span is discussed in "Raising a Million Dollars: Katharine Densford Dreves and the American Nurses Foundation" (Glass, 1985). This particular episode in history could be analyzed and recounted in a paper of reasonable length, unlike larger projects that require years of study and volumes to communicate. Located in the Dreves Papers was extensive correspondence with the American Nurses Foundation staff, state nurses' association members, foundation donors, and national nursing leaders. Dreves also kept brochures, press releases, financial reports, and internal organizational memos and reports. These items provided a wealth of information about the foundation and the roles played by Dreves and her husband. The archived records of the American Nurses Foundation (at the Nursing Archives, Boston University) contained little new information. Major activities also could be verified through nursing journals. In total, there was a 10- to 12-inch stack of usable material (about 2,000 pieces of paper). From this material it was possible to reconstruct the fund-raising campaign, identify the key players, ascertain Dreves's motivation and commitment to the campaign, and identify an emerging concern with nursing research. The significance of Dreves's work with the foundation is emphasized by the reputation and activities of the foundation today and by the fact that this was the first fund-raising campaign conducted for the American Nurses Foundation. The report of this project not only provides previously unknown information but also describes fund-raising methods that could be used today.

STRENGTHS AND WEAKNESSES OF THE METHOD

The historical method can be used to answer questions and to contribute to the solution of nursing problems. However, it rarely stops with nursing concerns, because the content dealt with must be considered within the context in which it occurred. Nursing's concerns do not occur in a vacuum but within societal, political, and economic arenas. Using the historical method to answer nursing questions also facilitates answering questions in other areas, such as women's activities, education, role development, and institutional development. The strength of the method lies in its applicability to diverse topics and the breadth of knowledge that can be discovered through its use.

The historical method relies on the critical examination and analysis of materials. The individual investigator is the sole finder and analyzer of the data. The analysis depends on the intellectual processes used by the investigator. To conduct a study, the investigator assumes there are adequate data to answer the question. The sources of data are classified, organized, and stored according to a system developed by an archivist. There is a certain amount of inflexibility to the data, because they may not be in the form that the investigator wants. Because they were created by someone else, the data exist in a form that was useful to the originator and not necessarily to the investigator. For example, the data may be in the form of annual statistics when the researcher desires monthly statistics, or the data might be located in committee minutes that are labeled and stored in an unusual manner.

Access to data also can be an item of concern. Archival data are located in public and private agencies. Each sector has rules regarding access to and use of the records for research. Access is more difficult to achieve in private agencies such as hospitals, visiting nurse associations, or professional associations because usage is controlled by the current executive officer unless policies have been established. The investigator might have to seek permission from the original donor or the chief administrator to review the documents. After the materials have been located and access ensured, the researcher needs to be concerned with policies concerning how the records may be used and the information retained. Variations on usage rules include allowing reading only, reading and note taking, and photocopying.

The historical method can be expensive and time-consuming. Because the investigator must travel to the data, transportation and lodging expenses can become a burden if the data are located in numerous cities. The researcher must also have blocks of time available in which to travel and review the data. When traveling to the data, the researcher must allow enough time to account for finding more data than was anticipated so that additional trips may be avoided.

Reviewing thousands of pieces of paper to determine the significance of the content is a time-consuming task. Because so much of the location and analysis of data is an intellectual process implemented by the investigator, it is not feasible to hire research assistants to help with the project during this phase.

Given sufficient time, funding, and data, the historical method can be an exciting and satisfying process for the nursing investigator. However, because records often are stored in out-of-the-way places and archives are often located in basements, pursuit of historical research is not for those with allergies to dust, dirt, or mold.

MODEL

The historical method is used primarily for descriptive studies and theory building. An inductive approach to data collection is used. In the case of theory building, the investigator presents an interpretation for confirmation or argument and criticism. The best examples of theory building in nursing history are those arguments presented by Ashley (1976) and Melosh (1982). Each investigator presents data and an inter-pretation of how the nursing profession has developed as a workforce. Ashley (1976) concluded that nursing's development was limited by oppressive and paternalistic environmental forces (primarily physi-cian-dominated hospitals). Melosh (1982) suggests that nursing's devel-opment was affected by a split between nursing leaders and the work-ing nurse. The conclusions of these authors are interestingly different and invite criticism.

SAMPLES

Samples and sampling techniques as traditionally defined are not com-monly used in historical research. If an investigator discovers a massive data set in an archival setting and determines that it is not necessary to analyze the entire field of data, he or she may choose to sample the data set. For example, if 2,000 wills are available, the investigator might choose every fifth will for content analysis. An investigator also might determine a unit of analysis if the data for the project are plentiful and cut across settings or groups. For example, an investigator may choose to review the nursing committee minutes for January 1945 for each hospital in Chicago to analyze working nurses' responses to a possible draft of nurses. In this instance, the unit of analysis would be each set of nursing committee minutes.

These examples represent rare occurrences in historical research. The investigator's concern is to locate sufficient primary data to answer the research questions. To do this, times, places, events, and people related to the research questions are identified. Indexes to manuscript collections and telephone calls or letters to organizations and people can be used to discover the actual physical location of relevant sources. In addition, journal indexes and books published near the time of interest might provide clues to sources of data. The research questions determine the quest for data. If the questions are specific to a person, place, or thing, the search for data sources may not be as extensive as for broad, general questions. In the study of an individual's life, data sources may be compact, or they may be spread about widely. The papers of Katharine Densford Dreves were located in one place because she was primarily associated with one institution. The papers of Laura Logan are located in seven different places because she tended to change jobs. Research may involve using all locatable data or collecting as many data as needed to answer the question. When the same information is found repeatedly in the data, the quest for additional data ceases.

METHODS OF DATA COLLECTION

The main method of data collection in historical research is the critical examination of documents. However, the investigator might also interview relevant people, review and analyze videotapes or films, visit sites of events, and examine artifacts.

Issues With Secondary Document Sources

Secondary sources are documents written by others about the research question or a related area. Items included in this category are books, journal articles, newspaper articles (including obituary notices), and films. To identify these sources, the researcher uses cumulative indexes to the published literature, reference lists in historically significant books, and computerized search programs such as HISLINE (National Library of Medicine medical history resource citations). Because the major cumulative indexes for nursing literature begin with the 1950s, a hand search through the pages of the journals published prior to this time may be the only reasonable way to locate pertinent articles. To do a thorough job of this, the investigator must be familiar with the journals published during the years of interest and must know the words used to describe the phenomena at that time. Language changes over time, as does the popularity of words, and both retrieval and recognition (during hand searches) are affected by language familiarity. Making a list of terms in bold print and keeping it visible during the search facilitates the recognition of significant items.

To review the secondary sources, the researcher may have to rely on interlibrary loan services, because older books and journals are not readily available in some libraries. Historical societies and used bookstores are also excellent resources for the location of old materials. Under the right circumstances (depending on availability and price) it is sometimes easier to buy a resource than to borrow it, because restraints are often placed on the usage of old materials that are valued.

Changing technology creates a special issue when the investigator is using films and audio recordings as data. Unless the film or audio recording is located in an organized archival setting, the equipment needed to view the film or listen to the recording may no longer be available. As technology changes, the ability to retrieve information that was collected with that technology changes. An excellent example of this is the 1935 recording of M. Adelaide Nutting and Florence Nightingale. Victrolas and record players that can play this record are now almost nonexistent. In one institution, the recording was transferred to cassette tape, so that it was usable. This was possible only because an Educational Communications Department employee searched until he discovered an old machine that could play the record.

Issues With Primary Document Sources

The issues related to primary sources include finding the sources, accessing the sources, and judging the sources. Primary sources can be identified and located through the use of indexes, such as the Library of Congress's (1959-1985) *National Union Catalog of Manuscript Collections* (NUCMC) or Hinding's (1980) *Women's History Sources: A Guide to Archives and Manuscript Collections in the United States*. Local or state guides may also be available. It might even be necessary to write to institutions that have a specific relationship to the research questions to inquire about records in their possession or about their knowledge of the location of such records.

Once the records have been located, basic questions must be asked before the investigator travels to the site of the data. Is permission needed to review the records? If so, from whom? Is there a special form to be used in requesting permission? How are records organized? Have the records been processed? This is particularly important because the degree of organization of the records directly affects the amount of time the investigator will need to plan on spending looking at the records. Is there an inventory of the collection? This file-by-file listing of the collection is an invaluable tool for locating specific material or at least providing direction for the hunt. Is someone else currently using the data? If someone else is using the collection, the researchers might want to discuss their mutual interests, possible duplication of efforts, or a team approach to their search for specific answers.

During the search for and use of primary sources, the investigator's best friend and ally is the archivist. These people who work profession-ally to collect, organize, and make accessible the records that provide us with a view of history can provide priceless assistance. Archivists know their collections and can suggest other collections where addi-tional information might be found. If the research questions involve a local problem or person, archivists know the local history and can provide information about people and organizations. Their experience with the organization of records and files can also facilitate problem solving when the researcher is trying to figure out where a certain piece of information might be located. The investigator will benefit from knowing the archivist and talking to the archivist about the research. As professionals, archivists adhere to a code of confidentiality for each researcher's work, so "trade secrets" are never discussed. However, they will refer one investigator to another if there is a crossover in the area of interest. Archivists want their collections to be used (it justifies the storage of all that paper), and generally will go out of their way to be of assistance.

During the actual data collection, the issues are twofold: Are these really usable data? Are these data significant? Each piece of possible evidence is analyzed. To make a decision about the data really being usable, the researcher must judge a document's authenticity and credi-bility. This is accomplished through external and internal criticism. External criticism questions the authenticity of the document. In other words, is this document really what it appears to be? This judgment is made based on where the document is found and on the handwriting, ink, type, or paper used. The scandal over the so-called Hitler diaries is an example of documents that failed to pass tests of external criticism.

Internal criticism questions the accuracy, meaning, and credibility of the content of the document. Is what it says really what happened? To establish credibility of a document, the investigator must find corroborating evidence to support what is said, for instance, by finding another account of an incident described and comparing the stories.

Recognizing data as significant requires in-depth familiarity with the topic and an alertness when going through the data that is strengthened by practice. Significance is determined by the fit of the data with the whole picture. However, if the data are spread out, the investigator may not initially recognize their significance. For example, in the Dreves Papers what appeared to be the publication of a rather routine nursing textbook on ethics later resurfaced as the source of great controversy. Detailed notes on the location of data facilitate the researcher's return to significant sources when this happens.

Historical researchers also develop a sense of their content when they are immersed in the data for long periods. This sense provides recognition of missing pieces, something that doesn't look quite right, or something that appears to be missing. With the zeal of a detective, the researcher pursues whatever is necessary to get the complete story.

Another clue to significance in data collection is the repetitious citing of a particular idea, act, or event. Repetition can be a sign that a trend or pattern is developing, that an individual's values are reflected in his or her behavior, or that the issue was of concern to a wide audience. The researcher needs to investigate the meaning behind the repetition.

When using primary sources, the researcher may encounter additional problems related to the fact that the data were created by other people. Missing data may mean that records were destroyed and that the data are not retrievable. The filing system and language may be something the investigator has never seen before. Files that may contain relevant and significant information may be restricted in usage or may be sealed until a date 20 years into the future. This is common practice when the records contain information about people who are still alive or when the records contain information judged to be damaging if released at this time.

Artifacts and Site Visits

A researcher may also find it helpful to examine nontextual items related to the topic. For example, photographs, certificates, medallions, clothing, and equipment can provide a sense of history and reveal interesting bits of information. A visit to the site of a home, meeting, grave, battle, or other event also can enhance the spirit with which an investigator writes about a topic. Because the names of towns and streets change, the researcher should check old city directories for correct locations. When the researcher visits a cemetery, the manager can provide specific information about the location of a grave and the family history at the time of the death.

DATA ANALYSIS

During data collection, the researcher analyzes each possible piece of evidence to determine if the document and information it contains is truly solid. This data analysis is different from, yet related to, the analysis that occurs after the primary data have been collected. The actual data analysis occurs through a process of synthesis. According to Austin (1958), "This process involves several problems, such as organization of the data according to some plan, their adequate documentation, the determination of the meaning of the facts, and the discovery of relationships among them—a creative process" (p. 9). The data are sorted into categories and examined for themes, trends, and patterns. The data are interpreted within the time and standards of the era in which they were created. That era may be compared to other eras, but the basic interpretation must be consistent with the time in which the data were generated. This becomes particularly important when analyzing data that are sociologically based, especially with topics such as women's roles and family.

The data might be analyzed and interpreted according to a conceptual framework or the framework formed by the research questions. Support is sought for the premise that led the investigation. It is through the analysis that the groundwork is laid for the argument presented. Unlike other methods, the analysis does not appear on paper. It is a process that goes on in the head of the researcher, who eventually puts ideas on paper in the form of a report. The visual aspect of the data analysis process jumps from the pile of notes to the story. As with a jigsaw puzzle, the pieces are assembled into a picture to communicate results.

The mechanics of historical research dictate that data analysis must occur at the same time as the exposition or writing of the report. Reports are narrative and make extensive use of footnotes. Footnotes are essential with this method. They are used to explain statements, to acknowledge cited sources, and to document the location of data. Because historians do not have the raw data in their possession and the "experiment" cannot be replicated, footnotes are the key to the verification of the research and the stimuli for additional investigations. Historical reports without footnotes are suspect because a reader cannot determine the validity of the data on which the interpretation was based.

RELIABILITY AND VALIDITY

Reliability and validity issues are pertinent to data collection and interpretation (analysis). The internal and external criticism of the documents during data collection represent an attempt to secure reliable and valid data. External criticism determines the validity or authenticity of the document. It answers the where, when, why, and by whom questions (Christy, 1975). Validity of the document must be ascertained before the reliability of the information contained in it is assessed. Internal criticism questions the reliability of the information contained in the document. Does the researcher understand what is being said? Is what is being said an accurate portrayal of what happened? Here, the researcher must be alert to possible misinterpretation—either by himself or herself or by the document's author. In his discussion of the principles of historical criticism, Hockett (1955) provides specific ways and means to review for external and internal criticism. External criticism includes determining authorship, finding evidence of dates, detecting spurious documents, and determining the original form. Internal criticism refers to understanding the meaning of the statements and establishing their dependability.

Reliability and validity issues in the data analysis refer to the interpretation made or the argument proposed. The reliability of an interpretation is based on the type of evidence that was found and whether there is enough evidence to support the interpretation. Were the data competently analyzed? Was the researcher aware of possible bias during the analysis? Is the interpretation as objective as it can be? Validity is harder to ascertain. It asks the question, How good an answer is this? The overall aim of historical research is to discover and understand a subject. Reliability and validity questions are related only to the internal consistency and goodness of fit within a study. Comparison between studies is not appropriate unless exactly the same question is being asked.

HUMAN SUBJECTS ISSUES

Historical research occurs primarily through document review. The use of human subjects in the usual sense of a committee review is not an issue unless interviews are scheduled as part of the data collection. Two related issues are particularly relevant to historical research and the involvement of other people.

The first issue revolves around who owns the documents that need to be used. If an archive, library, or business owns the documents that describe an event, this is not an issue. However, if the documents belong to a family and describe activities of family members, then permission is needed to use the documents, and the report might be requested for review by the family. This places the researcher in the position of being censored by family members, which is not conducive to scholarly research. The same type of situation might occur when a researcher is writing the history of an organization or institution.

The second issue is the use of information about people who are still alive or who do not know that their names can be found in someone else's archives. This issue is important in the use of papers that contain personal correspondence. If the person mentioned is still alive, the researcher should use professional judgment in detailing the specifics of a topic or disclosing information that may embarrass that individual. If there is any doubt as to whether or not disclosure is an issue, it is best to be conservative; if the information is not crucial to the topic, it should be omitted.

It can come as quite a shock to some individuals that their names exist in archived documents. If a long-standing correspondence between two people is archived without the knowledge of one correspondent, the researcher must use caution in quoting that individual. A basic decision rule for these issues is as follows: If the evidence is truly necessary for the research, the researcher should take the time to find out if the individual is alive and should review the literary property rights laws.

PROPOSAL FEATURES

The key features to be attended to in reviewing proposals for historical research are problem identification, the available sources, and the investigator's qualifications. The problem identified for the research should be delineated in the research questions. It should be specific enough to be answered and to provide a guide but general enough to be of significance to a broad audience. The problem should be limited in scope to fit within the time line of the investigation. Historical research is more time-consuming than it appears. The background and rationale for investigating the problem should also be stated. The investigator should report everything known about the topic and why the research should occur.

The proposal should indicate that relevant secondary sources have been read and integrated into the background information on the research topic. The proposal also should describe the location, amount, and type of primary sources available to answer the research question. Section headings for a proposal might include the following: Introduction and Background, Purpose, Research Questions, Parameters, Sources, Justification, Time Line, and References.

The investigator should be an experienced historical researcher. Because the historical research design is grounded in the review, analysis, and interpretation of documents by one person, it is important that the investigator be reputable. Formal education and research experience in the historical method establish credibility.

CRITIQUING A REPORT

In critiquing a published research report, the following points should be addressed:[1]

1. Do the research questions provide a guide or framework for the research? The questions should be specific enough for the reader to understand where the researcher is coming from and where the researcher will go.

2. What sources did the researcher use? Were sufficient primary sources available for the research? Have secondary sources been used to validate and substantiate the primary sources? The majority of the research should be based on primary sources. Is sufficient documentation presented in the footnotes to allow verification or an attempt at replication?

3. Are the facts reported satisfactorily to give an honest and clear message? Is the researcher's argument convincing? Is the evidence clearly and logically presented and related to other variables?

4. Does the writing style make the reader want to continue reading? Is it a smooth style that provides the reader with an enjoyable experience? Are any photographs, tables, or figures used appropriate?

5. Does the author have the credentials of a historical scholar? Does he or she provide evidence of educational qualifications and other studies?

Historical research reports require the use of the Turabian (1996) style of presentation or that laid out in the University of Chicago's (1993) *Manual of Style*. These styles allow for the inclusion of footnotes and the citation of unpublished sources, a necessity for this method.

Overall, the historical method can be used to explore many topics and to answer many research questions. In nursing, there are ample questions and sufficient primary resources to enable scholarly historical research. The method can be combined with other methods or it can stand alone. It provides an intellectual challenge for the researcher who doesn't mind dust, who likes old things, and who has the skills of an amateur detective.

NOTE

1. I would like to acknowledge as sources for this list the unpublished criteria for evaluating historical research by Janie Brown Novak (1984) and editorial review criteria by Eleanor Pajunen (1985).

REFERENCES

Ashley, J. A. (1976). *Hospitals, paternalism and the role of the nurse.* New York: Teachers College Press.

Austin, A. L. (1958). The historical method in nursing. *Nursing Research, 7,* 4-10.

Barritt, E. R. (1981). Critique: Historical study. In S. D. Krampitz & N. Pavlovich (Eds.), *Readings in nursing research* (pp. 161-163). St. Louis: C. V. Mosby.

Barzun, J., & Graff, H. F. (1985). *The modern researcher* (4th ed.). San Diego, CA: Harcourt Brace Jovanovich.

Brooks, P. C. (1969). *Research in archives: The use of unpublished sources.* Chicago: University of Chicago Press.

Christy, T. E. (1975). The methodology of historical research. *Nursing Research, 24,* 189-192.

Glass, L. K. (1984). Katharine Densford Dreves: Marching at the head of the parade (Doctoral dissertation, University of Illinois, 1983). *Dissertation Abstracts International, 44,* 3358B.

Glass, L. K. (1985). Raising a million dollars: Katharine Densford Dreves and the American Nurses Foundation. *Journal of* Nursing *History, 1,* 56-67.

Hinding, A. (Ed.). (1980). *Women's history sources: A guide to archives and manuscript collections in the United States.* Ann Arbor, MI: R. W. Bowker.

Hockett, H. C. (1955). *The critical method in historical research and writing.* Westport, CT: Greenwood.

Kalisch, P. A., & Kalisch, B. J. (1976). Nurses under fire: World War 11 experiences of nurses on Bataan and Corregidor. *Nursing Research, 25,* 409-425.

Krampitz, S. D. (1981). Research design: Historical. In S. D. Krampitz & N. Pavlovich (Eds.), *Readings in nursing research* (pp. 54-58). St. Louis: C. V. Mosby.

Library of Congress, Descriptive Cataloging Division. (1959-1983). *National union catalog of manuscript collections.* Washington, DC: Author url http://lcweb.loc.gov/coll/nucmc/.

Melosh, B. (1982). *The physician's hand: Work culture and conflict in American nursing.* Philadelphia: Temple University Press.

Notter, L. (1972). The case for historical research in nursing. *Nursing Research, 21,* 483.

Turabian, K. L. (1996). *A manual for writers* (6th ed.). Chicago: University of Chicago Press.

University of Chicago Press. (1993). *A manual of style* (14th ed.). Chicago: Author.

15

The Pilot Study: One Key to Research Success

NANCY R. LACKEY
ANITA L. WINGATE

Behind every successful piece of completed research stands a pilot study. In most basic research methodology courses, students are told of the importance of a pilot study, but they are given little information on how to do one. Rarely is the actual conduct of a pilot study included in their assignments. It is questionable as to how much credence experienced nurse researchers give to pilot studies. Prescott and Soeken (1989) state that pilot studies are "underdiscussed, underused and underreported" (p. 60). A review of current nursing textbooks showed that approximately half of the authors refer to the term *pilot study*, but do not go into detail about how to conduct one. In those textbooks that list the term in the index, the actual coverage of the topic ranges from a brief entry in the glossary (Abdellah, Levine, & Levine, 1986) to a chapter delineating the definition and detailing the actual conduct of a study (Treece & Treece, 1986). The purpose of this chapter is to explore the definitions, philosophies, purposes, and methods of conducting a pilot study.

Our experiences with pilot studies have convinced us that a wealth of information can be obtained from such studies. One such pilot study was to prepare for a larger study whose purpose was to determine the needs of noninstitutionalized cancer patients and their primary care-givers. The proposal included the statement that a pilot study would be completed before the actual study began. Little did we realize how much we would learn from our pilot study.

DEFINITION OF A PILOT STUDY

Our review of nursing research textbooks showed a number of terms that were used somewhat synonymously with the term *pilot study: pretest* (Fox & Ventura, 1983; Treece & Treece, 1986), *small-scale study* (Fox & Ventura, 1983), and *exploratory study* (Dempsey & Dempsey, 1986; Woods & Catanzaro, 1988). According to Hogstel and Sayner (1986), a pilot study is "a miniature version of the major research study and mimics or resembles the major research study in every detail" (p. 58). The terms *small-scale study, exploratory study,* and *preliminary study* are used synonymously with the term *pilot study* in most nursing research textbooks. When the term *preliminary study* is used, it most frequently refers to pilot study data incorporated into research grant proposals to "illustrate the investigators' competence to pursue the proposed project and relevant experience in studying the topic" (Woods & Catanzaro, 1988, p. 500). Reporting the results of the preliminary study or pilot study in a research grant application will not only help establish the competence of the investigator but will also strengthen the case for the study being proposed (Tornquist & Funk, 1990).

The term *pretest,* when used in reference to pilot studies, has a slightly different connotation. Treece and Treece (1986) define a pilot study as a preliminary small-scale trial run of the research study that includes pretesting, which is the process of measuring the effectiveness of the instrument. The purpose of this pretesting of the instrument is to evaluate factors such as the length, wording, and validity of the instru-ment. Similarly, Fox and Ventura (1983) state two definitions of pretest-ing, one of which refers to the process of measuring the effectiveness of the instrument used to gather data, checking for reliability and preliminary indications of validity. Both of these sources also use the term pretesting as it is commonly used, meaning to gather baseline data about a sample for later comparisons in a posttest.

PHILOSOPHIES OF CONDUCTING PILOT STUDIES

From a general review of the literature, two basic philosophies about pilot studies become apparent. Sidman's (1960) philosophy suggests that an experiment is designated as a pilot study only after it has been performed and has proved to have technical flaws. He believes that any proposed major research study should be rigorously designed and conducted. If at any time during the conduct of the study a technical inadequacy is found, then the experiment becomes a pilot study and should not be published. If no flaws or procedural difficulties are encountered during the data collection or final written report, the study is considered successful.

There are some advantages and disadvantages inherent in Sidman's (1960) philosophy. One advantage of this approach is that it allows the researcher to avoid spending time and money doing a pilot study that, because of its limited sample size, may not actually reveal lack of control over certain variables. Another advantage of this approach is that it allows the researcher to avoid depleting a limited population from which to draw a sample of participants, for example, amyelotropic lateral sclerosis patients. The use of this philosophy is almost inevitable in conducting studies that examine phenomena associated with speci- fied catastrophes such as the Coconut Grove fire or natural disasters, which, by their very nature, preclude the opportunity for pilot testing. A disadvantage of Sidman's philosophy is the expenditure of time, money, and effort in the execution of a major study that may prove to have serious flaws that might have been detected using a less costly pilot study. This becomes extremely problematic if grant funds have been used to conduct the large study.

A controversy related to this philosophy is whether or not a pilot study should be published. According to Sidman (1960), a study should be published only if no serious flaws have been recognized during the conduct of the study. He believes, however, that publication of a pilot study is justified if a technique is discovered that would be valuable to other researchers, if new insights are developed about the research topic that have been alluded to in previous literature. Brink (1988) suggests that because a pilot study's purpose is to serve the investigator by improving the larger proposed study, it is not meant to be published. She proposes that a study that describes a phenomenon or process not described before in the literature is actually an exploratory study, not necessarily a pilot study, and acknowledges that such findings might be publishable. Others hold that there are specific occasions when the total pilot study or selected parts of it should be published (Burns & Grove, 1997; Seaman & Verhonick, 1982).

A computerized search of CINAHL database for nursing research (using "pilot studies" as the key word) generated 136 articles published in 1994. Of those 136 articles, only 28 used the words "pilot studies" in the title. Of those 28 articles, the abstracts revealed a wide variety of topics and types of studies. Not all abstracts indicated the number of study participants, but those that did demonstrated a wide range (4-268). Of the 136 articles, 18 had references in the abstract to some aspect of instrument development as a purpose of the study.

The most commonly expressed philosophy about conducting a pilot study is that the whole major research proposal should be vigorously conducted on a small scale to search for defects in the methodology (Polit & Hungler, 1991; Treece & Treece, 1986). Other textbooks state that not only should methodology be pretested but so should all of the components of the major study, such as instruments, directions, selection of participants, and data recording forms (Hogstel & Sayner, 1986; Shelley, 1984; Van Ort, 1981). This philosophy is based on the assumption that the data collected during the pilot study will not be included in the analysis of the major study.

Advantages of this approach are that flaws in the large study may be detected without a large expenditure of time and money, and subsequent changes may improve the major proposal substantially. Nevertheless, it must be recognized that doing a pilot study with a limited sample may not, in fact, reveal all the flaws in the design, instruments, or methodology and will deplete the available population of potential participants.

It has been our experience that a more plausible philosophy combines elements of both of the above. For example, if the researcher is experienced with the instruments and methodology used with a specific population, certain parts of a pilot study may be unnecessary. Many sources emphasize pretesting the instrument or its administration but may not advocate doing an entire pilot study (Fox & Ventura, 1983; Treece & Treece, 1986). Every researcher needs to evaluate diligently the major research study being proposed to determine which areas, if not all, need a "trial run." One pilot study may not be adequate; changes resulting from a completed pilot study may, in themselves, need to be "piloted" again. We believe that the main advantage of this philosophy is the eventual savings in time, effort, and expense. The main disadvantage in piloting is the possibility of overlooking major flaws that could seriously impair the outcome of a major study.

PURPOSE OF A PILOT STUDY

According to Van Ort (1981, p. 49), there are five basic purposes for conducting a pilot study:

1. To determine the feasibility of the major study
2. To identify problems in the research design
3. To refine the data collection and analysis plan
4. To test the instrument to be used in the major study
5. To give the researcher some experience with the participants, methodology, and instruments

In addition, Prescott and Soeken (1989) state that the purposes of a pilot study are these:

1. To assess the feasibility of the planned study
2. To assess the adequacy of the instrumentation
3. To assess problems in data collection and proposed methods (p. 60)

Burns and Grove (1997) identify six purposes:

1. To develop or refine a research instrument
2. To develop a protocol for the implementation of a treatment
3. To determine whether the sample is representative of the population or whether the sampling technique is effective
4. To examine the reliability and validity of the research instruments
5. To develop or refine data collection instruments
6. To try out data analysis techniques (pp. 52-53)

CONDUCTING THE PILOT STUDY

Before the pilot study is undertaken, the entire major research proposal should be prepared and should have the approval of the institution's research review (human subjects) committee. Plans for the pilot study can either be included in the proposal that goes to the human subjects committee or written up separately and then submitted to the committee. Participants in the pilot study must be guaranteed confidentiality and anonymity, just as they would in the major study.

Research Questions and Hypotheses

The research questions and/or hypotheses should be stated exactly as they will be for the proposed major study. The issue to be addressed here is whether or not the research questions/hypotheses will elicit the type of data the researcher desires. Actual data will be collected during the pilot study and should be analyzed carefully to ascertain whether or not they answer the research questions.

Participants

Participants selected for the pilot study should come from the same population from which the participants in the proposed major study will be selected, although individuals included in the pilot study should not be included in the major study. The sample size will depend on the overall size of the population, the amount of time the researcher has for the pilot study, and the cost. A pilot study can provide some basic information about a sample that is drawn from a specific population. It can help the researcher determine participant availability, possible percentage of participant enrollment into the study, and possible attrition rate (Talbot & Davis-Lagrow, 1995). Nieswiadomy (1993) says that there is no set number of participants needed for a pilot study. The sample must be large enough to detect flaws or weaknesses in the methodology. It is recommended that the pilot study sample be one tenth the size of the sample proposed for the major study (Treece & Treece, 1986). For example, if the sample size proposed for the major study is 60, the sample size in the pilot study should be 6.

Instruments

Periodically, a researcher will find two or more instruments that appear suitable for collection of data regarding a specific concept or intervention. A pilot study can be used to determine which of these instruments would be more appropriate and feasible to use in collecting the data. Also, the results from the pilot study can help the researcher decide if the selected instrument(s) needs to be refined before use in a major study (Jacobson, 1997). Wilson (1985) states that pilot testing should be used to (a) determine the amount of time it takes to complete the instrument(s) (b) establish if the instructions are clear, and (c) identify if study participants found anything objectionable or inappropriate about the instrument (p. 314).

A pilot study can be very useful in establishing the reliability and validity of an instrument. Specific tests can be built into the pilot study that measure the reliability and validity of an instrument. Also, the time it takes respondents to complete a questionnaire, survey, or research tool can be established in the pilot study (Burns & Grove, 1997). The researcher should ask participants to complete the instruments used in the study and to include comments about the instruments.

In our study, we used the Object Content Test, an unstructured, self-administered, paper-and-pencil test that can be administered to respondents either in a group or individually (Garretson, 1967). We structured our question after the examples accompanying the instrument. Initially, the wording was, "When I see the phrase 'needs of the cancer patient,' to me it means . . ." During our pilot study, we learned that the way this was stated was confusing to the respondents. We changed it to read, "What are the needs of the noninstitutionalized cancer patient?" Our second pilot study demonstrated that the revised question elicited the types of responses that were appropriate for the research question. The instructions on the questionnaire asked the respondents to "go along fairly fast." During our pilot study, we were reminded that patients receiving radiation treatments or chemotherapy are frequently fatigued and can do few things fast. We removed this statement from our directions, because the responses were more important than the time element.

A quick survey of published pilot studies reveals that investigators use pilot studies to refine instruments. For example, a series of pilot studies were used by one group of investigators to refine a scale measuring children's responses to bone marrow transplantation. This scale's content was refined, and its psychometric properties (internal consistency, interrater reliability, and validity) were established in the series of pilot studies (Phipps, Hinds, Channell, & Bell, 1994). Another article described the development of a 17-item instrument that measures the level of functioning of chronically mentally ill persons living in the community. A pilot study was used to examine the scale's interrater and test-retest reliability and its validity (Barker, Barron, McFarland, & Bigelow, 1994).

Methodology

While conducting our pilot study, we became aware of a problem in the actual procedure. After selecting our participants, we contacted them by phone, explained the study, and asked them if they would participate. If they consented, we set up an appointment to deliver the questionnaire, demographic data sheets, and a self-addressed, stamped envelope in which they were to return the materials. During this visit to the home, the study was again explained and instructions were given about return of the completed materials.

During the pilot study, it became evident that the return rate was far below our expectations, even after telephone calls to the participants to answer their questions and encourage them to complete and mail the materials. Three weeks into the pilot study, we realized that we were going to have inadequate responses with this procedure. Our revised procedure was to place an initial call to the respondents, as before, describe the study, and ask them to participate. If they consented, we mailed the questionnaires, demographic data sheets, and instructions to them. We also informed them that we would call again in 5 days to make an appointment to come to their residence to collect their complete materials. We pilot tested these changes and learned that this procedure was more successful than the previous one. There was one flaw: The U.S. mail moved more slowly than we had anticipated. Therefore, we allowed a week rather than 5 days to establish the appointment for pickup of completed materials.

During the first pilot study, we realized that our record-keeping form was insufficient, because we were trying to match patients' data with those of their primary caregivers. This required a precise coding system, so we revamped and enlarged our form and established a better coding system. These changes were then pilot tested to make sure they would meet our needs with a large number of participants.

Testing the methodology (the research design) in the pilot study can answer questions about many aspects of the study. If the researcher wishes to know which threats to internal validity are likely and how they might be controlled, he or she can assess whether random assignment of participants can actually be implemented in the intended setting. Whatever the sampling plan, pilot testing can evaluate the appropriateness and feasibility of it. Pilot testing can help in determining the appropriate sample size to represent the population of interest, by providing a critical element, the relative variance of the dependent variable in the sample (Prescott & Soeken, 1989).

Data Analysis

The pilot work represents the opportunity to try out the intended data analysis techniques. Potential problems with the proposed analysis may be uncovered in time to avoid time-consuming errors in data analysis techniques (Prescott & Soeken, 1989).

Because the proposed statistical test should be included in the major proposed research study, the researcher should be able to tell if the proposed analysis is appropriate to either answer the research question or accept or reject the hypothesis. The researcher should be able to speculate from the data collected in the pilot study whether or not the statistical test will do this. The kind of data generated in the pilot study may suggest the need for additional or different kinds of data analysis.

EVALUATING THE RESULTS OF THE PILOT STUDY

The researcher must remember that not all of the flaws of a major proposed research study will show up in a pilot study, because a pilot study uses a small sample size, is an artificial situation, and has a limited scope (Hogstel & Sayner, 1986; Treece & Treece, 1986). In evaluating the results of the pilot study, the researcher must identify the weaknesses and strengths of the research questions/hypotheses, methodology, and analysis. The results elicited in the pilot study should be given careful consideration.

Some of the major questions the researcher should ask at this time are as follows: What weaknesses have appeared in the proposed major research study prior to its implementation? Based on the results of the pilot study, is the proposed major research study warranted? Will the results of the proposed major research study justify the proposed cost and time involved? If the evaluation of the results of the pilot study determines that a number of changes or a major methodological change needs to be made in the larger study, it is advisable to conduct a second pilot study that incorporates these changes.

Because pilot studies are often not reported and discussed, benefits of pilot work are not always apparent to novice investigators. Hinds and Gattuso (1991) present an organized and articulate description of the pilot work they conducted with adolescent cancer patients whose adaptation they were interested in studying. The purpose of their pilot study was to determine how well the design, methods, and sampling procedures would allow the investigators to describe adaptation experienced by the adolescents during the first 6 months of chemotherapy. The investigators were able to correct serious flaws related to data collection points, improve the coding plan and the data analysis computer program, and actually alter the focus of the major study slightly as the result of unexpected findings in the pilot study.

As Lindquist (1991) puts it, even failed pilot investigations may be valuable because they "provide insight into problems and generate important questions" (p. 92). For example, one pilot study that was intended to prepare the ground for a randomized, controlled clinical trial instead revealed that the methodology, involving patient-kept diaries, contained major flaws (Read & George, 1994). Recognition of the problems led to abandonment of the plan to conduct a clinical trial and directed the researchers to explore the research questions in a different way.

SUMMARY

Many researchers do not conduct pilot studies, mainly because of the time involvement they require. However, more grant applications are now requiring evidence of a pilot study. No matter how diligent a researcher is in planning a proposed major research study, there will always be unanticipated flaws. If these flaws are corrected before the initiation of the major research study, the researcher's time, money, and efforts are more likely to be rewarded with meaningful findings in the larger project.

REFERENCES

Abdellah, F. G., Levine, E., & Levine, B. S. (1986). *Better patient care through nursing research*. New York: Macmillan.

Barker, S., Barron, N., McFarland, B., & Bigelow, D. (1994). A community ability scale for chronically mentally ill consumers: Reliability and validity, Part 1. *Community Mental Health Journal, 30*(4), 363-383.

Brink, P. (1988). The pilot study (editorial). *Western Journal of Nursing Research, 10*(3), 237-238.

Burns, N., & Grove, S. K. (1997). *The practice of nursing research: Conduct, critique and utilization* (2nd ed.). Philadelphia: W. B. Saunders.

Dempsey, P. A., & Dempsey, A. D. (1986). *The research process in nursing*. Boston: Jones & Bartlett.

Fox, R. N., & Ventura, M. R. (1983). Small-scale administration of instruments and procedures. *Nursing Research, 32*(2), 122-125.

Garretson, W. S. (1967). The consensual definition of social objects. In J. G. Morris & B. N. Meltzer (Eds.), *Symbolic interaction* (pp. 337-342). Boston: Allyn & Bacon.

Hinds, P., & Gattuso, J. (1991). From pilot work to a major study in cancer nursing research. *Cancer Nursing, 14*(3), 132-135.

Hogstel, M. O., & Sayner, N. C. (1986). *Nursing research*. New York: McGraw-Hill.

Jacobson, S. F. (1997). Evaluating instruments for use in clinical nursing research. In M. Frank-Stromberg & S. J. Olsen (Eds.), *Instruments for clinical health-care* (2nd ed., pp. 3-19). Boston: Jones & Bartlett.

Lindquist, R. (1991). Don't forget the pilot work! *Heart & Lung, the Journal of Critical Care, 20*(1), 91-92.

Nieswiadomy, R. M. (1993). *Foundations of nursing research* (2nd ed.). Norwalk, CT: Appleton & Lange.

Phipps, S., Hinds, P., Channell, S., & Bell, G. (1994). Measurement of behavioral, affective, and somatic responses to pediatric bone marrow transplantation: Development of the BASES Scale. *Journal of Pediatric Oncology Nursing, 11*(3), 109-119.

Polit, D. F., & Hungler, B. P. (1991). *Nursing research*. Philadelphia: J. B. Lippincott.

Prescott, P., & Soeken, K. (1989). The potential uses of pilot work. *Nursing Research, 38*(1), 60-62.

Read, S., & George, S. (1994). Nurse practitioners in accident and emergency departments: Reflections on a pilot study. *Journal of Advanced Nursing, 19*(4), 705-716.

Seaman, C., & Verhonick, P. (1982). *Research methods.* Norwalk, CT: Appleton-Century Crofts.

Shelley, S. I. (1984). *Research methods in nursing and health.* Boston: Little, Brown.

Sidman, M. (1960). Pilot studies. In M. Sidman, *Tactics of scientific research* (pp. 217-223). New York: Basic Books.

Talbot, L. A., & Davis-Lagrow, P. A. (1995). The research topic and problem statement. In L. A. Talbot (Ed.), *Principles and practice of nursing research.* St. Louis, MO: Mosby Year Book.

Tornquist, E., & Funk, S. (1990). How to write a research grant proposal *Image: Journal of Nursing Scholarship, 22*(1), 44-51.

Treece, E. W., & Treece, J. W. (1986). *Elements of research in nursing.* St. Louis: C. V. Mosby.

Van Ort, S. V. (1981). Research design: Pilot study. In S. D. Krampitz & N. Pavlovich (Eds.), *Reading for nursing research.* St. Louis, MO: C. V. Mosby.

Wilson, H. S. (1985). *Research in nursing.* Menlo Park, CA: Addison-Wesley.

Woods, N. F., & Catanzaro, M. (1988). *Nursing research: Theory and practice.* St. Louis, MO: C. V. Mosby.

Author Index

387

Subject Index

About the Authors

Joan L. Bottorff, R.N., Ph.D., is Associate Professor at the School of Nursing, University of British Columbia, Vancouver, Canada. Her research interests include the interactions between health professionals and the recipients of care or service and health promotion.

Pamela J. Brink, R.N., FAAN, received her B.S. from Mount St. Mary's College in Los Angeles, her M.S.N. in psychiatric nursing from Catholic University, and her Ph.D. in cultural anthropology from Boston University. She has published two books (*Transcultural Nursing*, 1976; *Basic Steps in Planning Nursing Research*, 1978, 1982, 1988, 1994, with Marilynn J. Wood) and numerous articles and book chapters, and is the Founder and Executive Editor of the *Western Journal of Nursing Research*. She is currently Professor in the Faculty of Nursing, University of Alberta, Edmonton, Canada.

Kathleen C. Buckwalter, R.N., Ph.D., FAAN, is a geriatric mental health nurse and is currently Professor and Associate Director, Office for Nursing Research Utilization and Development, University of Iowa College of Nursing, Iowa City, Iowa, and geropsychiatric consultant, Abbe Center for Community Mental Health, Cedar Rapids, Iowa. After completing her doctorate at the University of Illinois at the Medical Center, Chicago, in 1980, she was a Geriatric Mental Health Academic

Awardee from the National Institute of Mental Health, Mental Disorders of the Aging Research Branch. She is presently on the DHHS Advisory Panel on Alzheimer's Disease and the NIA Advisory Council, where she serves as council liaison to the Special Care Unit Initiative. She is active in geriatric mental health education, practice, and research.

Laurie K. Glass, R.N., Ph.D., FAAN, is Professor of Nursing and Director of the Center for Nursing History at the University of Wisconsin—Milwaukee School of Nursing. She received her Ph.D. in nursing research and nursing history from the University of Illinois at Chicago in 1983. Her specific interest is the historical analysis of nursing leaders and their impact on issues and events. She is a member of various national committees that focus on nursing history and is a past president of the Wisconsin Nurses Association. She also is Adjunct Associate Professor at the University of Illinois at Chicago College of Nursing.

Joy L. Johnson, R.N., Ph.D., is Assistant Professor at the School of Nursing, University of British Columbia, Vancouver, Canada. Her research interests include health promotion, heart health, and women's health with a focus on theory development and testing.

Nancy R. Lackey is Professor of Nursing at the University of Missouri-Kansas City School of Nursing. She holds a B.S.N. from Indiana University, a M.S.N. from Marquette University, and a Ph.D. in Nursing from Texas Women's University. She completed a 2-year postdoctoral fellowship at the University of Utah College of Nursing in family theories, issues, and research methods. Her research interests include needs of noninstitutionalized cancer patients, their primary caregivers, and families and adolescent caregivers of adults with chronic illnesses. She has authored a number of book chapters and has had articles published in *Cancer Practice, Oncology Nursing Forum, Cancer Nursing, Western Journal of Nursing Research,* and *Journal of Post Anesthesia Nursing.*

Janice Lander is Professor and Associate Dean for Research in the Faculty of Nursing at the University of Alberta, Edmonton, Canada. She received her Ph.D. in psychology from the University of Manitoba, Winnipeg, Canada. Her interests include research methods and pain management. She is currently conducting research on children's pain.

Meridean L. Maas, R.N., Ph.D., FAAN, is Professor of Nursing at the University of Iowa College of Nursing. She has authored numerous journal articles and book chapters and several books. She and Kathleen Kelly, Ph.D., R.N., received the *American Journal of Nursing* Book of the Year Award for Volume VI of the Series on Nursing Administration. Her clinical and research interests include classification of nursing diagnoses, interventions, and outcomes, testing nursing interventions for the institutionalized elderly, and the design and evaluation of organization and management interventions that facilitate professional nursing practice and the achievement of quality patient outcomes.

Janet C. Meininger, R.N., Ph.D., FAAN, is Professor of Nursing and Epidemiology at the University of Texas–Houston Health Science Center. She received her B.S.N. from St. Louis University, an M.S.N. from Case Western Reserve University with a specialty in public health nursing, and a Ph.D. in epidemiology from the University of North Carolina, Chapel Hill. Her interests include cardiovascular risk factors in children and adolescents, behavioral factors, health services research, and family health. She has published research papers on these topics as well as articles on research methodology in journals such as *Nursing Research, Journal of Chronic Diseases,* and *Social Science and Medicine.*

Merle H. Mishel is Kenan Professor of Nursing at the University of North Carolina at Chapel Hill, School of Nursing. She holds a Ph.D. in social psychology from Claremont Graduate School and has authored numerous papers in the area of instrument development and testing that have appeared in several scholarly nursing research journals. Her interests include the development of instruments to index nursing concepts and the development of the theory of uncertainty in illness.

Patricia L. Munhall, ARNP, Ed.D., Psy A, FAAN, is Professor of Nursing and Director of the Ph.D. Program in Nursing at Barry University. She has published and presented papers extensively on phenomenology and qualitative research. She is coeditor, with Carolyn J. Oiler, of the AJN award-winning textbook *Nursing Research: A Qualitative Perspective.* In addition, she is the author of *Revisioning Phenomenology;* Volume I and Volume II of *In Women's Experience,* a collection of phenomenological studies, including her own; *The Emergence of the 21st Century Woman,* and the forthcoming *The Emergence of the 21st Century Family.*

Pamela A. Ratner, Ph.D., R.N., is Assistant Professor at the School of Nursing, and a Postdoctoral Fellow at the Institute of Health Promotion Research, University of British Columbia, Vancouver, Canada. Her research interests have focused primarily on women's health, including the health consequences of violence within intimate relationships, smoking cessation, and health promotion. She has a particular interest in structural equation modeling.

David Reed received his B.A., M.A., and Ph.D. degrees in Sociology from Indiana University. He is Project Director of Family Involvement in Care Research at the University of Iowa College of Nursing. He currently manages a research project using a quasi-experimental design. The project, for which Meridean Maas is principal investigator, is testing an intervention to increase participation by family members in the care of their relatives who have been institutionalized with Alzheimer's disease or a related disorder. He has also participated in research on the attitudes of physicians toward children with mental retardation, the influence of social support on sobriety for veterans who completed an alcoholism treatment program, and the impact of job training programs on earnings. His research interests are in occupational socialization and health care delivery systems.

Janet K. Pringle Specht, R.N., M.A., Ph.D., is Program Assistant and Investigator, Alzheimer's Family Role Trial Grant, at the University of Iowa College of Nursing, and a postdoctoral fellow at the University of Iowa Center on Aging. She has co-authored a number of book chapters and has published and presented numerous papers on gerontological nursing and long-term care.

Bonnie Wakefield, R.N., M.A., is a Ph.D. candidate at the University of Iowa College of Nursing. Her clinical and research interests include quality-of-care issues for the elderly, such as the diagnosis and treatment of acute confusion in hospitalized elderly and health status assessment of elderly populations.

Anita L. Wingate, is Associate Professor and Academic Coordinator at the University of Kansas School of Nursing. She holds a B.S.N. in nursing and a Ph.D. in anatomy, both from the University of Kansas.

Her research interests are fatigue and quality-of-life issues in oncology patients, especially those with breast and prostate cancer.

Marilynn J. Wood is Dean of the Faculty of Nursing at the University of Alberta, Edmonton, Canada. Her doctorate is from the School of Public Health at UCLA, in gerontology and biostatistics. She is coauthor of a basic nursing research text, coeditor of *Clinical Nursing Research,* and was recipient of an American Journal of Nursing Book of the Year Award in 1984. Her current research is in the area of health promotion for seniors.